Fundamentals of
Anatomy *&* Movement
A Workbook and Guide

Anatomy

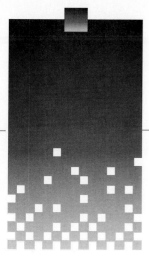

Fundamentals of
Anatomy & Movement
A Workbook and Guide

Carla Z. Hinkle, BS, RPTA

Instructor, Tulsa Community College
Tulsa Oklahoma

with 328 illustrations

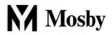 **Mosby**

St. Louis Baltimore Boston
Carlsbad Chicago Naples New York Philadelphia Portland
London Madrid Mexico City Singapore Sydney Tokyo Toronto Wiesbaden

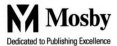

Mosby

Dedicated to Publishing Excellence

A Times Mirror
Company

Publisher: Don Ladig
Executive Editor: Martha Sasser
Developmental Editor: Kellie F. White
Project Managers: Dana Peick and Gayle Morris
Manufacturing Manager: Betty Mueller
Designer: Dana Peick
Cover: David Ziellinski

Printed in the United States of America
Composition by GraphCom Corporation
Illustrations by Accu Color, Inc.
Printing and binding by R.R. Donnelley

Mosby–Year Book, Inc.
11830 Westline Industrial Drive
St. Louis, Missouri 63146

International Standard Book Number 0-8151-2210-0

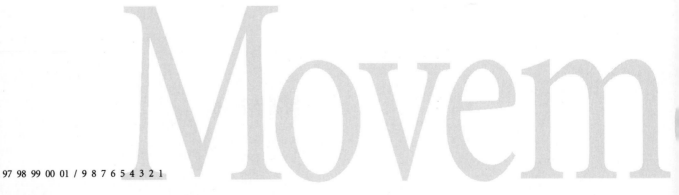

To my Monkie,
whose patience and strength sustains me,
and to my family,
who cheers me on.

nt

Foreword

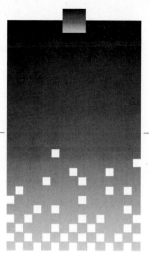

Foreword

A working knowledge of the musculoskeletal system and related aspects of the cardiovascular and nervous systems is critical to the success of every student of physical therapy, as well as students of many other health professions. This criticality is evidenced by the fact that anatomy is usually the first course offered in physical therapy educational programs, laying the foundation for future work. It is equally important that students share a common perspective of the human body to communicate effectively with their colleagues about the function or dysfunction of the musculoskeletal system.

Because of the nature of the anatomy and the demand for detail in learning it, college courses often incorporate laboratories that involve cadaver dissection or dissection of other closely related mammals, affording students experiential learning opportunities. After all, anatomy is not just the memorization of muscles and bones; it is the understanding of how they all work together.

Many health educational programs, especially those at 2-year colleges, do not have the luxury of offering intensive and expensive learning opportunities to their students. Therefore the instructors at these institutions must rely on other activities to make anatomy come alive for their stu-

dents. *Fundamentals of Anatomy and Movement: A Workbook and Guide* by Carla Hinkle, BS, PTA, offers such an opportunity. The laboratory activities in this text are innovative, interactive, and help fulfill this critical need.

Ms. Hinkle, who we are privileged to have as an instructor of anatomy for the students of physical therapy at Tulsa Community College, has developed teaching methods that allow students to effectively and efficiently study anatomic functions and relationships. Her laboratory sessions have evolved over the past 4 years from a lecture format into a series of wonderful collaborative learning activities that allow students to direct their own learning experiences and exercise their capacities for inquiry. This textbook is the product of this evolution.

Ms. Hinkle is precise and thorough in her authorship of this text. The mastery of the information presented will serve the physical therapist assistant, occupational therapy assistants, massage therapists, recreational therapists, and other paraprofessionals in their education. I am honored and pleased to have the opportunity to recommend this textbook as a valuable resource to all past, current, and future students of anatomy.

Suzanne Reese, MS, PT
Program Director
Physical Therapist Assistant Program
Tulsa Community College
Tulsa, Oklahoma

Preface

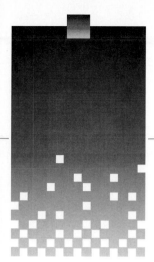

Preface

What started out as a few study assignments for homework has grown into a textbook. All educators try to convince their students of the importance of study time outside the lecture hall or laboratory, but the argument often falls on deaf ears and closed book covers. The challenge is to convince and sell the student on a level of commitment to an area of study in a way that will draw them into the very heart of the course content.

On the surface, a subject such as musculoskeletal anatomy often appears to be a collection of minutiae and trivial detail, thus many students approach the material with the intent of committing endless lists to short-term memory. For those of us who are practitioners in the fields of health care and athletics, these sundry details become the difference between critical or routine conditions, effective or ineffective treatment, or perhaps successful performance or repeated injury. Thus short-term memory storage involving bone, muscle, connective tissues, and vital organs is not the best functional manner for later application in the assessment and determination of injury, disease, treatment approach, appropriate exercise and activity, as well as equipment design and fit.

Although anatomy texts are not in short supply, this unique book focuses on the musculoskeletal aspects of anatomy, including organ systems immediately necessary for performing physical activity. The text has been written so that the student can spell out the content through exercises, once the initial reading has been accomplished. In this manner the student can retrieve, relive, and hopefully recall the assembly of their own body. The exercises have been inserted into the text so that the student has an immediate opportunity to apply the information they have read and achieve immediate success. An answer key is provided for comparison. Once an exercise is completed, it continues to serve as its own piece of reference material—one written by the student, not an absent author. Thus the student is making a direct contribution to their own learning.

Since there are many professions around which musculoskeletal anatomy and the systems related to human movement revolve, this text has something to offer on a broad scale. Professional and paraprofessional levels of physical, occupational, recreational, respiratory, and massage therapy, as well as rehabilitation engineering and chiropractic medicine, will find applications for this text. This book may also be beneficial to athletic trainers, exercise physiologists, coaches, personal trainers, and athletes themselves. Any person interested in exploring the nature of their own movement can gain insight from the material as it is presented. When it comes to physical dysfunction, a sound familiarity of anatomy is, in itself, a tool of prevention.

Carla Z. Hinkle

Acknowle

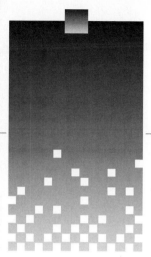

Acknowledgments

I am indebted to many individuals who contributed to my ideals of setting up and striving for high standards in education and health care. Most frequently, the motivation for pushing on comes from students and patients who want to know more.

Colleagues and mentors in many forms are gathered at Tulsa Community College and at the Oklahoma Physical Therapy Association. The stars among the group are Rita Zeman, who convinced me that anatomy is "our bread and butter," and Suzanne Reese and Kathy Johnson who have been superbly supportive and patient.

Authorship would not have been attained without the direction and assistance provided by many at Mosby–Year Book in St. Louis. Out front to lead the way and also stay by my side were Martha Sasser, Dana Peick, Kellie White, Laura MacAdam, and Leah Hiner. Without these professionals and their teamwork, this project could not have been!

Special thanks to Sue Minshall for her ever-present encouragement and for pressing the work schedule onward. Thanks also to Karen LeFlore for letting me take her photo! To Mom, Pop, Carlton and Kathy, and Joanie and Freddie—your support and faith were always present.

dgments

Contents

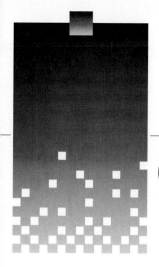

Contents

Preface, vii

Acknowledgements, ix

I General Anatomic Terminology, I

Introduction, 1
    Anatomic position, 1
    Directional terminology, 2
    Practice makes permanent, 3
    Anatomic regions, 3
    Cardinal planes, 4
Key Words, 8

2 Human Skeleton, 9

Bone as a Living Tissue, 9
Basic Compounds Found in Bone, 9
Prenatal Development of Bone, 9
Types of Bone Tissue, 10
    Compact bone, 10
    Spongy bone, 10
Function of Bone, 11
    Force-resistant framework, 11
    Mineral storage, 12
    Muscle attachment, 12
    Protection, 12
    Fat storage and blood cell production, 12
    Filtration, 12
Terminology of Bone Shapes, 14
    Long bones, 15
    Short bones, 15

Irregular bones, 15
Flat bones, 15
Sesamoid bones, 15
Terminology of Skeletal Landmarks, 15
Axial Skeleton, 17
    Bones of the cranium, 17
    Bones of the face, 23
    Maxillary bones, 23
    Vertebral column, 24
    Thoracic cage, 33
Appendicular Skeleton, 35
    Pectoral girdle, 35
    Upper extremity, 37
    Pelvic girdle, 41
    Lower extremity, 46
Summary, 53
Key Words, 53

3 Joints, 55

Structure and Movement of Joints, 55
    Fibrous joints, 55
    Cartilaginous joints, 56
    Synovial joints, 56
Terminology of Movement, 62
Principle Joints of the Pectoral Girdle and Upper Extremity, 65
    Sternoclavicular joint, 65
    Acromioclavicular joint, 65
    Glenohumeral joint, 65
    Scapulothoracic joint, 66
Pelvic Girdle and Lower Extremity, 71

Hip, 71
Knee, 72
Ankle, 73
Intervertebral Joints, 77
Key Words, 78

4 Skeletal Muscle Contraction, 79

Movement, 79
Types of Muscle Tissue, 79
Components of Muscle Tissue, 80
Skeletal Muscle Fiber Contraction, 80
Muscle Fiber Innervation, 82
Slow Twitch and Fast Twitch Muscle Fibers, 82
Musculoskeletal Line of Pull, 83
Musculoskeletal Lever System, 83
   First class levers, 83
   Second class levers, 84
   Third class levers, 84
Methods of Skeletal Muscle Contraction, 84
Prime Movers, Synergists, Fixators, and Antagonists, 86
Summary, 86
Key Words, 88

5 Muscles and Movement of the Shoulder and Upper Extremity, 89

Nomenclature of Skeletal Muscles, 89
Analysis and Application, 89
Muscles of Scapular Stability, 90
   Functional significance, 91
Muscles of the Shoulder, 92
   Functional significance, 96
Muscles of the Elbow and Forearm, 98
   Functional significance, 99
Muscles of the Wrist and Muscles Extrinsic to the Hand, 103
Muscles Intrinsic to the Hand, 107
   Functional significance, 107
Summary, 107
Key Words, 114

6 Muscles and Movement of the Hip and Lower Extremity, 115

Muscles of the Hip, 115
   Muscles of the anterior hip, 115

Muscles of the gluteal group, 116
Lateral rotator muscles of the hip, 116
Adductor muscles of the hip, 118
Hamstring muscles of the posterior hip and knee, 118
Functional significance, 119
Muscles of the Knee, 122
   Functional significance, 125
Muscles of the Ankle, 131
   Extrinsic muscles of the foot, 131
   Intrinsic muscles of the foot, 132
   Functional significance, 133
Key Words, 142

7 Muscles and Movement of the Abdomen, Vertebral Column, Face, and Temporomandibular Joint, 143

Muscles of the Abdomen, 143
   Functional significance, 144
Muscles of the Vertebral Column, 144
   Functional significance, 147
Muscles of Primary Respiration, 150
Muscles of the Face and Temporomandibular Joint, 152
Summary, 152
Key Words, 158

8 Nervous System, 159

Function and Structure of a Neuron, 159
Impulse Transmission, 161
Saltatory Conduction, 162
Central Nervous System, 165
   Brain, 165
   Spinal cord, 167
   Meninges, 168
Peripheral Nervous System, 170
   Cranial nerves, 170
   Spinal nerves, 171
Autonomic Nervous System, 174
Somatic Nervous System, 175
Neuromuscular Regulation of Movement, 175
   Muscle spindles, 175
   Golgi tendon organs, 175
   Proprioception, 175
   Reflex arc, 175
Key Words, 178

9 Cardiovascular System, Blood, and Lymphatic System, 179

Internal Anatomy of the Heart, 179
    Heart chambers, 179
    Heart valves, 180
Pathway of Blood through the Heart, 181
Monitoring the Activity of the Heart, 181
    Heart rate, 181
    Blood pressure, 182
    Heart sounds, 182
Cardiac Muscle Fibers, 184
Electrical Stimulation of Cardiac Muscles, 184
Blood Vessels, 188
    Blood supply to the cardiac muscle, 190
Blood, 192
    Red blood cells, 192
    White blood cells, 192
    Platelets, 193
    Blood plasma, 193
Lymphatic System, 193
Key Words, 195

10 Respiratory System, 197

Anatomy of the Respiratory System, 197
Mechanical Principles of Air Exchange, 202
Skeletal Muscles of Respiration, 202
Cycle of Respiratory Air Volumes, 203
Control of Respiration, 204
Key Words, 207

11 Functional Movement, 209

Movement and Function, 209
Movement Identification, 209
Functional Muscle Activity, 213
Components of functional activity: more exercises, 216
Key Words, 228

Bibliography 229

Glossary, 231

Answer Key, 241

Index, 275

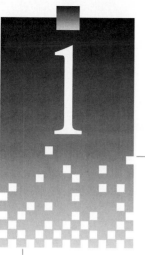

General Anatomic Terminology

❝ *This chapter will enable you to develop a vocabulary of general anatomic terminology that is related to the orientation of the human body and to the general locations on and about the body.* ❞

Chapter objectives

The student will be able to:

1. Describe the anatomic position of the human body as it exists in space for consistent reference.

2. Describe locations on and about the body using directional terminology.

3. Describe various anatomic regions.

4. Identify and define cardinal planes that describe various views of the human body or parts of the human body.

5. Practice using directional terminology, anatomic regions, and cardinal planes individually and with a study partner.

Introduction

In this text the human body is discussed as a structure, a physical tactile object, or, in a sense, a machine. Beyond the scope of this text, more consideration should be given to behavior, injury, disease processes, and therapeutic treatment techniques.

Individuals must each have the same perspective of an object to discuss it accurately. Even then, individuals can accurately communicate with one another *only if* their terminology and language are the same. For example, the mention of an automobile may bring to mind the image of a sports car to one person, whereas another may think of a pickup truck. Therefore a uniform starting point must be created. Even when the original object is well identified, if those conversing do not speak the same language, errors may occur during translation without warning. A set pattern must be established to ensure consistency in the terminology used.

When a person comes into contact with an unknown object, it may be described according to individual perceptions. This brings to mind the age-old story of several visually challenged individuals and the elephant. In this story the person holding the tail of the elephant describes it as a thin, snakelike creature with hair. The person holding the trunk describes the elephant as thick, very flexible, and moist. The person holding the foot describes the animal as built similar to a tree trunk—thick skinned and flat on one end. The last person sitting on top of the elephant describes a bony, coarse body, far too large to reach around. Those of us who have seen an elephant know that each of these descriptions is relative to bits and pieces, but not one does justice to the enormous size, strength, agility, and skill of the entire animal. Similarly, it is necessary to first reference our study of anatomy to a healthy, fully developed, adult human being.

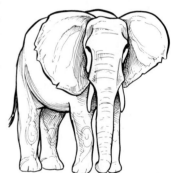

Anatomic position

When discussing the human anatomy, the model must be referenced in the upright **anatomic position,** that is, standing on two feet with back straight, head erect, and facing forward; the arms are outstretched and hang down to each side, the palms are forward, and the fingers are straight and pointing toward the ground.

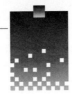

In the medical context, all references to the human anatomy are based on this anatomic position unless a different position is otherwise indicated. Similarly, in this text a patient's body is always discussed as if it is upright, regardless of whether he or she is lying on a bed or sitting in a chair. All measurements and movements are described from this upright anatomic position (Fig. 1-1).

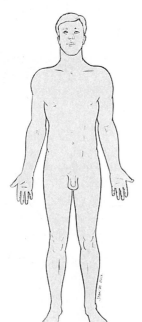

Figure 1-1. Anatomic position.
From Thibodeau: Structure & function of the body, *ed 9, St Louis, 1992, Mosby.*

Directional terminology

Beginning with the upright anatomic position, the human body can be described with respect to its top, bottom, sides, front, or back, but these words are too general. There must be a known **reference point** where specific anatomic terminology is used to describe a direction, location, region, or microscopic point. It is not proper to look at a human body and label something as "top," or "bottom." Written and verbal descriptors must be more specific. Box 1-1 provides a list of terms that describe location or direction.

Box 1-1. Directional terminology

Anterior—in front
Posterior—in back

Cephal—toward the head
Caudad—toward the tail

Ventral—toward the belly
Dorsal—toward the back

Superior—above
Inferior—below

Box 1-1. Directional terminology—*cont*

Medial—toward midline
Lateral—away from midline

Proximal—closer to the head
Distal—farther from the head

Superficial—near the surface
Deep—below the surface

These terms are paired, each having an opposite. If one object is **superior,** the implication is that there is another object that is **inferior.** It is incorrect to refer to an object as existing "above" if there is no "below."

A term must be used in reference to a known location, or **landmark,** that does not change. For example, if the location of the left knee cap is identified, another point may be described as either above (superior to) or below (inferior to) this landmark. An accurate reference cannot be made without first locating the starting point. For medical reference and documentation, words such as "above," "below," "in back," or "in front" are not sufficient (Fig. 1-2). A **directional**

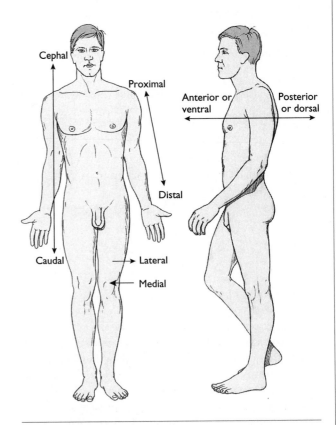

Figure 1-2. Directional terminology.
From Mathers et al: Clinical anatomy principles, *St Louis, 1996, Mosby.*

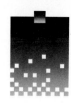
term is used to describe a location as it exists in relation to a known point. If no reference point is given, you cannot get there from here!

How about a few examples? Rather than say, "My nose is superior," it is more correct to say, "My nose is superior *to my chin.*" Two reference points appear in the latter statement. Instead of saying, "My knee cap is proximal," it is more accurate to say, "My knee cap is proximal *to my foot.*" Again, two references make this statement anatomically specific. Box 1-2 lists examples of how a directional term can be used to describe a location.

Box 1-2. Use of directional terms

The face is **anterior to** the back of the head.
The back of the head is **posterior to** the face.
The chest is **ventral to** the shoulder blades.
The shoulder blade is **dorsal to** the chest.
The nose is **superior to** the lips.
The lips are **inferior to** the nose.
The navel is **medial to** the elbow.
The elbow is **lateral to** the navel.
The elbow is **proximal to** the hand.
The hand is **distal to** the elbow.
Hair is **superficial to** skin.
Skin is **deep to** hair.

Anatomic references do not always have to be pinpoint specific. Often, the portion being discussed is a region or an entire limb. Obviously, the more precise a description, the more accurate the description will be.

It is possible to combine several directional terms to describe two points that lie in an angular orientation to one another (Box 1-3). Of course, one would never combine two opposing terms. Correct spelling is vital to the accuracy of all medical documentation (see Fig. 1-2).

Box 1-3. Combining directional terms

Superolateral—above and away from midline
Superomedial—above and toward midline
Inferolateral—below and away from midline
Inferomedial—below and toward midline

Also possible:

Anterolateral—to the front of and away from midline
Anteromedial—to the front of and toward midline
Posterolateral—to the back of and away from midline
Posteromedial—to the back of and toward midline

Practice makes permanent

It is commonly thought that "practice makes perfect." However, if one should incorrectly learn a concept or skill and then repeat the inaccuracy, the knowledge or performance will consistently be inaccurate. Therefore it is best to consider that **"practice makes permanent."**

The following exercise shows figures in anatomic position and provides opportunities to exercise your understanding of directional terminology. Be sure to check your work for accuracy of terminology *and* spelling!

Exercise I-I. Directional terms

Provide the appropriate directional term for the paired labels as listed in this exercise (see Fig. 1-3 on page 4).

1. A is _____ to B.

2. B is _____ to A.

3. C is _____ to D.

4. D is _____ to C.

5. E is _____ to F.

6. F is _____ to E.

7. G is _____ to H.

8. H is _____ to G.

9. I is _____ to J.

10. J is _____ to I.

11. K is _____ to L.

12. L is _____ to K.

13. M is _____ to N.

14. N is _____ to M.

15. O is _____ to P.

16. P is _____ to O.

Anatomic regions

As previously mentioned, references are often made to certain regions of the human body. It is important to be familiar with these regional terms because they are often named for more specific structures or functions that occur in the area. Study each **anatomic region** listed in Box 1-4, and observe how it corresponds to Figure 1-4.

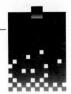

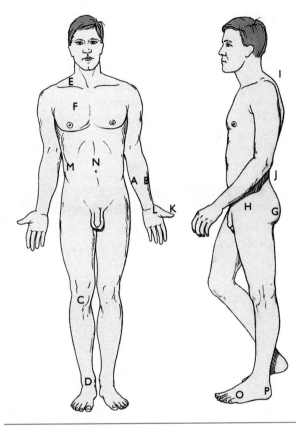

Figure 1-3. Directional terminology.
From Mathers et al: Clinical anatomy principles, *St Louis, 1996, Mosby.*

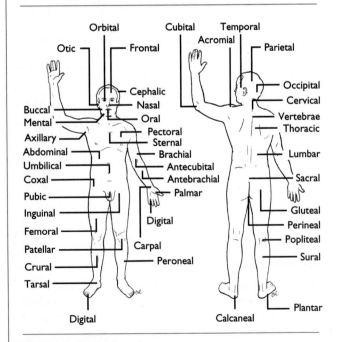

Figure 1-4. Anatomic regions.
From Fritz: Fundamentals of therapeutic massage, *St Louis, 1995, Mosby.*

Box 1-4. Anatomic regions

Cranial region

Cephalic	Occipital	Temporal
Frontal	Parietal	

Facial region

Orbital	Oral	Buccal
Nasal	Otic	Mental

Spine and trunk region

Vertebral	Lumbar	Sternal
Cervical	Sacral	Umbilical
Thoracic	Pectoral	Abdominal

Shoulder and arm region (upper extremity)

Acromial	Antecubital	Carpal
Axillary	Cubital	Palmar
Brachial	Antebrachial	Digital

Hips and pelvis region

Inguinal	Pubic	Coxal
Gluteal	Perineal	

Leg region (lower extremity)

Femoral	Sural	Plantar
Popliteal	Peroneal	Digital
Patellar	Tarsal	
Crural	Calcaneal	

Cardinal planes

The human body can be divided into sections. This is often done to discuss structures inside the body and to accurately describe the movement of a body part. A plane is simply created by slicing completely through an object in a straight line. The human body is commonly described in terms of three **cardinal planes,** each perpendicular to one another.

The **sagittal plane** slices through the full length of the body from **anterior** to **posterior.** Thus the sagittal plane cuts the body into right and left portions, longitudinally. If these portions are equal in size, the plane is called **midsagittal plane,** or median sagittal plane. It is not necessary for a sagittal plane to create two equal portions. This plane can separate right from left, and it can separate the **medial** portion from the **lateral.**

The **frontal plane** slices through the full length of the body from left to right. This plane cuts the body into anterior and posterior portions, also longitudinally. Often called the coronal plane, the frontal plane separates the anterior portion from the posterior (Fig. 1-5).

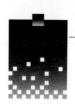

The **transverse plane** slices through the full width of the body from right to left, as well as from anterior to posterior. The transverse plane cuts the body into superior and inferior portions horizontally and thus is also called the **horizontal plane.** This plane separates the superior portion from the inferior.

It is important to reference the body from its correct anatomic position before identifying a plane. The terms sagittal, frontal, and transverse are only valid when considering the body in its anatomic position. To change the orientation of the body or body part in space, a plane must be correctly identified by its appropriate definition.

When considering the division of a body part by a plane, it is important to consider the definition of the plane and determine whether the plane divides the body part into right and left portions, anterior and posterior portions, or superior and inferior portions. For example, even though the arm may not hang straight down from the shoulder, it is possible to divide the arm longitudinally into its own sagittal or frontal plane and observe the portions of the limb.

To view interior structures such as inside blood vessels, bones, or organs, it may be necessary to slice through the body in a **cross section.** A cross section can lie in any of the three cardinal planes but most often follows the transverse plane of a body or body part. If, however, the plane lies at an angle that is perpendicular to another plane, it is referred to as an **oblique plane** (Fig. 1-6).

Exercise 1-2. Anatomic regions

Now test the accuracy of your knowledge of anatomic regions. Be sure to correct yourself before permanence sets in where inaccuracy exists! Identify the anatomic regions labeled in Figure 1-7 on page 6.

1. _____   23. _____

2. _____   24. _____

3. _____   25. _____

4. _____   26. _____

5. _____   27. _____

6. _____   28. _____

7. _____   29. _____

8. _____   30. _____

9. _____   31. _____

10. _____   32. _____

11. _____   33. _____

12. _____   34. _____

13. _____   35. _____

14. _____   36. _____

15. _____   37. _____

16. _____   38. _____

17. _____   39. _____

18. _____   40. _____

19. _____   41. _____

20. _____   42. _____

21. _____   43. _____

22. _____   44. _____

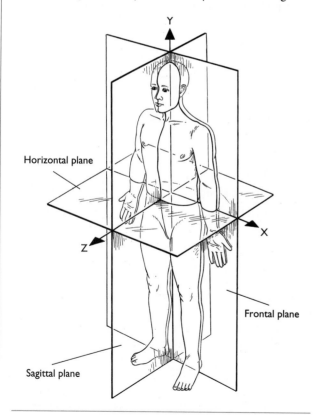

Figure 1-5. Cardinal planes.
From Greenstein: Clinical assessment of neuromusculoskeletal disorders, St Louis, 1997, Mosby.

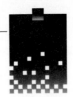

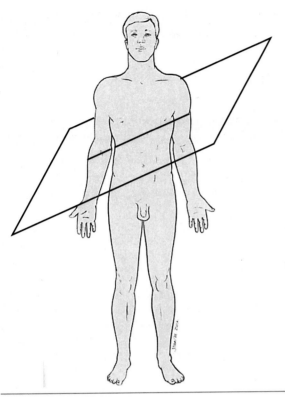

Figure 1-6. Oblique plane.
From Thibodeau: Structure & function of the body, ed 9, St Louis, 1992, Mosby.

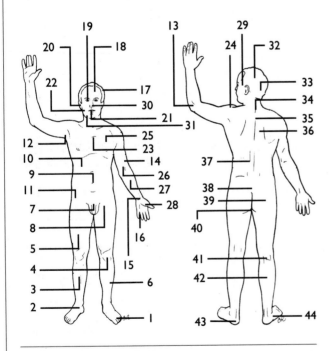

Figure 1-7. Anatomic regions.
From Fritz: Fundamentals of therapeutic massage, St Louis, 1995, Mosby.

Exercise 1-3. Cardinal planes

Identify the body planes as labeled in Figure 1-8. Consider which pair of directional terms is separated by each plane.

1. _____

2. _____

3. _____

4. _____

Exercise 1-4. Directional terminology

Give the directional term that best completes each sentence.

1. The ears are _____ to the nose.

2. Body hair is _____ to muscle.

3. The shoulder blade is _____ to the chest.

4. The knee cap is _____ to the hip.

5. The eye is _____ to the eyebrow.

6. The little finger is _____ to the thumb.

7. The navel is _____ to the buttocks.

8. Bone is _____ to skin.

9. The nose is _____ to the lips.

10. The shoulder is _____ to the wrist.

11. The occipital region is _____ to the mental region.

12. The brachial region is _____ to the axillary region.

13. The crural region is _____ to the sural region.

14. The sacral region is _____ to the thoracic region.

15. The buccal region is _____ to the frontal region.

16. The inguinal region is _____ to the gluteal region.

17. The perineal region is _____ to the peroneal region.

18. The inguinal region is _____ to the pubic region.

19. The antecubital region is _____ to the carpal region.

20. The plantar region is the most _____ of all the body regions.

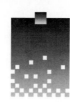

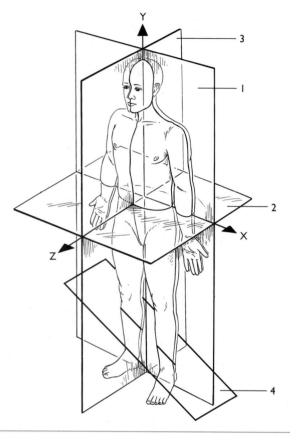

Figure 1-8. Anatomic planes.
From Greenstein: Clinical assessment of neuromusculoskeletal disorders, *St Louis, 1997, Mosby.*

■ Exercise 1-5. Cardinal planes defined

Complete the following statements.

1. The plane that divides the body into unequal left and right halves, anterior to posterior, is the _____ plane.

2. The only horizontal plane is the _____ plane.

3. The plane that divides the body into equal left and right halves, anterior to posterior, is the _____ plane.

4. The plane that divides the anterior and posterior portions of the body is the _____ plane.

5. The plane needed to view a cross section within the body is the _____ plane.

6. Two vertical planes of the body are the _____ and _____ planes.

7. The nose, umbilicus, and palm of the hand all lie within the _____ plane.

■ Exercise 1-6. Anatomic locations

Perform the following steps with a study partner.

1. Each study partner should cut five small pieces of tape and label them *A, B, C, D,* and *E.*

2. Attach each label to various parts of the body but all on the right side. (Do not cross the midsagittal plane with your labels.)

3. Each student should describe the locations of the labels on their study partner using correct directional terminology.

NOTE: When describing the locations, use the second label in a pair as the fixed reference. For example, if you are describing *A in relationship to B,* then *B* would be the fixed reference. Try the opposite; locate *B,* and describe the location of *A* using correct directional terminology. Correct anatomic position must be maintained if this exercise is to be accurately completed. It may be necessary to use combinations of directional terms for points that lie in an oblique plane.

Partner 1	Partner 2
A is _____ to B	A is _____ to B
B is _____ to C	B is _____ to C
C is _____ to D	C is _____ to D
D is _____ to E	D is _____ to E
E is _____ to A	E is _____ to A

■ Exercise 1-7. Anatomic locations by region

Without removing the labels from the previous exercise, list the anatomic region in which each label is located.

Partner 1	Partner 2
A _____	A _____
B _____	B _____
C _____	C _____
D _____	D _____
E _____	E _____

Exercise I-8. Anatomic directions

Using a tape measure and two small pieces of tape, follow the instructions given. The tape must be a metric measure since most medical measurements are performed using the metric system. In this exercise, measure from a known point and mark each resulting point, continuing through each step until the last point is marked with a separate piece of tape. Identify each location by its correct anatomic region. This exercise must be completed with the subject in anatomic position.

Instructions	Anatomic region
1. Measure 51 cm along the surface of the body in an inferior direction starting from the tip of the nose.	_____
2. From the last point, measure 40 cm laterally.	_____
3. From the last point, measure 60 cm inferiorly again.	_____
4. From the last point, measure 15 cm medially.	_____
5. From the last point, measure 20 cm superomedially.	_____
6. Measure the distance from the last point to the center of the knee cap. This distance is _____ cm.	_____

Key Words

It is important to periodically review each term listed to ensure familiarity with its definition, spelling, and location. Remember, practice makes permanent!

abdominal	dorsal	perineal
acromial	facial	peroneal
anatomic position	femoral	plantar
anatomic region	frontal	popliteal
antebrachial	frontal plane	posterior
antecubital	gluteal	posterolateral
anterior	horizontal plane	posteromedial
anterolateral	inferior	proximal
anteromedial	inferolateral	pubic
axillary	inferomedial	reference point
brachial	inguinal	sacral
buccal	landmark	sagittal plane
calcaneal	lateral	sternal
cardinal planes	lower extremity	superficial
carpal	lumbar	superior
caudal	medial	superolateral
cephalad	mental	superomedial
cephalic	midsagittal plane	sural
cervical	nasal	tarsal
coxal	oblique plane	temporal
cranial	occipital	thoracic
cross section	oral	transverse plane
crural	orbital	umbilical
cubital	otic	upper extremity
deep	palmar	ventral
digital	parietal	vertebral
directional term	patellar	
distal	pectoral	

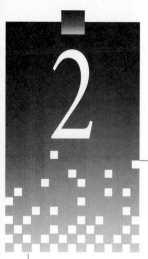

Human Skeleton

66 *This chapter will enable you to identify the primary elements of the skeletal system, including bone tissue, individual bones, and their landmarks.* 99

Chapter objectives:

The student will be able to:

1. Describe the essential elements of bone tissue.

2. Describe bones by classification as it applies to shape.

3. Describe basic terminology as it applies to bony landmarks of the skeleton.

4. Identify the bones of the axial skeleton and its specific landmarks.

5. Identify bones of the appendicular skeleton and its specific landmarks.

6. Palpate superficial skeletah landmarks on study partner.

7. Practice recognition and the use of bone and landmark terminology by completing exercise individually or with a study partner.

Bone as a Living Tissue

With the human body oriented in space, it is possible to discuss the specific elements that are responsible for achieving shape and movement. The most elemental framework of the human body is provided by the skeleton through the collection of rigid, interlocking pieces. Though bone appears to be a lifeless material, it is in fact a very active tissue and must be carefully observed at the microscopic level to fully understand its structure.

Basic Compounds Found in Bone

Bone is a living, growing, changing tissue; therefore it requires the same factors as any living organism—nutrients, oxygen, heat, and pressure. These elements enable bone tissue to grow, to produce much needed blood cells, to repair itself, and to serve as the body's structural support system.

The most abundant compounds required to build bone fall into two categories: **calcium salts** and **organic matrix.** Calcium is the most abundant mineral in the body, and as a chemical it is also vitally necessary to sustain a normal heartbeat, regular nerve impulses, and muscle tissue contraction. Other minerals found in the body are magnesium, sodium, and potassium.

The organic matrix is a living framework, a complex network of semiflexible **collagen fibers** made up of chains of protein molecules. The network of these fibers provides shape and yet is flexible. Its covering is a collection of tiny flat plates, which are actually calcium salts. The calcium attaches and interlocks in layers onto the collagen framework, just as bricks form the walls of a house. The calcium is hard and provides strength to the collagen framework.

The organic matrix allows bone to bend slightly without breaking. This flexibility is referred to as **tensile strength.** Calcium provides the ability of bone to withstand **compressive forces** without being crushed. Therefore a healthy, active person must have the appropriate combination of collagen fiber and calcium to withstand the force of their own body weight while standing erect, as well as to resist the repeated trauma of moving about.

Prenatal Development of Bone

During prenatal development, the initial structures that later become bone are composed of **hyaline cartilage.** Hyaline carti-

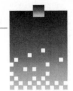

lage is a firm but flexible tissue made primarily of collagen fibers. Early in prenatal development the cells of the hyaline cartilage multiply and enlarge at a rapid rate. Later, hyaline cartilage is replaced by **osteoblasts,** or bone-forming cells. The osteoblasts bring about the development of the collagenous organic matrix. Calcium is then deposited onto the matrix, and blood vessels grow into the tissues providing nutrients and oxygen. These tissues, which begin as hyaline cartilage and evolve into bone, are called **endochondral bone.** The depositing of calcium onto the organic matrix is referred to as **ossification.**

Types of Bone Tissue

Every bone in the human body is a collection of several different combinations of the organic matrix laden with calcium. The outer covering of bone is called the **periosteum,** a layer of tough, fibrous tissue with a vascular network that provides nutrients to the bone. Beneath the periosteum layer, bone tissue is arranged in two distinct patterns—**compact (cortical) bone** and **spongy (cancellous) bone.** Each bone type has different properties that contribute to the specific needs of the body with respect to its location and abundance (Fig. 2-1).

Individual bones of the skeleton possess both compact and spongy bone tissue. The walls and strong shaft of a bone are made up of compact bone tissue, whereas the irregularly shaped, round portions of a bone and the distal ends of a

long bone are composed of spongy bone tissue. Thus a single bone has the benefits of firmness and the ability to resist bending (derived from the outer compact bone tissue), as well as the ability to resist compressive forces (derived from the inner spongy bone tissue). Without the mineral and organic matrix in each type of bone tissue, the integrity of the bone is compromised, and an injury or disease is more likely.

Compact bone

Microscopically, compact, or cortical bone, consists of a circular pattern where **osteocytes** (bone cells) are surrounded by **lacuna,** which are open spaces. Together, osteocytes and lacuna form layers that are called **lamellae** and are "wrapped" around one another, similar to the concentrically arranged rings in a tree trunk. **Canaliculus** are tiny passages that connect the lamellae to one another. At the center of the circular lamellae, there is a hollow, vertical opening known as the **haversian canal,** or central canal. The haversian canal is hollow and contains a complex network of blood and lymph vessels and nerves. Each haversian canal is interconnected with other haversian canals via **Volkmann's canals.** These canals are horizontal openings through which the blood and lymph vessels and nerves branch out to all portions of the bone tissue (Fig. 2-2). This group of structures—the lamellae, their osteocytes and lacuna, and the haversian and Volkmann's canals and adjoining canaliculi–is referred to as the **haversian system** or **osteon structure.** Countless osteon structures, each tightly packed lying side by side, give compact bone its resistance to bending.

Spongy bone

Spongy, or cancellous, bone differs from compact bone in its lack of density. Spongy bone tissue has a breadlike appear-

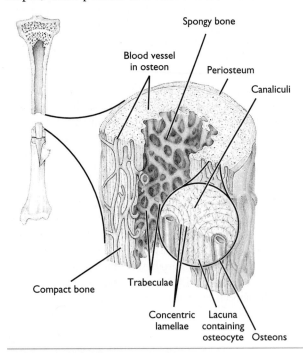

Figure 2-1. Microscopic structure of bone.
Drawing by Laurie O'Keefe, John Daugherty. From Thibodeau, Patton: Structure & function of the body, ed 10, St Louis, 1997, Mosby.

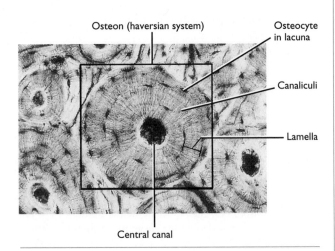

Figure 2-2. Compact bone.
From Thibodeau, Patton: Structure & function of the body, ed 10, St Louis, 1997, Mosby.

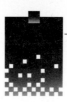
ance with many small openings surrounded by a tiny intricate web of irregular cancellous branches called **trabeculae.** The value of spongy bone lies in its ability to resist compressive forces that occur while bearing weight through the length of a bone or stepping down forcefully.

Some bones have a hollow tube at their center known as the **medullary cavity** in which **bone marrow** is found. The wall of the medullary cavity is called the **endosteum** (Fig. 2-3).

■ Exercise 2-1. Bone tissue

Match each definition to the correct term.

_____ 1. Lacks density; breadlike tissue
_____ 2. Hollow tube; contains marrow
_____ 3. Primary mineral of bone tissue
_____ 4. Flexible portion of organic matrix
_____ 5. Horizontally connects haversian canals
_____ 6. Web of cancellous branches
_____ 7. Made of collagen fibers
_____ 8. Against which calcium resists
_____ 9. Vertical opening within a canaliculus
_____ 10. Existing bone cells
_____ 11. Lining of medullary cavity
_____ 12. Open spaces in bone tissue
_____ 13. Another name for spongy bone
_____ 14. Layers formed by osteocytes and lacuna
_____ 15. Allows bone to bend, not break
_____ 16. Premature bone made of cartilage
_____ 17. Depositing of calcium onto organic matrix
_____ 18. Complex interconnecting structure of bone
_____ 19. Tiny passages between lamellae
_____ 20. Flexible tissue preceding bone
_____ 21. Bone-forming cells
_____ 22. Tough vascular exterior of bone
_____ 23. Another name for compact bone
_____ 24. Material found in medullary cavity

a. Endochondral bone
b. Canaliculus
c. Compressive forces
d. Cortical bone
e. Calcium
f. Trabeculae
g. Periosteum
h. Osteoblasts
i. Tensile strength
j. Lacuna
k. Spongy bone
l. Volkmann's canal
m. Haversian canal
n. Lamellae
o. Bone marrow
p. Collagen fibers
q. Haversian system (osteon)
r. Hyaline cartilage
s. Organic matrix
t. Cancellous bone
u. Ossification
v. Medullary cavity
w. Endosteum
x. Osteocytes

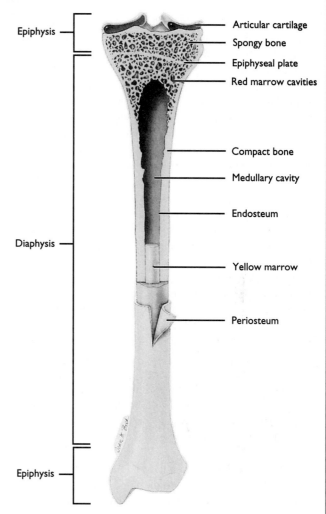

Epiphysis

Diaphysis

Epiphysis

Articular cartilage
Spongy bone
Epiphyseal plate
Red marrow cavities

Compact bone
Medullary cavity
Endosteum

Yellow marrow

Periosteum

Figure 2-3. Longitudinal section of a long bone.
Drawing by Joan Beck. From Thibodeau, Patton: Structure & function of the body, ed 10, St Louis, 1997, Mosby.

Functions of Bone

The skeleton serves many purposes in its role in human physiology and mobility. Bones, as living structures, interact with the systems and organs around them and perform several vital functions without which human life would be impossible. Understanding the makeup of bone tissues is necessary to apply appropriate treatment techniques to the patient with a bone disorder or injury.

Force-resistant framework

The obvious function of the skeleton is to give the body its shape and posture. Our height and ability to stand erect are possible because of the solid interlocking bones of the trunk and extremities. A foundation of bone and cartilage contributes to the contours of the entire body. Other tissues surround and attach to bone without which the body would become a soft mass. An injury to a bone can affect the use of a limb or the posture of the entire body.

As the framework of the human body, bone resists many forces—bending and stretching (tensile strength), the pull of gravity on all body tissues (compression forces), and the response to contact with outside objects that may occur in walking, running, lifting, and any other movement.

According to Julius Wolff, an eighteenth-century German anatomist, bones will grow and develop in response to the activities in which they participate.* This is called **remodeling,** a process in which the makeup of the bone tissue changes its composition in response to the demands placed on it. In effect, a bone consistently used in strenuous activity will maintain its size and shape and calcium content. The cellular makeup and percentage of calcium in an inactive bone that has not been regularly stressed will change. Removal of calcium from a bone is called **resorption,** and if this process continues over time, the result is a weakening of the bone and a higher potential for injury or fracture.

Mineral storage

As previously stated, calcium is one of the most abundant minerals found in the body. Its molecular composition makes it capable of combining easily with other elements, creating a wide variety of chemical compounds. The presence of calcium in bone, as well as in other physiologic processes of the body, is essential to human life.

Calcium is found in teeth, blood, muscle, and many other soft tissues. The presence of calcium in these areas is not a constant occurrence but a transient one, ever changing and adjusting to the immediate needs of the body. When organs such as the heart or muscles need calcium to function, the body draws the required levels from the blood stream and bone. Calcium does not permanently exist in any one place, but it is frequently exchanged with many body systems. It can be deposited in bone or absorbed from bone by the blood stream and transported to other areas. The skeleton is a storage area for calcium currently not in use by other organs. If, however, the stored quantity is not sufficient to provide the rigidity needed in bone, the bone may break or become deformed in response to excessive outside pressures. Other minerals stored in bone are potassium, sodium, magnesium, sulphur, and copper.

Muscle attachment

The only contractile tissue of the body is muscle, and it must anchor itself to a bone to move it. The skeleton is a platform that allows a person to voluntarily move body parts. This movement is accomplished with the help of the **tendon,** a rigid connective tissue. Without this bony attachment, muscles would not be able to effect change in the position of the body or body parts.

Voluntary movement can only take place in areas where two bones come together to form a joint. Movement cannot occur in the middle of a solid bone but is allowed by specialized structures occurring in areas intended for mobility according to the human design. Thus movement is possible where joints exist.

Protection

The vital and vulnerable internal organs (brain, heart, and lungs), depend on the skeleton to provide shelter and protection from outside forces. Similar to a coat of armor, the bones of the skull, chest, and shoulders effectively serve this purpose.

Fat storage and blood cell production

Bone marrow is a collection of very specialized cells whose responsibility it is to store fat and, more importantly, manufacture several types of blood cells. Blood-producing red bone marrow can be found in the open areas of some spongy bone tissue. Fat-storing yellow bone marrow is primarily found in the medullary cavity. The process of blood cell production by the bone marrow is called **hematopoiesis.** If the bone and bone marrow are damaged, as can occur from radiation or chemical exposure, the body cannot create the cells required for transporting oxygen in the body.

Filtration

Finally, bones with their intact circulatory structures form a sort of filter through which some contaminants can be collected. For instance, lead is all too often a contaminant in our environment, and if ingested or absorbed, it is deposited and stored in the skeleton via the blood stream.

■　　**Exercise 2-2. Functions of bone tissue**

List seven primary functions of bone tissue. Provide a brief description of each function.

Function 1: _____

　Description: _____

_____

_____

Function 2: _____

　Description: _____

_____

_____

*Gamble: *The musculoskeletal system: physiological basics,* New York, 1988, Raven Press.

Exercise 2-2. *Functions of bone tissue*–cont

Function 3: _____

Description: _____

_____

_____

Function 4: _____

Description: _____

_____

_____

Function 5: _____

Description: _____

_____

_____

Function 6: _____

Description: _____

_____

_____

Function 7: _____

Description: _____

_____

_____

Exercise 2-3. *Bone tissue*

Identify bone tissue on Figures 2-4, 2-5, and 2-6.

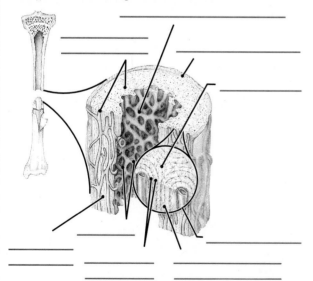

Figure 2-4. Microscopic structure of bone.
Drawing by Laurie O'Keefe, John Daugherty. From Thibodeau, Patton: Structure & function of the body, ed 10, St Louis, 1997, Mosby.

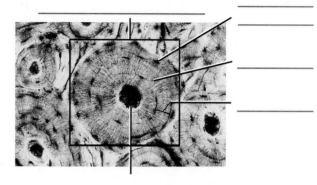

Figure 2-5. Compact bone.
From Thibodeau, Patton: Structure & function of the body, ed 10, St Louis, 1997, Mosby.

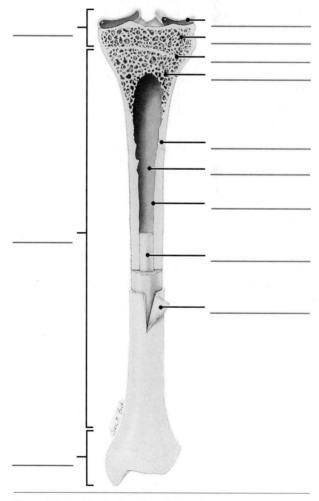

Figure 2-6. Longitudinal section of a long bone.
Drawing by Joan Beck. From Thibodeau, Patton: Structure & function of the body, ed 10, St Louis, 1997, Mosby.

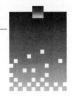

Terminology of Bone Shapes

Each bone has a distinct form that is directly related to the overall size and age of the body and its location in the body. Many bones are mirror images of themselves, providing right and left components of the same bone. The location and function of each bone can be correctly identified by its shape. The common terms used to describe the shape of a bone are long, short, irregular, flat, and sesamoid (Fig. 2-7).

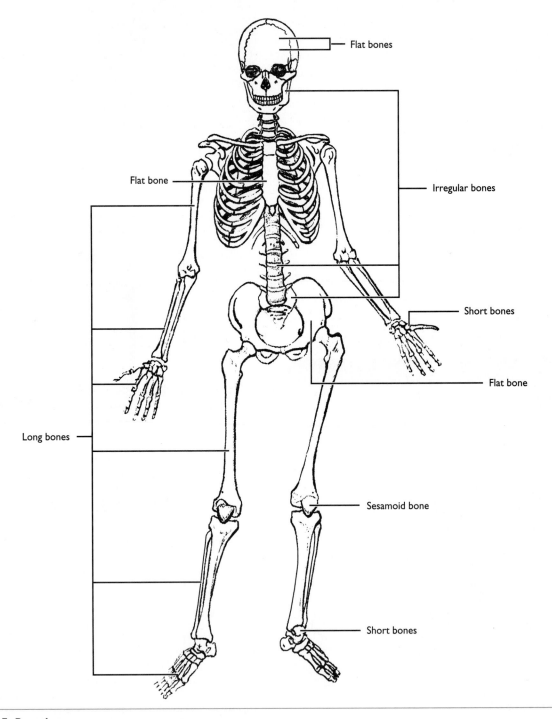

Figure 2-7. Bone shapes.
From Fritz: Fundamentals of therapeutic massage, *St Louis, 1995, Mosby.*

Long bones

As its name implies, the **long bone** has a long shaft known as the **diaphysis.** The end of a long bone is called the **epiphysis,** and it is usually wider than the diaphysis. During the growing years the diaphysis and epiphysis are separated by a cartilaginous plate called the **epiphyseal plate,** or growth plate (see Fig. 2-3). It is here that the growth process takes place at a rapid rate while the bone gradually increases in length. Once the growth is complete and the bone has achieved its full size, the epiphyseal plate undergoes ossification and the cartilage becomes solid bone. The long bone possesses both cortical and cancellous bone tissue. The diaphysis is constructed from cortical, or compact, bone for its tensile strength. A thin cortical outer shell over a cancellous core makes up the epiphysis and provides the long bone its resistance to compressive forces. Most long bones are located in the femoral, crural, brachial, antebrachial, and digital anatomic regions. Specific names of these bones are the femur, the tibia and fibula, the humerus and ulna, the radius, and the metacarpals and phalanges.

Short bones

The **short bone** does not have a diaphysis or epiphysis and is often called a round bone. The short bone has a smooth curving surface and is usually small compared with the long bone. It is composed of a superficial layer of cortical bone over a cancellous bony core. The **carpals** and **tarsals** are short bones and are found in the anatomic regions of the same name.

Irregular bones

An **irregular bone** does not have a simple or common pattern. Each irregular bone is adapted to its particular location and function. Some irregular bones have jagged or blunt edges, holes, or unusual branching or sloping characteristics. Samples of irregular bones can be located in the facial, vertebral, and sacral regions. Specific names are the mandible and maxilla, the individual vertebrae, and the sacrum.

Flat bones

The **flat bone** has a broad, smooth surface and is generally platelike in shape. The border of this bone may have a variety of forms. A flat bone is often called irregular, based on the contours of its edge. The most significant characteristic of a flat bone is its wide, smooth area. Similar to short and irregular bones, the flat bone has a cancellous core covered by a cortical shell. Flat bones are located in the cranial, thoracic, and coxal regions. Specific names are the frontal, parietal, and occipital bones, the scapulae, and the coxal bones.

Sesamoid bones

The **sesamoid bone** is quite small and usually round. It is similar to the short bone in shape. It, too, is usually cancellous and covered with a layer of cortical bone. The difference between a sesamoid bone and short bone is its location, function, and size. It is found adjacent to an existing bone, usually in the feet and hands, does not bear weight or resist heavy forces, and is usually small. Individual sesamoid bones are generally embedded inside tendons. The well-known sesamoid bone is the *patella,* or kneecap. Aside from the patella, the presence of sesamoid bones varies from individual to individual.

Exercise 2-4. Terminology of bone shapes

Match the bone shape with the correct description.

____ 1. Has a diaphysis and an epiphysis

____ 2. Has adapted to its particular location and function

____ 3. Has a wide, smooth surface

____ 4. Has a round, smooth, curving surface

____ 5. Is found adjacent to other bones; is small

a. Flat bone
b. Sesamoid bone
c. Short bone
d. Long bone
e. Irregular bone

Exercise 2-5. Bone identity by shape

Label each bone according to its correct shape on Figure 2-8 found on the following page.

Terminology of Skeletal Landmarks

Each bump, groove, hole, and edge on every bone has a name. This terminology is necessary to provide a consistent map of the human skeleton, which can be used to describe the specific location of every bone. These landmarks are the same from one healthy person to another with only slight variations caused by body size or growth patterns. In this text a list of commonly used landmark terms will be first identified; second, these terms will be assigned to a variety of locations over the entire human skeleton. Table 2-1 lists fourteen common landmark terms and a brief description of each.

As individual bones are discussed, particular attention is paid to the significant landmarks of each. Most bony landmarks are the points where muscles attach to the skeleton, making movement possible. Other landmarks are the points where two or more bones unite, or **articulate,** to form a joint.

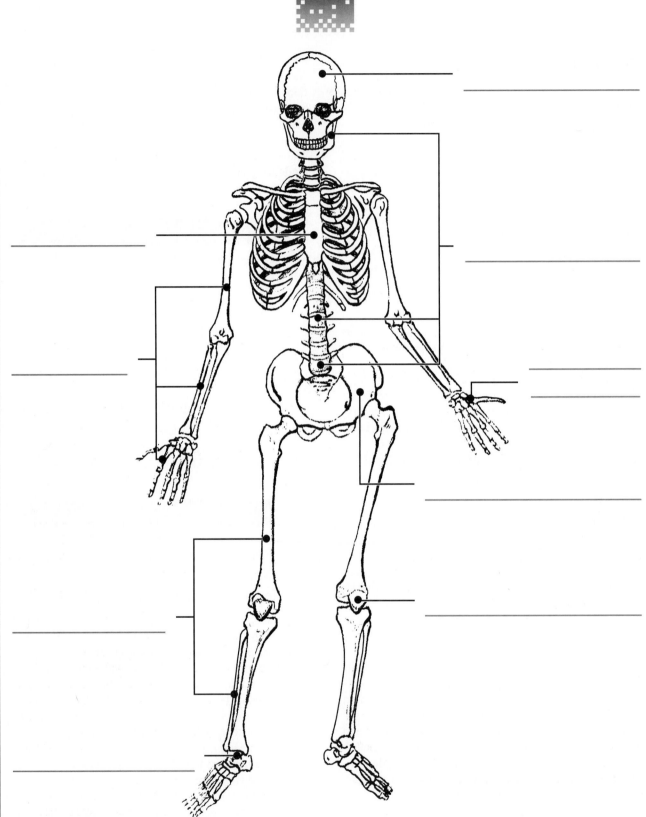

Figure 2-8. Bone shapes.
From Fritz: Fundamentals of therapeutic massage, *St Louis, 1995, Mosby.*

Table 2-1. Common landmark terms

Landmark	Definition	Skeletal location
Condyle	Round projection on the epiphysis	Femur
Crest	Angular ridge on the diaphysis or on the edge of an irregular bone	Ilium
Epicondyle	Raised and usually rough area; proximal to a wide epiphysis of a long bone	Femur, humerus
Facet	Small, flat face; smooth and usually circular	Vertebrae, rib
Foramen	Round hole completely through a bone	Coxal bone Occipital bone
Fossa	Round, cuplike depression	Scapula, coxal bone
Groove	Long, shallow depression or trough	Humerus
Head	Blunt, hammerlike protrusion, often round and smooth	Radius, humerus, femur, rib
Ramus	Flat bridge between two bones	Coxal bones
Sinus	Enclosed cavern	Facial bones
Tubercle	Small, rough, bulblike protrusion	Vertebrae, rib
Tuberosity	Large, rough, bulblike protrusion	Radius, ulna

Axial Skeleton

The human skeleton can be divided into two sections—**axial skeleton** and **appendicular skeleton.** The axial skeleton is the portion that creates an axis, or central framework, on which the arms and legs are attached. The axial skeleton consists of the bones of the head, face, vertebral column, and thoracic region (Fig. 2-9).

Bones of the cranium

The head is referred to as the **cranium,** or skull, and is made up of eight bones. As discussed in the previous sec-

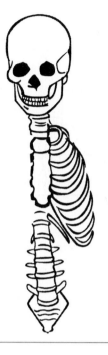

Figure 2-9. Axial skeletal.
From Brister: Mosby's comprehensive board review, *St Louis, 1996, Mosby.*

tion, a joint is formed where two or more bones unite, or articulate. Bones of the cranium knit together along their edges. The following is a discussion of the bones in the cranium, as oriented from anterior to posterior (Figs. 2-10, 2-11, 2-12, 2-13).

Frontal bone

The **frontal bone** is a flat bone that makes up the forehead area; its significant landmarks are the **superior portions of the right and left orbits,** which house the eyes. The second landmark is the **supraorbital foramen,** a small hole located just superior to each orbit. The frontal bone articulates with the parietal, sphenoid, ethmoid, and several facial bones.

Sphenoid bone

Just inferior to the frontal bone is the **sphenoid bone,** which resembles a butterfly with outstretched wings. It is best viewed from the floor of the interior of the cranium. The sphenoid bone articulates anteriorly with the zygomatic bone, frontal bone, and maxilla of the face and articulates with the temporal and occipital bones of the cranium. A portion of the sphenoid bone forms the deepest part of the **orbit,** which contains the eye.

Parietal bones

The two **parietal bones** make up the most superior portion of the cranium. They are large, flat bones that articulate with the frontal, occipital, sphenoid, and temporal bones, as well as with each other. There are no significant landmarks on these bones.

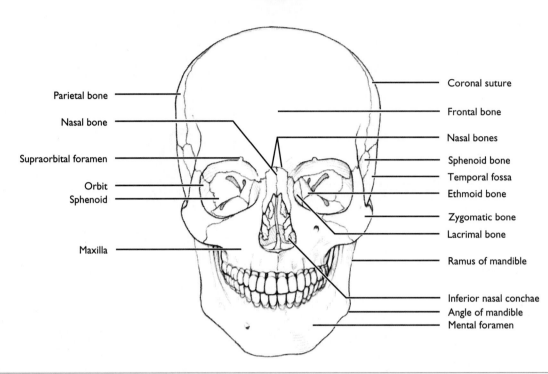

Figure 2-10. Anterior or frontal view of the skull.
From Mathers et al: Clinical anatomy principles, *St Louis, 1996, Mosby. (C.L.A.S.S. series, Stanford Project.)*

Parietal bone
Nasal bone
Supraorbital foramen
Orbit
Sphenoid
Maxilla

Coronal suture
Frontal bone
Nasal bones
Sphenoid bone
Temporal fossa
Ethmoid bone
Zygomatic bone
Lacrimal bone
Ramus of mandible
Inferior nasal conchae
Angle of mandible
Mental foramen

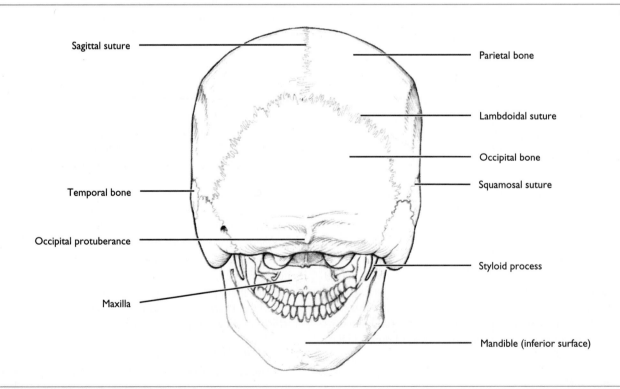

Sagittal suture
Temporal bone
Occipital protuberance
Maxilla

Parietal bone
Lambdoidal suture
Occipital bone
Squamosal suture
Styloid process
Mandible (inferior surface)

Figure 2-11. Posterior view of the skull.
From Mathers et al: Clinical anatomy principles, *St Louis, 1996, Mosby. (C.L.A.S.S. series, Stanford Project.)*

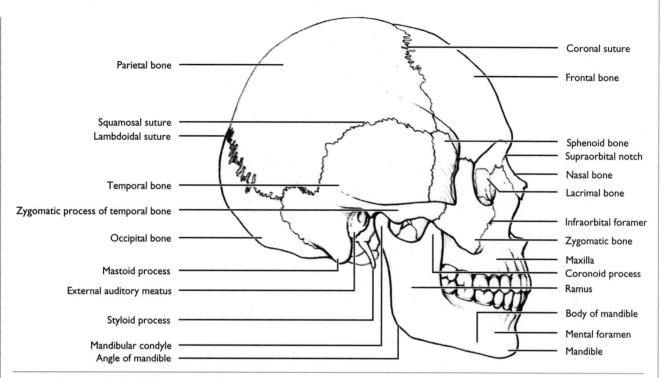

Figure 2-12. Lateral view of the cranium and face.
From Mathers et al: Clinical anatomy principles, St Louis, 1996, Mosby. (C.L.A.S.S. series, Stanford Project.)

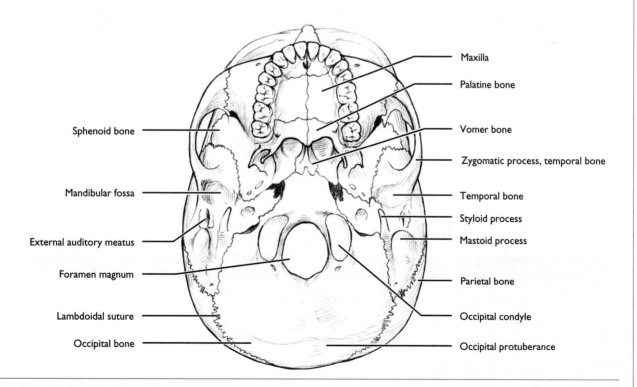

Figure 2-13. Inferior view of the skull.
From Mathers et al: Clinical anatomy principles, St Louis, 1996, Mosby. (C.L.A.S.S. series, Stanford Project.)

Temporal bones

The two **temporal bones** are irregular bones that make up the area surrounding both ears. The most prominent of these bones is the **external auditory meatus,** which is a portal to the inner ear. From this significant and easily located landmark, several others can be referenced. The **mastoid process** is a palpable, blunt process that lies just posterior and slightly inferior to the external auditory meatus. Directly inferior to the external auditory meatus is the **styloid process**, a landmark very different from the mastoid process; it is a long, thinly pointed bony projection. Moving directly anterior to the external auditory meatus is the **mandibular fossa**, the place where the bone of the lower jaw articulates. Just superior to the external auditory meatus is the base of a bony projection, which forms a bridge from the temporal bone to the zygomatic bone of the face. This bridgelike piece is called the **zygomatic process** of the temporal bone.

Occipital bone

The most posterior of all the cranial bones is the **occipital bone.** It articulates with the parietal bone, with both temporal bones, and with the sphenoid bone. The large opening is called the **foramen magnum** where the brain stem becomes the spinal cord. Externally and just laterally to the foramen magnum are two oval raised processes called the **occipital condyles.** These articulate with the first vertebra. The **occipital protuberance** is the most distinct palpable landmark, which is generally easy to locate on most individuals and is the raised area along the same transverse plane as the external auditory meatus.

Ethmoid bone

The **ethmoid bone** lies deep to other bones of the cranium and face and cannot be seen by either an exterior or interior view of the cranium. This bone articulates anteriorly to the sphenoid bone and inferiorly with the frontal bone in the small midline region.

Sutures of the cranium

Bones of the cranium are attached to one another by very irregular borders that form interlocking grooves and spaces. Each of these borders is called a **suture** and has a specific anatomic name. On close examination of a suture, tiny bones may be found, which only fill in spaces and are not actually part of either adjacent cranial bone. These are sutural bones, or wormian bones, and they vary from one individual to another. Significant sutures of the cranium are the **coronal, sagittal, squamosal, and lambdoidal sutures.**

■ Exercise 2-6. Bones of the cranium

Complete the following table.

Bones of the cranium	Quantity	Significant landmarks	Type of bone (shape)
Frontal	_____	_____	_____
Ethmoid	_____	_____	_____
Sphenoid	_____	_____	_____
Parietal	_____	_____	_____
Temporal	_____	_____	_____
Occipital	_____	_____	_____

■ Exercise 2-7. Sutures of the cranium

Provide two adjacent articulating cranial bones for each cranial suture.

Coronal _____

Sagittal _____

Squamosal _____

Lambdoidal _____

■ Exercise 2-8. Cranium

Identify the bones, landmarks, and sutures of the cranium on Figures 2-14 through 2-17 on pages 21 and 22.

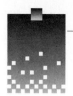

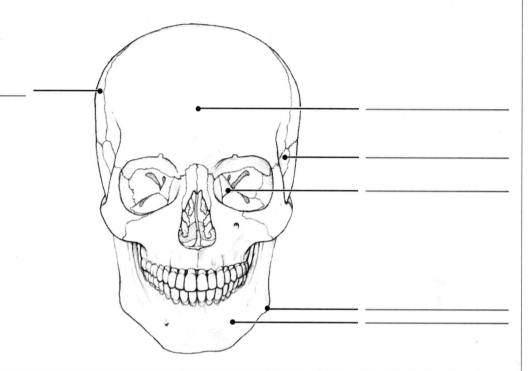

Figure 2-14. Anterior or frontal view of the skull.
From Mathers et al: Clinical anatomy principles, *St Louis, 1996, Mosby. (C.L.A.S.S. series, Stanford Project.)*

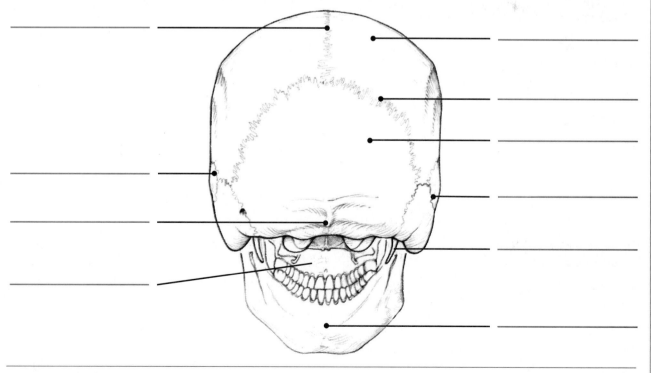

Figure 2-15. Posterior view of the skull.
From Mathers et al: Clinical anatomy principles, *St Louis, 1996, Mosby. (C.L.A.S.S. series, Stanford Project.)*

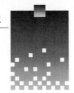

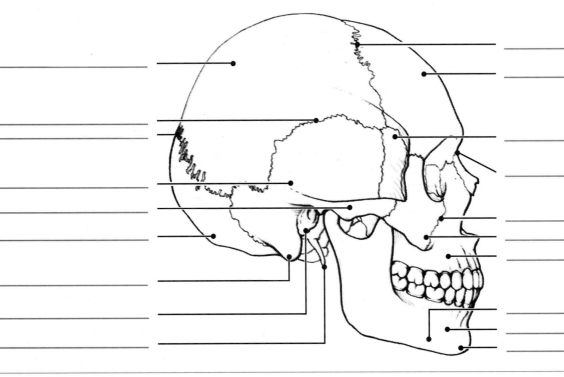

Figure 2-16. Lateral view of the cranium and face.
From Mathers et al: Clinical anatomy principles, *St Louis, 1996, Mosby. (C.L.A.S.S. series, Stanford Project.)*

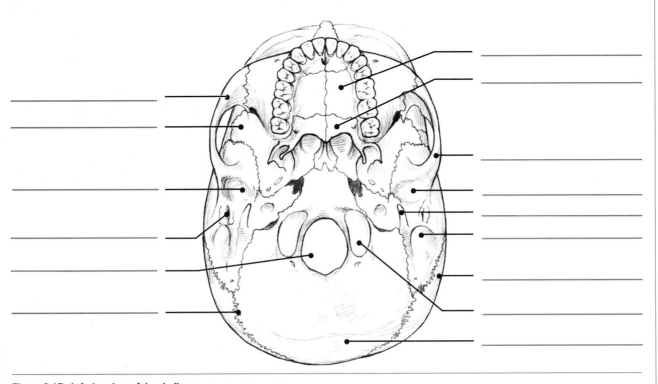

Figure 2-17. Inferior view of the skull.
From Mathers et al: Clinical anatomy principles, *St Louis, 1996, Mosby. (C.L.A.S.S. series, Stanford Project.)*

Study Note

Consider an important point. When discussing landmarks of specific bones of the human skeleton, it is important to identify the bone being discussed *along with* the landmark to provide clarity and continuity in communication. Occasionally, it is possible that a landmark name will be the same on another bone in the body. In these cases, discussing the landmark without the specific bone may cause confusion. Remember that ***practice makes permanent.*** When studying the bones and their landmarks, mention (either silently or aloud) the landmark and the bone together; the information will more quickly become familiar. For example, consider the following:

- External auditory meatus *of the temporal bone*
- Mastoid process *of the temporal bone*
- Styloid process *of the temporal bone*
- Zygomatic process *of the temporal bone*

By the way, there are several styloid processes on the skeleton; to delete the name of the specific bone in a discussion may lead to inaccuracy!

Bones of the face

There are fourteen different bones of the face (Box 2-1), some of which articulate with the bones of the cranium. Each is highly irregular in shape, and only one of the facial bones—the mandible—is movable (see Figs. 2-10, 2-11, 2-12, 2-13).

Box 2-1. Bones of the face

Maxilla	(2)
Zygomatic	(2)
Nasal	(2)
Vomer	(1)
Lacrimal	(2)
Palatine	(2)
Inferior nasal conchae	(2)
Mandible	(1)

Maxillary bones

Two **maxillary bones** form the upper jaw—the lower portion of the orbit and the base of the nose. An extension of these bones forms the **hard palate,** or the roof of the mouth.

Zygomatic bones

The cheek bones are called the **zygomatic bones** and form the inferolateral portion of the orbit. This is a bridgelike process that attaches to the zygomatic process of the temporal bone via the **temporal process** of the zygomatic bone to form the **zygomatic arch.** The connection of the two is the attachment between two bones and processes.

Nasal, vomer, lacrimal, and palatine bones and inferior nasal conchae

Two **nasal bones** lie alongside one another and form the bridge of the nose. Visible from an inferior view of the cranium and face, the **vomer bone** forms the nasal septum at the point where it connects to the ethmoid bone at the perpendicular plate. The two **lacrimal bones** are very small and form the lateral wall of the nasal cavity and the medial wall of the orbit. The **palatine bones** make up part of the hard palate and the floor of the nasal cavity. The **inferior nasal conchae** is separate from the middle and superior nasal conchae of the ethmoid bone, positioned appropriately just below it. This is a long, curved, fragile bone covered by nasal membranes.

Mandible

The **mandible** is the heavy, lower jawbone and is the only facial bone that is movable. This is a U-shaped bone with a broad, flattened area at each end, providing a wide surface for muscle attachment, known as the **mandibular ramus** (see Fig. 2-12). A ramus is a branch or a part that divides a larger structure.

The heavier area near the places where the teeth are seated is the **body of mandible,** and the curved area where the ramus and body meet is the **angle of mandible.** On the most superior portion high on the ramus of the mandible are two more significant landmarks. The first blunt rounded projection is the **mandibular condyle**—right and left. The mandibular condyle articulates with the mandibular fossa of the temporal bone. The second landmark is the flat, yet more pointed **coronoid process of mandible,** serving as the primary area for muscle attachment needed for closing and opening the jaw.

Hyoid bone

The **hyoid bone** is a very unique bony structure that is not included in any other group of bone. It is found in the anterior cervical region (the throat). The hyoid bone is shaped like a small horseshoe, serves as an anchor for muscles of the tongue and mouth, and is held in place by a ligament. It does not directly articulate with any other bone in the skeleton and is classified as irregular in shape (Fig. 2-18).

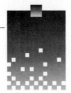

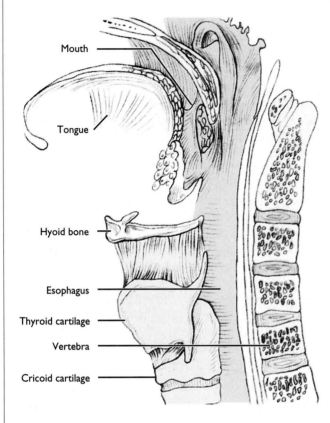

Mouth

Tongue

Hyoid bone

Esophagus

Thyroid cartilage

Vertebra

Cricoid cartilage

Figure 2-18. Hyoid bone.
From Mathers et al: Clinical anatomy principles, St Louis, 1996, Mosby.
(C.L.A.S.S. series, Stanford Project.)

Exercise 2-9. Bones and landmarks of the face

Identify the bones and landmarks of the face on Figures 2-19 through 2-21 on pages 25 and 26.

Exercise 2-10. Bones of the face

Complete the following table.

Bone of the face	Quantity	Significant landmarks
Maxilla	_____	_____
Nasal	_____	_____
Vomer	_____	_____
Lacrimal	_____	_____
Zygomatic	_____	_____
Palatine	_____	_____
Inferior nasal conchae	_____	_____
Mandible	_____	_____

Vertebral column

The **vertebral column** is a complex stack of 28 irregular bony structures that interlock with the pieces above and below it. The vertebral column is divided into four primary sections, based on the structure of the individual vertebra and the body region in which it exists. These sections are the **cervical, thoracic, lumbar,** and **sacral** areas. (In discussing these structures the spelling of *vertebra* is singular, whereas *vertebrae* is plural (see Figs. 2-22, 2-23, 2-24 on page 27).

Individual vertebrae are separated by **intervertebral disks.** These disks are constructed of fibrous connective tissue and filled with clear fluid. They serve as cushions, absorbing pressure between the vertebral bodies.

Cervical vertebrae

The first seven vertebrae, counting from the most superior (C_1) to the most inferior (C_7), are the smallest of all the vertebrae and are also the most varied in shape. In the adult the alignment of this group forms a **convex curve** when facing anteriorly and a **concave curve** when facing posteriorly.

The first cervical vertebra is named **Atlas,** since it carries the entire cranium (see Fig. 2-25 on page 28). The circular shape of Atlas attaches to the cranium via the two **superior articulating facets,** which directly correspond to the occipital condyles. It articulates with the second cervical vertebra via two inferior articulating facets. This vertebra has an **anterior arch** and **tubercle** but no significant vertebral body; it has a **posterior tubercle** but no spinous process projecting posteriorly, like all other vertebrae.

Along the anterior midline of this vertebra, there is a flattened lip facing the **vertebral canal** known as the **odontoid facet,** which articulates with the similar process on C_2. This facet prevents a cervical vertebra from slipping off the next cervical vertebra. Atlas has two lateral bony projections known as **transverse processes,** which serve as

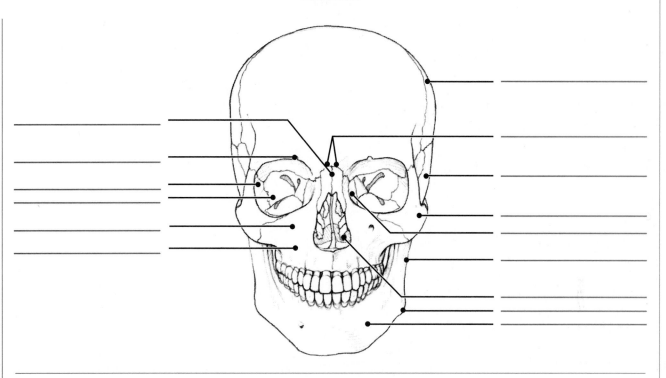

Figure 2-19. Anterior or frontal view of the skull.
From Mathers et al: Clinical anatomy principles, *St Louis, 1996, Mosby. (C.L.A.S.S. series, Stanford Project.)*

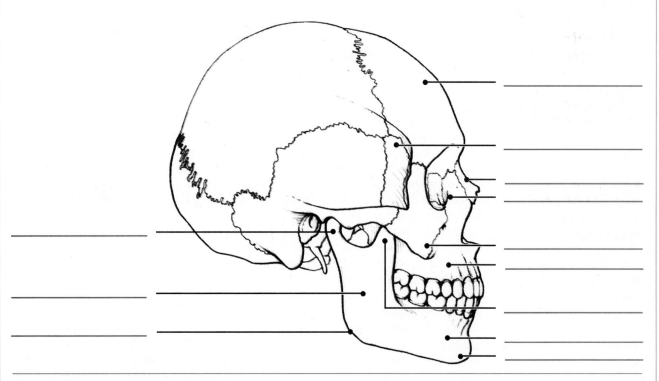

Figure 2-20. Lateral view of the cranium and face.
From Mathers et al: Clinical anatomy principles, *St Louis, 1996, Mosby. (C.L.A.S.S. series, Stanford Project.)*

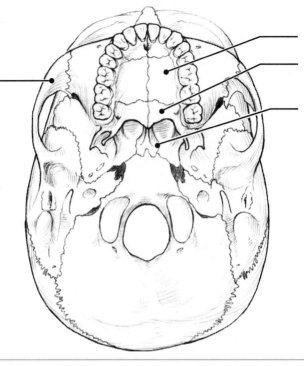

Figure 2-21. Inferior view of the skull.
From Mathers et al: Clinical anatomy principles, *St Louis, 1996, Mosby. (C.L.A.S.S. series, Stanford Project.)*

attachments for ligament and muscle. Just between the transverse processes and superior articulating facets, the **transverse foramen** is found, a pathway for the **vertebral artery.** Atlas, as do all cervical vertebrae, has two **inferior articular facets** that receive the superior facets from the second cervical vertebra.

    Axis, also known as C_2, is a thicker vertebra on which Atlas pivots. This pivotal point is called the **odontoid process** and is an extension of the thick anterior *body* of C_2. The two **superior articulating facets** of Axis articulate with the inferior articulating facets of Atlas. Like Atlas, Axis has two laterally oriented transverse processes and two transverse foramen. New, however, is the **spinous process,** which projects posteriorly. The tip of the spinous process of C_2 through C_5 is forked, or **bifid.** The spinous processes of all other vertebrae end in a single edge.

    The remaining five cervical vertebrae are all similar in structure and have similar landmarks. First, the thick vertebral *body* is located anteriorly; second, a large vertebral canal is found. Moving in a circle around the vertebrae, the landmarks are identified in order—transverse processes (2), superior articulating facet, inferior articulating facet, lamina (bony bridge), and spinous process. The spinous processes of C_6 and C_7 have a single tip and are also longer and angled downward. The spinous process of C_7 is a common landmark that can be palpated at the base of the neck on most individuals.

Thoracic vertebrae

There are twelve thoracic vertebrae that are similar in structure. As each vertebra is examined, the body of each appears progressively larger in diameter and thicker in depth; the overall vertebral column gets larger as the vertebral canal becomes smaller. All vertebrae will have one pair each of superior articulating facets and inferior articulating facets. The alignment of this group is opposite that of the cervical vertebrae with its convex curve posteriorly and its concave curve anteriorly (see Fig. 2-22).

    A thoracic vertebra has a rounded *body;* along the lateral aspect are two paired *facets for the head of the rib.* Each side of the thoracic vertebral body has one pair of these facets. The head of a single rib attaches between two vertebral bodies, thus contacting a single vertebral body inferiorly and superiorly simultaneously.

    From the body of the vertebra, a very short bridge called a **pedicle** is found, followed by the **superior articular facet,** which is now somewhat raised and facing posteriorly. The transverse processes can then be examined, which is longer than the cervical vertebrae and is also pointed in a posterolateral direction. At the end of the transverse process is the *facet for the tubercle of the rib.* The bridge from the transverse process to the spinous process is called the **lamina.** Thoracic spinous processes are long and slender and

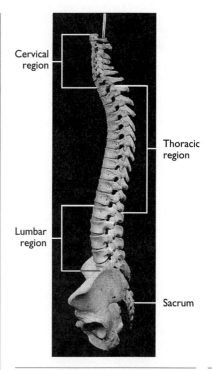

Cervical region

Thoracic region

Lumbar region

Sacrum

Figure 2-22. Vertebral column and pelvis, lateral view.
From Cramer, Darby: Basic & clinical anatomy of the spine, spinal cord, and ANS, St Louis, 1995, Mosby.

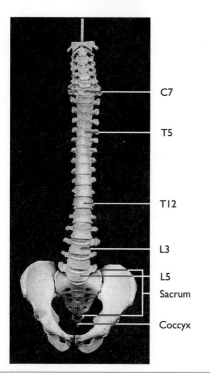

C7

T5

T12

L3

L5

Sacrum

Coccyx

Figure 2-23. Vertebral column and pelvis, anterior view.
From Cramer, Darby: Basic & clinical anatomy of the spine, spinal cord, and ANS, St Louis, 1995, Mosby.

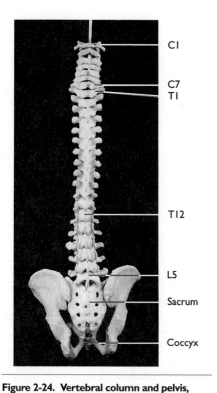

CI

C7
TI

T12

L5

Sacrum

Coccyx

Figure 2-24. Vertebral column and pelvis, posterior view.
From Cramer, Darby: Basic & clinical anatomy of the spine, spinal cord, and ANS, St Louis, 1995, Mosby.

pointing in an inferior direction, providing a long surface for muscle attachment in this region of the body. Inferiorly, one vertebra attaches to the next via an **inferior articulating facet** (Fig. 2-26).

To summarize, there are five pairs of facets on the thoracic vertebrae:

- ◼ 1 pair—superior articular facets
- ◼ 2 pairs—costal facets for the head of the rib
- ◼ 1 pair—costal facets for the tubercle of the rib
- ◼ 1 pair—inferior articular facets

Note the presence of the intervertebral disk between the vertebral bodies. This helps maintain the size of the **intervertebral foramen** found between the pedicles of two adjacent vertebrae. Through this foramen, the spinal nerve roots pass.

Lumbar vertebrae

The five **lumbar vertebrae** are the largest individual vertebrae, each with a heavy, oval vertebral *body* (Fig. 2-27). Since there are no ribs in this region, no facets are found on their bodies. The lumbar pedicle is thicker than its counterpart in the thoracic region, and the transverse processes are shorter and point in a lateral direction; it, too, has no rib facets. Two superior articulating facets are vertical and face posteromedially. Two

inferior articulating facets are also vertical and face anterolaterally. The lamina is also thicker than in the thoracic region. The lumbar spinous process is broad, significantly shorter than that of the thoracic vertebrae and pointing in a posterior direction, as opposed to inferior. This process creates a wider surface area on which the large low back muscles attach. Again, the vertebral canal is smaller than all preceding vertebrae since the spinal cord itself becomes progressively smaller in diameter as it moves farther from the brain.

The alignment of the lumbar vertebrae is similar to the cervical vertebrae, whereas it is opposite of the thoracic vertebrae. Here the curve is concave anteriorly and convex posteriorly.

Sacrum

The **sacrum** is actually five vertebral bodies that have fused together to form one bone (Fig. 2-28). Though it does not have the same landmarks as individual vertebrae, the sacrum has a structure similar to a vertebral body that enables it to receive the weight of the entire vertebral column. This structure is known as the **sacral promontory;** it has a *surface for articulation with L_5.* Near the sacrum are the last two superior articular facets, which receive the inferior articulating facets from L_5. Posterior to the sacral promontory is the **sacral canal,** which is the sacral portion of the vertebral foramen.

27

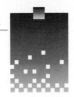

From the anterior view, the entire sacrum is approximately the size of an outstretched hand, wider proximally and coming to a point distally. The proximal winglike structures are called the **ala of sacrum.** The lateral, rough surfaces of each ala are the articular surfaces, or **sacroiliac facets,** which attach to the bones of the pelvis on the appendicular skeleton.

There is a series of four pairs of **sacral foramen** that exit both anteriorly and posteriorly through the sacral canal where nerves and blood vessels also exit. Posteriorly the sacral canal opens into the **sacral hiatus.**

Coccyx

The vertebral column comes to an end with the tiny bones of the **coccyx.** Technically, these four bones fuse together during early adulthood (see Figs. 2-23, 2-24).

Exercise 2-11. Vertebrae and vertebral landmarks

Complete the following table.

Vertebra	Quantity	Vertebral landmarks
C$_1$ (Atlas)	_____	_____
		_____
		_____
		_____
		_____
		_____
		_____

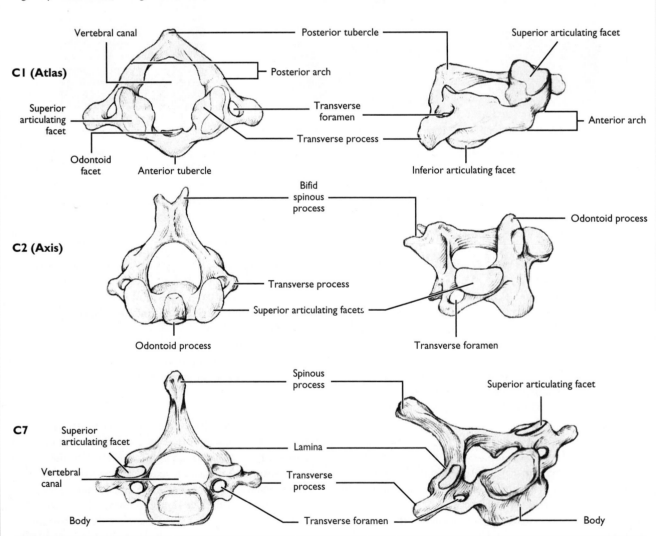

Figure 2-25. Cervical vertebrae, C$_1$, C$_2$, and C$_7$.
From Mathers et al: Clinical anatomy principles, St Louis, 1996, Mosby.

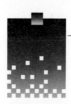

Exercise 2-11. Vertebrae and vertebral landmarks–*cont*

Vertebra	Quantity	Vertebral landmarks	Vertebra	Quantity	Vertebral landmarks
C$_2$ (Axis)	_____	_____	Cervical	_____	_____
		_____			_____
		_____			_____
		_____			_____
		_____			_____
		_____			_____
		_____			_____
		_____	Lumbar	_____	_____
Thoracic	_____	_____			_____
		_____			_____
		_____			_____
		_____			_____
		_____			_____
		_____			_____
		_____	Sacrum	_____	_____
		_____			_____
		_____			_____
		_____			_____
		_____			_____
		_____			_____
			Coccyx	_____	_____

Superior view

Spinous process —
Lamina
Vertebral canal —
Transverse process
Pedicle —
Facet for the head of rib —
Facet for the tubercle of rib
Body
Superior articulating facet

Intervertebral foramen

Two articulating vertebrae

Intervertebral disk

Lateral view

Facet for the head of rib —
Body —
Transverse process
Vertebral notch —
Combined articulating surface for the head of one rib
Inferior articulating facet —
Spinous process

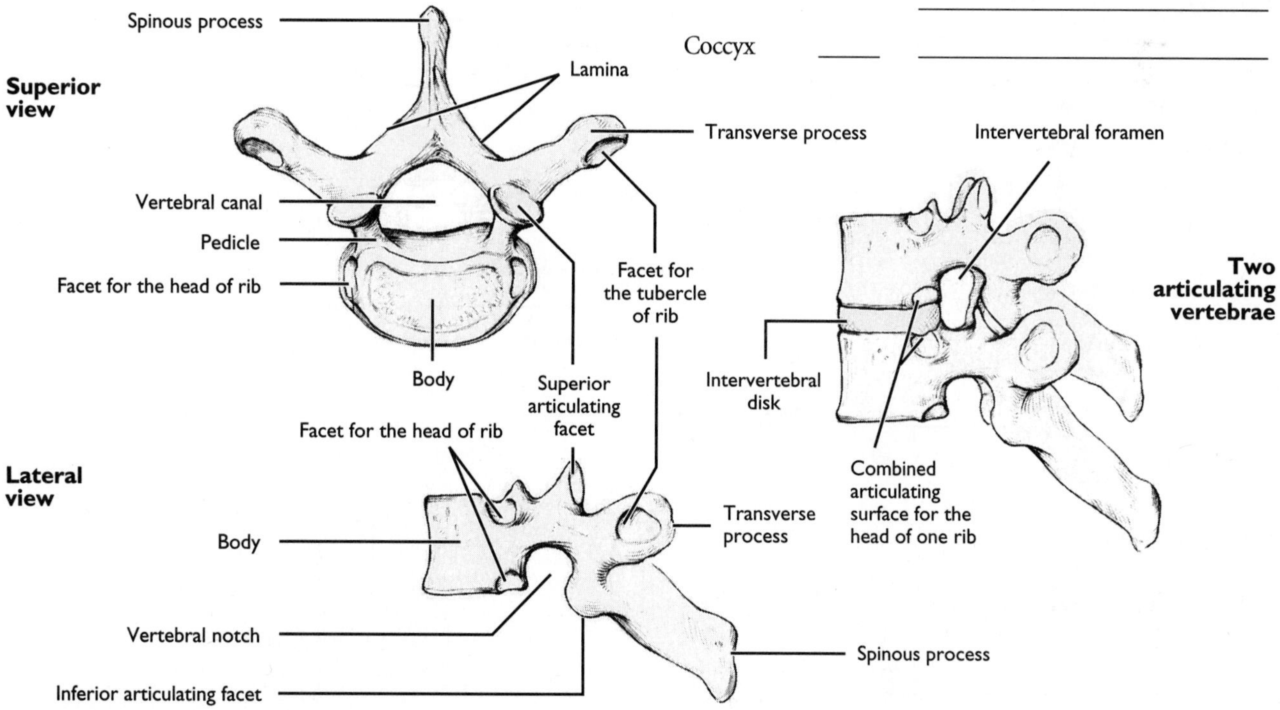

Figure 2-26. Thoracic vertebrae.
From Mathers et al: Clinical anatomy principles, *St Louis, 1996, Mosby.*

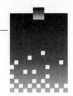

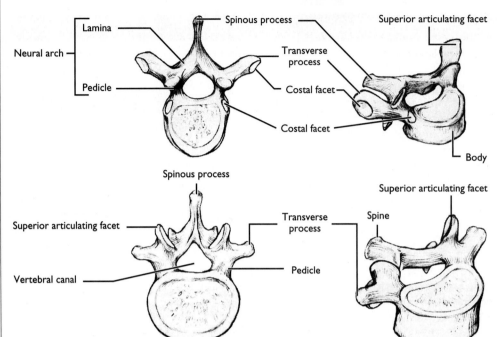

Figure 2-27. Typical thoracic and lumbar vertebrae (T$_7$ and L$_4$).
From Mathers et al: Clinical anatomy principles, *St Louis, 1996, Mosby.*

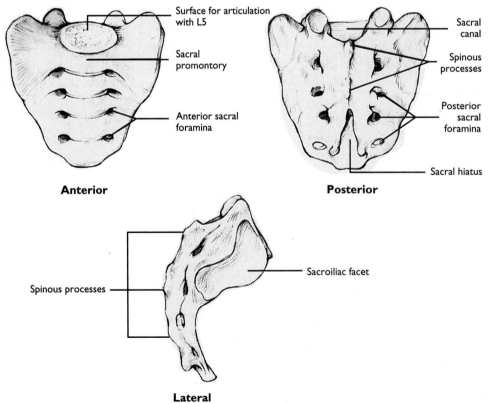

Anterior

Posterior

Lateral

Figure 2-28. Sacrum.
From Mathers et al: Clinical anatomy principles, *St Louis, 1996, Mosby.*

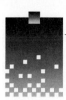

■ ■ ■ **Exercise 2-12. Vertebrae and vertebral landmarks**

*Identify the vertebrae and vertebral landmarks on Figures 2-29
through 2-32 on pages 31 through 33.*

■ ■ ■ **Exercise 2-13. Vertebral comparison**

*Review the characteristics and landmarks of the vertebrae.
Answer the following questions.*

1. What type of vertebra has the
   largest body?   _____

2. What type of vertebra has the
   smallest body?   _____

3. What landmark is found only on
   a typical cervical vertebra?   _____

4. What landmark is found only on
   a typical thoracic vertebra?   _____

5. What vertebral landmark is smallest
   on the lumbar vertebrae and largest _____
   on the cervical vertebrae?

6. What is significant about the spinous _____
   process of the cervical vertebrae?   _____

7. What is significant about the spinous _____
   process of the lumbar vertebrae?   _____

8. What is the difference in the   _____
   alignment of the superior and   _____
   inferior articulating facets of the   _____
   cervical vertebrae as compared   _____
   with those of the thoracic and   _____
   lumbar vertebrae?   _____

9. What is the difference in the shapes   _____
   of the transverse process of the cerv- _____
   ical, thoracic, and lumbar vertebrae? _____

10. What are alternative names for   _____
    C_1 and C_2?   _____

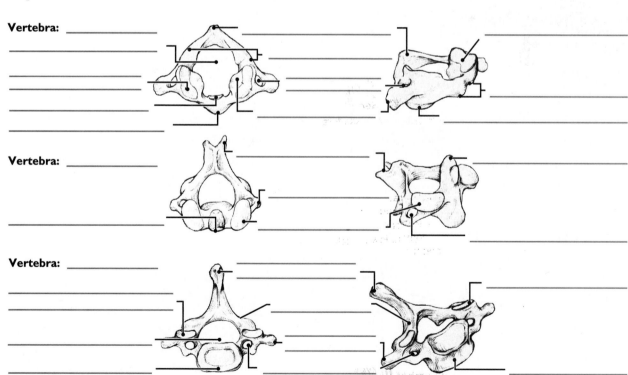

Vertebra: _____

Vertebra: _____

Vertebra: _____

Figure 2-29. Vertebral landmarks.
From Mathers et al: Clinical anatomy principles, *St Louis, 1996, Mosby.*

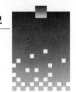

Vertebra: _____

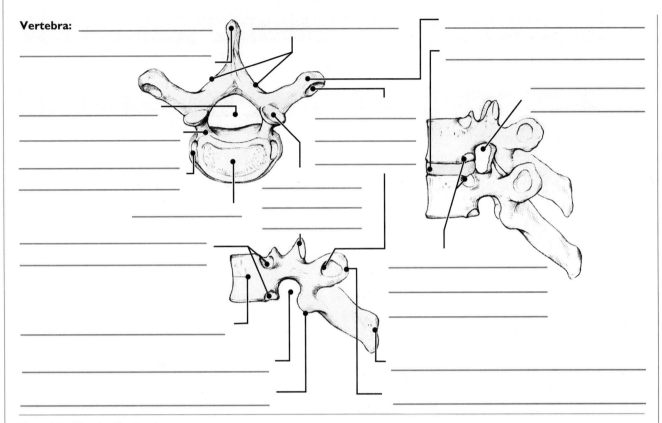

Figure 2-30. Vertebral landmarks.
From Mathers et al: Clinical anatomy principles, *St Louis, 1996, Mosby.*

Vertebra: _____

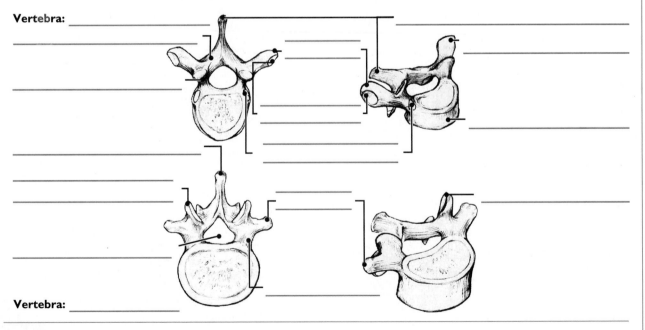

Vertebra: _____

Figure 2-31. Vertebral landmarks.
From Mathers et al: Clinical anatomy principles, *St Louis, 1996, Mosby.*

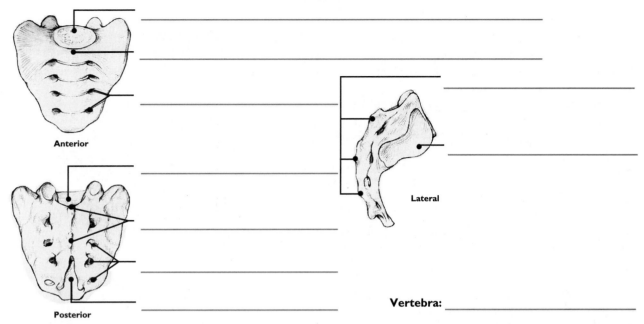

Anterior

Lateral

Posterior

Vertebra: _____

Figure 2-32. Vertebral landmarks.
From Mathers et al: Clinical anatomy principles, St Louis, 1996, Mosby.

Thoracic cage

Ribs

Typically, there are twelve pairs of **ribs,** although some individuals may have an extra pair or two. All ribs originate on the vertebral column at the thoracic vertebrae with two points of attachment. The blunt *head* of each rib, which articulates with the costal facets on the vertebral bodies that lie directly above and below one another, is the first point of attachment. The second vertebral attachment is at the **tubercle** of each rib, which corresponds to the costal facets located on the transverse processes of the thoracic vertebrae (Fig. 2-33).

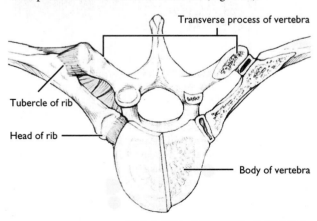

Transverse process of vertebra

Tubercle of rib

Head of rib

Body of vertebra

Figure 2-33. Thoracic vertebrae and ribs.
From Mathers et al: Clinical anatomy principles, St Louis, 1996, Mosby. (C.L.A.S.S. Series, Stanford project.)

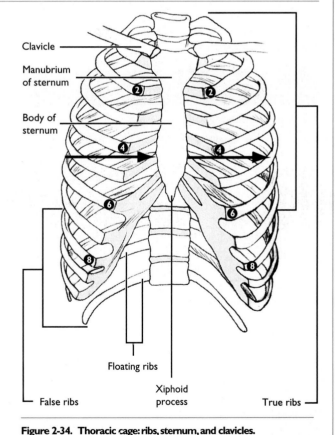

Clavicle

Manubrium of sternum

Body of sternum

Floating ribs

Xiphoid process

False ribs

True ribs

Figure 2-34. Thoracic cage: ribs, sternum, and clavicles.
From Mathers et al: Clinical anatomy principles, St Louis, 1996, Mosby. (C.L.A.S.S. Series, Stanford project.)

The most proximal seven pairs of ribs then attach *directly* onto the sternum anteriorly and are known as **true ribs.** The next five pairs (ribs 8 through 12) attach onto the vertebrae posteriorly and onto the sternum anteriorly via heavy costal (rib) cartilages; these are called **false ribs** (Fig. 2-34).

The proximal three pairs of false ribs are interconnected via **costal cartilage,** which attaches *indirectly* onto the sternum. The last two pairs of false ribs end short of any sternal attachment and thus are called **floating ribs.** All ribs are classified as flat bones.

Sternum

The **sternum** is a structure originally made up of three individual bones. The most proximal bone, the **manubrium,** is almost rectangular and articulates with the clavicle superiorly, with the first pair of ribs laterally, and with the **body of sternum** distally. The body of the sternum articulates with the remaining ribs via costal cartilages. The sternum ends with the **xiphoid process** (pronounced *zifoid*). These three bones fuse to become one piece during adult life; however, the xiphoid process can be broken away from the body of the sternum with a blow to the chest. The manubrium and the body of the sternum are generally referred to as flat bones, whereas the xiphoid process is referred to as irregular.

Exercise 2-14. Components of the ribs and sternum

Complete the following table.

Bone	Quantity	Landmarks
True ribs	____	_____
		_____
		_____
False ribs	____	_____
		_____
		_____
Floating ribs	____	_____
		_____
		_____
Sternum	____	_____
		_____
		_____

Exercise 2-15. Identify components of the ribs and sternum

Identify the components of the ribs and sternum on Figures 2-35 and 2-36.

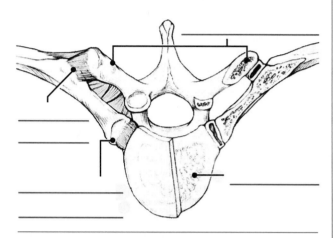

Figure 2-35. Landmarks of the ribs and vertebrae.
From Mathers et al: Clinical anatomy principles, *St Louis, 1996, Mosby.*

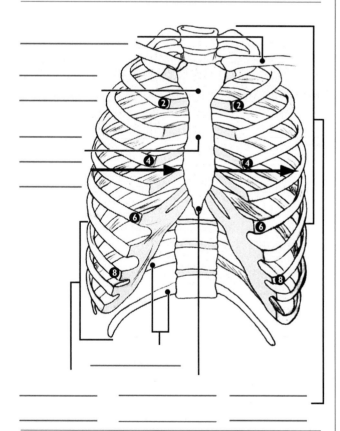

Figure 2-36. Landmarks on the ribs and vertebrae.
From Mathers et al: Clinical anatomy principles, *St Louis, 1996, Mosby.*

Exercise 2-16. Components of the axial skeleton

Complete the following table.

Category	Bones
Cranium	_____ _____
	_____ _____
	_____ _____
Face	_____ _____
	_____ _____
	_____ _____
	_____ _____
Anterior cervical region	_____
Vertebrae	_____ _____
	_____ _____
	_____ _____
	_____
Thoracic cage	_____ _____

Exercise 2-17. Palpating landmarks of the axial skeleton

Bony landmarks will feel differently on each individual. Practice your palpation skills on a partner; identify each bony landmark. With washable color markers or tape, label the following palpable skeletal landmarks on the body of your lab partner.

- Orbit
- Zygomatic arch
- Occipital bone
- Mastoid process of temporal bone
- Angle, ramus, and body of mandible
- Spinous processes of cervical vertebrae
- Seventh cervical spinous process
- Thoracic and lumbar spinous processes
- Sacrum
- Ribs
- Sternum

Appendicular Skeleton

The division of the human skeleton into its axial and appendicular sections helps discern which bones are associated with the trunk and which are related to the extremities. Movement is more readily demonstrated by the extremities. The appendicular skeleton includes the pectoral girdle and upper extremity and the pelvic girdle and lower extremity (Fig 2-37.)

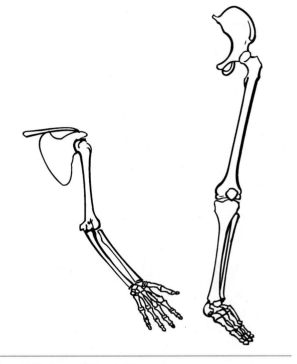

Figure 2-37. Appendicular skeleton.
From Brister: Mosby's comprehensive board review, *St Louis, 1996, Mosby.*

Pectoral girdle

The pectoral girdle is located in the acromial region of the body and is actually divided into right and left halves, separated by the sternum. This girdle consists of two clavicles and two scapulae (plural).

Clavicles

The two clavicles are the only means by which the pectoral girdle and entire upper extremity attach to the axial skeleton via articulating bones. The **clavicle** is classified as a long bone with a diaphysis and two epiphyses. It is a curved bone with a blunt, rounded **sternal** (proximal) **end** that articulates with the manubrium of the sternum. The **acromial** (distal) **end** is flat and articulates with the **acromion process of scapula** (Fig. 2-38).

Scapula

The two **scapulae** are flat bones, though quite irregular as a result of their unique landmarks; they are often called the *shoulder blades.* Perhaps it would be easiest to become familiar with the fifteen landmarks of each scapula by categorizing them by shape as listed in Box 2-2 (Fig. 2-39).

Observing the right scapula from the posterior view, it is somewhat triangular in shape. The angle at the upper medial side is the **superior angle,** whereas the bottom por-

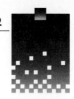

Anterior

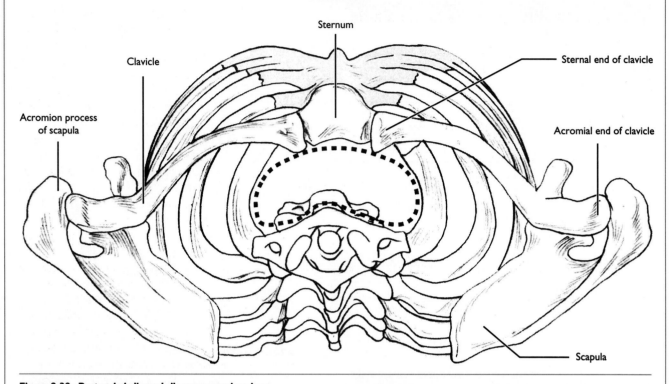

Figure 2-38. Pectoral girdle and rib cage, superior view.
From Mathers et al: Clinical anatomy principles, St Louis, 1996, Mosby. (C.L.A.S.S. series, Stanford Project.)

tion of the bone is the **inferior angle.** Two borders correspond to the two angles as the **vertebral** (medial) **border of scapula** lies between the superior and inferior angles. The **axillary** (lateral) **border of scapula** lies to the right of the inferior angle or toward the axillary region.

Box 2-2. Landmarks of the scapulae

Angles	*Processes*
Superior angle	Acromion process
Inferior angle	Coracoid process

Borders	*Fossa*
Vertebral (medial) border	Glenoid fossa
Axillary (lateral) border	Infraspinous fossa
	Supraspinous fossa
	Subscapular fossa

Root of the spine of scapula	*Spine of scapula*

Tubercles	*Scapular notch*
Supraglenoid tubercle	
Infraglenoid tubercle	

About one third the distance from the superior angle down the vertebral border, the **root of the spine of scapula** arises and gradually increases in height and thickness forming a heavy ridge. This ridge is the **spine of scapula.** It ends in a broad, flat projection, referred to as the **acromion process of scapula,** which is the largest process of the two on this bone. The other is the **coracoid process of scapula** (not to be confused with the coro*n*oid process of the mandible). The coracoid process looks like a hook and is located anterior to the acromion process of scapula.

The cuplike process at the most superior end of the axillary border is the **glenoid fossa,** which articulates with the largest bone of the arm, the humerus. Just above the spine of scapula is the **supraspinous fossa;** the larger indention below the spine of scapula is the **infraspinous fossa of scapula.** The **subscapular fossa** is a large, shallow indention located on the anterior (ventral) side of scapula and articulates indirectly with the ribs by gliding over them as the scapula moves. The *sub* prefix indicates a location that can be considered beneath or under the bone as it lies against the body. The subscapular fossa is the only landmark to be identified on the anterior aspect of scapula.

The two tubercles of scapula can both be referenced from the glenoid fossa. The **supraglenoid tubercle** is slightly

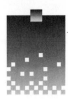

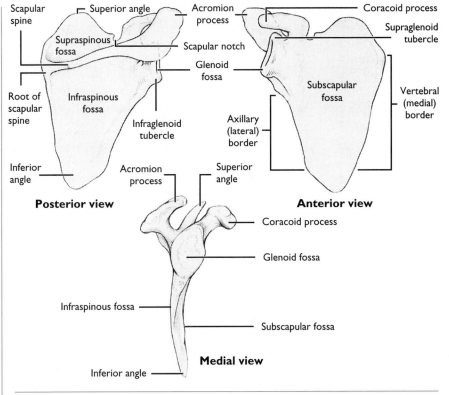

Scapular spine — Superior angle — Acromion process — Coracoid process
Supraspinous fossa — Scapular notch — Supraglenoid tubercle
Glenoid fossa
Root of scapular spine — Infraspinous fossa — Subscapular fossa — Vertebral (medial) border
Infraglenoid tubercle — Axillary (lateral) border
Inferior angle — Acromion process — Superior angle

Posterior view   **Anterior view**

Coracoid process
Glenoid fossa
Infraspinous fossa
Subscapular fossa

Medial view

Inferior angle

Figure 2-39. Scapula.
From Mathers et al: Clinical anatomy principles, *St Louis, 1996, Mosby. (C.L.A.S.S. series, Stanford Project.)*

superior, whereas the **infraglenoid tubercle** is slightly inferior. Finally, the **scapular notch** is a small indention medial to the base of the coracoid process of scapula.

Upper extremity

The upper extremity consists of the bones of the arm and hand—the humerus, ulna, radius, carpals, metacarpals, and phalanges.

Humerus

The **humerus** is the only bone of the upper arm. It is distal to the acromion and axillary regions and proximal to the cubital and antecubital regions. It is a long bone with definite epiphyses and a strong diaphysis. There are 16 significant landmarks on the humerus that correspond to both muscle attachments and articulations with other bones (Fig. 2-40).

Most proximally lies the smooth **head of humerus,** which fits directly into the glenoid fossa of scapula. In reality, this landmark is covered by hyaline cartilage for a smooth articulating surface. The ridge that surrounds the head is the **anatomic neck,** whereas the **surgical neck** is the area where the epiphysis narrows into the diaphysis of humerus. Fractures of the humerus will more likely occur and surgical

repair or replacement will more often be performed in the surgical neck.

Just beyond the anatomic neck, more superior to the head of humerus, is a large process known as the **greater tubercle of humerus.** The **lesser tubercle of humerus** is a second, smaller process on the anterior and more inferior aspect of humerus. The method for identifying a right humerus from a left is to confirm that the greater tubercle is oriented laterally from the head of the humerus; the head will then fit into a glenoid fossa, thus toward the trunk.

Between these two tubercles is a depression that runs in an inferior direction and is called the **bicipital groove**—named for the tendon that lies here. Moving almost half the distance distally along the diaphysis, a small raised area is located on the posterolateral aspect; the area is called the **deltoid tuberosity.**

The remaining nine landmarks of the humerus can be located on its distal epiphysis. First, the bone must be oriented so that two distal fossa face anteriorly and only one faces posteriorly. This is a second method to accurately identify a right humerus from a left. Of the two anterior fossa, the **radial fossa of humerus** is along the same side of the bone as the greater tubercle (proximally); the **coronoid fossa of humerus** is along the other side. (Do not confuse this process with the coronoid process of mandible or the coracoid process of scapula!) Thus the radial fossa is most lateral, whereas the coronoid fossa is oriented medially to its counterpart. Both these fossa will articulate with processes on the bones of the lower arm.

Distal to the two anterior fossa are the **capitulum of humerus** (lateral) and the **trochlea of humerus** (medial). Posteriorly, the large single fossa is the **olecranon fossa of humerus.** It is possible to correctly identify the **medial and lateral epicondyles of humerus** where the distal epiphysis of humerus is the widest. There are no condyles on the humerus. The **medial and lateral supracondylar ridges** are proximal to the epicondyles.

Ulna

The **ulna** is the longest of the two parallel bones of the forearm and lies medial to its counterpart, the radius. (Any body part should be oriented to the anatomic position when

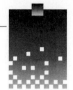

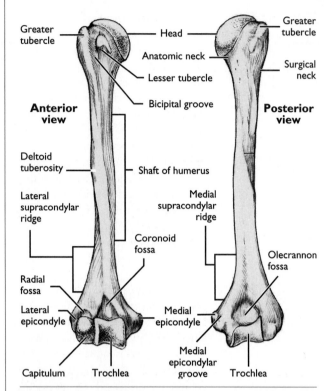

Greater tubercle

Head

Anatomic neck

Lesser tubercle

Bicipital groove

Greater tubercle

Surgical neck

Anterior view

Posterior view

Deltoid tuberosity

Shaft of humerus

Lateral supracondylar ridge

Medial supracondylar ridge

Coronoid fossa

Olecrannon fossa

Radial fossa

Lateral epicondyle

Medial epicondyle

Capitulum

Trochlea

Medial epicondylar groove

Trochlea

Figure 2-40. Humerus.
From Mathers et al: Clinical anatomy principles, *St Louis, 1996, Mosby.*
(C.LA.S.S. series, Stanford Project.)

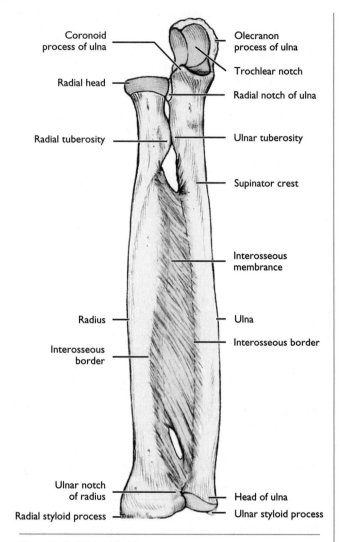

Coronoid process of ulna

Radial head

Radial tuberosity

Olecranon process of ulna

Trochlear notch

Radial notch of ulna

Ulnar tuberosity

Supinator crest

Interosseous membrane

Radius

Interosseous border

Ulna

Interosseous border

Ulnar notch of radius

Radial styloid process

Head of ulna

Ulnar styloid process

Figure 2-41. Ulna and radius.
From Mathers et al: Clinical anatomy principles, *St Louis, 1996, Mosby.*
(C.LA.S.S. series, Stanford Project.)

attempting to discern medial versus lateral or right versus left.) It is often helpful to relate the ulna to the little finger and the radius to the thumb. The ulna is also a long bone, though its epiphyses are not exceptional in size. Nine landmarks are identified on this bone (Fig. 2-41).

Beginning proximally, the **olecranon process of ulna** is the landmark that fits into the olecranon fossa of humerus. Considering the anterior view first and from the olecranon process, the ulna forms what resembles an ice cream scoop, with the deepest portion of the scoop being the **trochlear notch,** which fits over the trochlea of humerus. The medial orientation of the ulna and its trochlear notch, which articulates with the trochlea of humerus, can prevent confusion between the position of trochlea and the capitulum of humerus.

Moving distally across the trochlear notch is another raised edge, the **coronoid process of ulna,** which fits into the coronoid fossa of humerus. (Remember, there is also a coronoid process of mandible!) The **radial notch of ulna** is on the lateral edge of the coronoid process; the head of radius rests here.

Still on the anterior aspect of the ulna, the **ulnar tuberosity** is a raised and roughened area just distal to the coronoid process. Lateral to the tuberosity is a short ridge called the **supinator crest.** Moving laterally toward the bor-

der of the shaft of the ulna is a rather sharp ridge that runs almost the length of the ulna and is labeled the **interosseous border of ulna.** Heavy fibrous tissue will attach this landmark to the corresponding interosseous border of radius.

Finally, the **head of ulna** is the largest of two projections at the distal end of this bone; the other is the **styloid process of ulna,** which is more posteriorly oriented. (Do not forget there is also a styloid process on the temporal bone!)

Radius

The **radius** differs from the ulna in that it has a smaller proximal epiphysis and a much larger distal epiphysis. The proximal **head of radius** is round in diameter and quite blunt, articulating with the capitulum of humerus proximally and

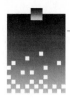

with the radial notch of ulna medially. This bone narrows slightly at the **neck of radius;** it then widens on the anterior aspect at the **radial tuberosity.** When placed alongside one another in proper alignment, the radial and ulnar tuberosities are in the same transverse plane (see Fig. 2-41).

The **interosseous border of radius** begins slightly posterior to the radial tuberosity and continues down the medial border toward the distal epiphysis. The most distal portion of the radius is its **styloid process of radius,** a much heavier structure than the styloid process of ulna. Both, however, are away from one another or lateral to the midline of the forearm. The ulna articulates with the radius distally at the **ulnar notch of radius.** The **dorsal tubercle** is on the radius, posteriorly.

Carpal bones

The eight **carpal bones** make up the wrist and are all short bones with rounded edges, enabling them to articulate easily with one another, as well as with the radius, ulna, and five metacarpals. This group of bones should be studied in reference to its alignment with surrounding bones (Box 2-3). The only significant landmark is the **hook of hamate,** which is visible on the anterior or palmar view of the hand (Figs. 2-42, 2-43).

Box 2-3. *Carpal bones (listed from radial to ulnar)*

Proximal row	Distal row
Scaphoid	Trapezium
Lunate	Trapezoid
Triquetrum	Capitate
Pisiform	Hamate

Hand

The **hand** is made up of both **metacarpals** in the palmar region and phalanges in the fingers, or **digits.** A **ray** is the full component of a metacarpal and its corresponding phalanges associated with an entire finger.

Metacarpal bones

The five **metacarpal bones** in each hand are long bones by virtue of their diaphyses and epiphyses at each end. These bones do not have individual names but are discussed by number; the metacarpal of the thumb is the *first* and the little finger is the *fifth.* The proximal epiphysis is the *base,* and it articulates with the carpals. The distal epiphysis is the *head,* and it articulates with the next phalanx of the finger.

Phalanges

A phalanx is also a long bone, even though its length is not substantial. The first digit has two phalanges—the proximal and distal. Each of the remaining four digits have three phalanges–proximal, middle, and distal. There are fourteen phalanges in each hand.

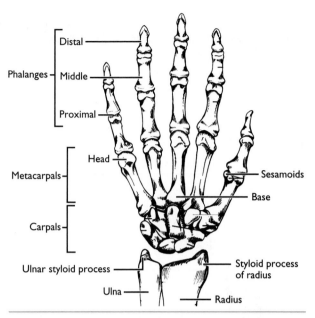

Figure 2-42. Anterior view of the hand.
From Malone, McPoil, Nitz: Orthopedic & sports physical therapy, ed 3, *St Louis, 1997, Mosby.*

Exercise 2-18. Pectoral girdle and upper extremity

Name the bones that best complete the following sentences.

1. The _____ and _____ make up the pectoral girdle.
2. The pectoral girdle articulates proximally to the
   _____.
3. The pectoral girdle articulates distally to _____.
4. The _____ and _____ articulate with the long bone of the upper arm distally.
5. The _____ is a long bone that lies proximal to the elbow.
6. The _____ is a bone of the forearm that lies medial to the extremity.
7. The _____ is a bone of the forearm that lies lateral to the extremity.
8. The _____ is the most proximal bone of the thumb.
9. The individual carpal bones are _____, _____, _____, _____, _____, _____, _____, and _____.
10. The _____ are the bones of the hand that lie distal to the carpals.

Exercise 2-19. Landmarks of pectoral girdle and upper extremity

Provide landmarks of the pectoral girdle and upper extremity.

Clavicle: ____________ ____________

Scapula: ____________ ____________
____________ ____________
____________ ____________
____________ ____________
____________ ____________
____________ ____________
____________ ____________
____

Proximal humerus: ____________ ____________
____________ ____________
____________ ____________
____

Distal humerus: ____________ ____________
____________ ____________

Distal humerus: ____________ ____________
(cont) ____________ ____________
____

Proximal ulna: ____________ ____________
____________ ____________
____________ ____________
____

Distal ulna: ____________ ____________

Proximal radius: ____________ ____________
____

Distal radius: ____________ ____________

Carpals: ____________ ____________
____________ ____________
____________ ____________
____________ ____________

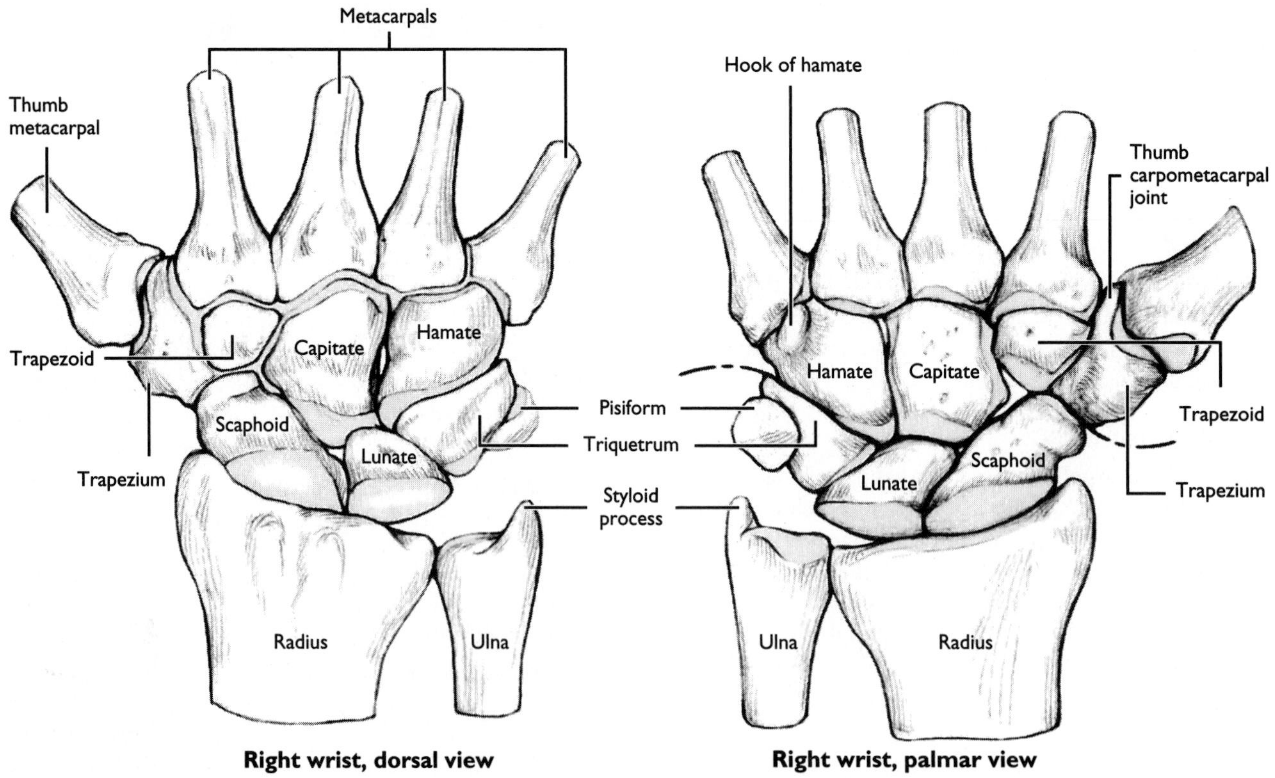

Metacarpals
Thumb metacarpal
Trapezoid
Capitate
Hamate
Scaphoid
Lunate
Trapezium
Radius
Ulna
Pisiform
Triquetrum
Styloid process
Hook of hamate
Thumb carpometacarpal joint
Hamate
Capitate
Trapezoid
Scaphoid
Lunate
Trapezium
Ulna
Radius
Right wrist, dorsal view
Right wrist, palmar view

Figure 2-43. Carpal bones.
From Mathers et al: Clinical anatomy principles, *St Louis, 1996, Mosby. (C.L.A.S.S. series, Stanford Project.)*

Exercise 2-20. Landmarks and directional terms

Complete the following sentences.

1. The scapula is _____ to the clavicle.

2. The coracoid process is _____ to the acromion process.

3. The vertebral border is _____ to the glenoid fossa.

4. The clavicle is _____ to the humerus.

5. The greater tubercle of humerus is _____ to the coronoid fossa of humerus.

6. The surgical neck of humerus is _____ to the anatomic neck of humerus.

7. The infraspinous fossa of scapula is _____ to the spine of scapula.

8. The acromion process of scapula is _____ to the glenoid fossa of scapula.

9. The subscapular fossa of scapula is _____ to the spine of scapula.

10. The lesser tubercle of humerus is _____ to the greater tubercle of humerus.

11. The bicipital groove is _____ to the lesser tubercle of humerus.

12. The deltoid process of humerus is _____ to the bicipital groove of humerus.

13. The head of radius is _____ to the head of ulna.

14. The coronoid fossa is _____ to olecranon fossa.

15. The trochlea of humerus is _____ to the capitulum of humerus.

16. The radial tuberosity is _____ to the trochlear notch of ulna.

17. The styloid process of radius is _____ to the head of radius.

18. The coronoid process of ulna is _____ to trochlear notch of ulna.

19. Pisiform is _____ to the hamate.

20. Trapezium is _____ to first metacarpal.

21. The hook of hamate is _____ to the hamate.

22. Triquetrum is _____ to the ulna.

23. Capitate is _____ to the lunate.

24. Scaphoid is _____ to the trapezoid.

25. The base of a metacarpal is _____ to the head of a metacarpal.

Exercise 2-21. Bones & landmarks of pectoral girdle & upper extremity

Identify the bones and landmarks of the pectoral girdle and upper extremity on Figures 2-44 through 2-49 on pages 42, 43, and 44.

Exercise 2-22. Palpate landmarks of the pectoral girdle & upper extremity

With washable color markers or tape, label the following palpable skeletal landmarks on the body of your lab partner.

- Sternal end of clavicle
- Acromion process of scapula
- Vertebral and axillary borders of scapula
- Spine of scapula
- Inferior and superior angles of scapula
- Greater tubercle of humerus
- Medial and lateral epicondyles of humerus
- Olecranon process of ulna
- Styloid process of radius
- Head of ulna
- Styloid process of ulna
- Carpal region
- Base of first metacarpal
- Head of metacarpal
- Proximal, middle, and distal phalanges

Pelvic girdle

The pelvic girdle is the group of bones that makes up the coxal, gluteal, and inguinal regions of the body and includes two **innominate bones** by which the lower extremities are attached. Innominate actually refers to something that has no name and is often used to describe the irregular shape of the bones attaching laterally to the sacrum. More commonly, these large structures are called the **os coxae,** (*os* for *bone* and *coxae* for *hips*). The attachment between the os coxae and sacrum is the **sacroiliac joint** (see Fig. 2-50 on page 45).

Each **coxal bone** is actually made up of three individual bones that are fused together early in life. These are the ilium, ischium, and pubis (see Fig. 2-51 on page 45). The fusion occurs at a landmark called the **acetabulum,** which forms the socket portion of the hip joint. The acetabulum is circular; the ilium, ischium, and pubis share equal thirds of its shape. The acetabulum is helpful when identifying the right and left halves of the pelvis because the acetabulum always faces posterolaterally. More important landmarks will be identified as the three coxal bones are assembled to form one half of the pelvis (see Figs. 2-52, 2-53 on page 45).

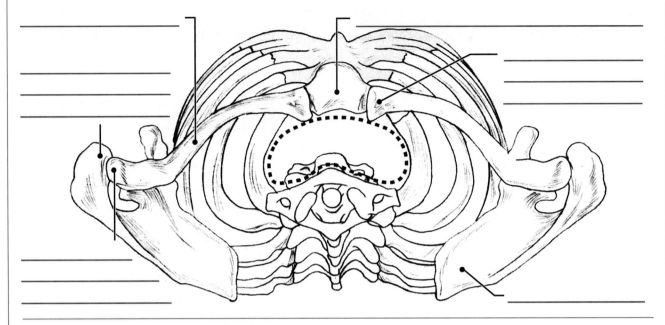

Figure 2-44. Landmarks of the pectoral girdle.
From Mathers et al: Clinical anatomy principles, *St Louis, 1996, Mosby. (C.L.A.S.S. series, Stanford Project.)*

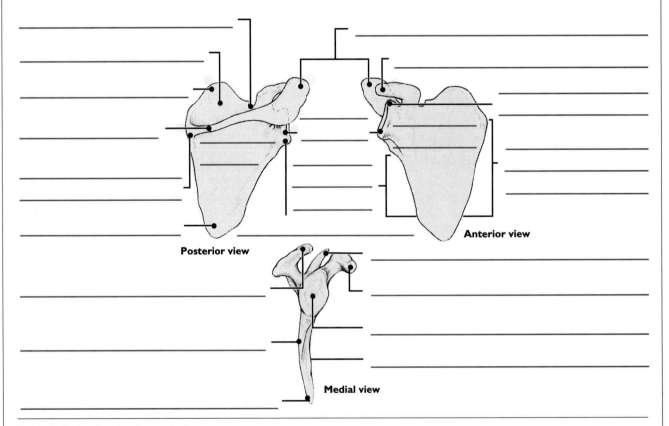

Posterior view

Anterior view

Medial view

Figure 2-45. Landmarks of the scapula.
From Mathers et al: Clinical anatomy principles, *St Louis, 1996, Mosby. (C.L.A.S.S. series, Stanford Project.)*

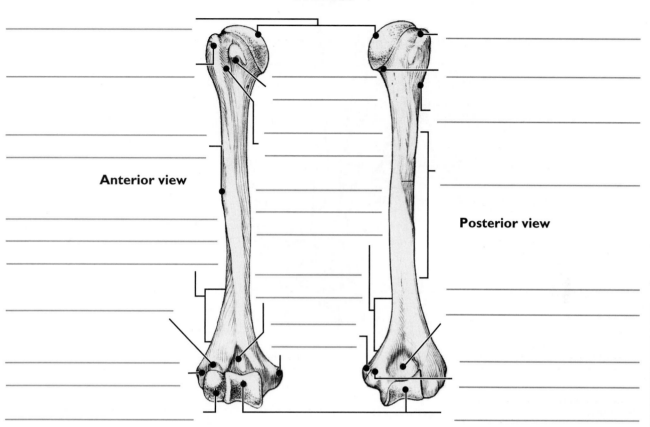

Figure 2-46. Landmarks of the humerus.
From Mathers et al: Clinical anatomy principles, *St Louis, 1996, Mosby. (C.L.A.S.S. series, Stanford Project.)*

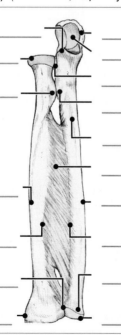

Figure 2-47. Landmarks of the ulna and radius.
From Mathers et al: Clinical anatomy principles, *St Louis, 1996, Mosby. (C.L.A.S.S. series, Stanford Project.)*

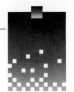

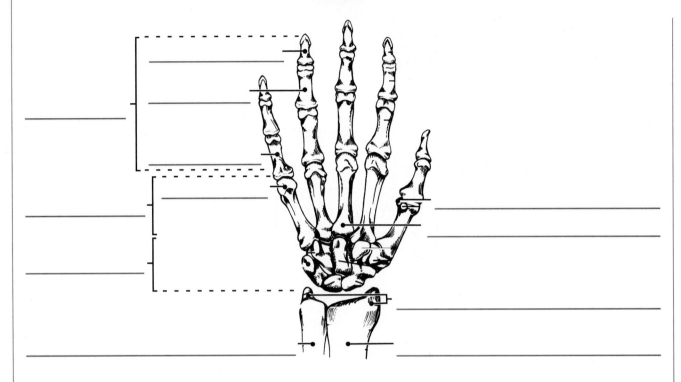

Figure 2-48. Landmarks of the hand.
From Malone, McPoil, Nitz:: Orthopedic & sports physical therapy, *ed 8, St Louis, 1997, Mosby.*

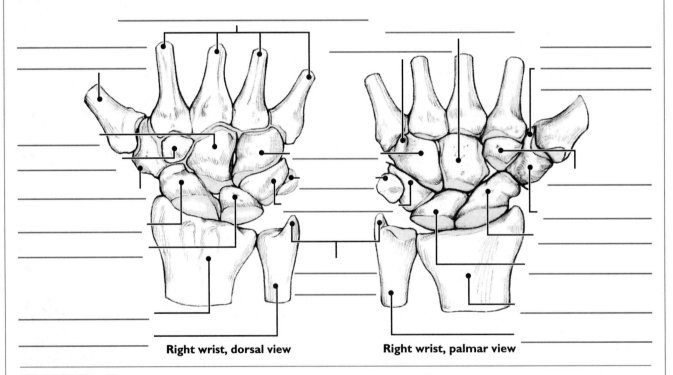

Right wrist, dorsal view   **Right wrist, palmar view**

Figure 2-49. Carpal bones.
From Mathers et al: Clinical anatomy principles, *St Louis, 1996, Mosby.   (C.L.A.S.S. series, Stanford Project.)*

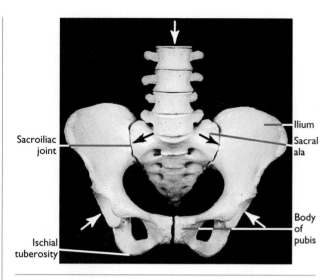

Sacroiliac joint

Ilium

Sacral ala

Body of pubis

Ischial tuberosity

Figure 2-50. Pelvis and sacrum.
From Mathers et al: Clinical anatomy principles, *St Louis, 1996, Mosby.*

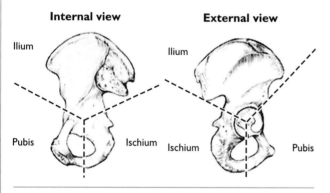

Internal view   **External view**

Ilium

Ilium

Pubis   Ischium   Ischium   Pubis

Figure 2-51. Coxal bones, internal and external views.
From Mathers et al: Clinical anatomy principles, *St Louis, 1996, Mosby.*

Ilium

The **ilium** is the large wing or fanned portion of the acetabulum that is palpable when the hands are on the *hips,* just below the waist. Similar to the sacrum, this wing portion is called the **ala of ilium.** The various landmarks on the halves of the pelvis or coxal bones are important for both surface palpation and reference, as well as for references to muscle attachment. The first of these landmarks is the **iliac crest,** the thick superior rim of the ilium that is palpated by placing the hands just below the waist in the coxal region.

Following this iliac crest anteriorly, a rather sharp point is found where the ilium abruptly turns downward. This point is the **anterior superior iliac spine** (ASIS); the **posterior superior iliac spine** (PSIS) is the corresponding landmark found in the opposite direction. Both the ASIS and PSIS are palpable on most individuals.

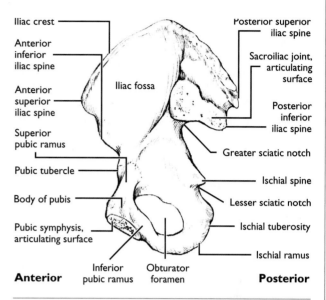

Iliac crest

Anterior inferior iliac spine

Anterior superior iliac spine

Superior pubic ramus

Pubic tubercle

Body of pubis

Pubic symphysis, articulating surface

Iliac fossa

Posterior superior iliac spine

Sacroiliac joint, articulating surface

Posterior inferior iliac spine

Greater sciatic notch

Ischial spine

Lesser sciatic notch

Ischial tuberosity

Ischial ramus

Anterior   Inferior pubic ramus   Obturator foramen   **Posterior**

Figure 2-52. Landmarks of the coxal bones, internal view.
From Mathers et al: Clinical anatomy principles, *St Louis, 1996, Mosby.*

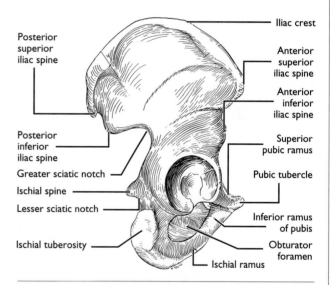

Posterior superior iliac spine

Posterior inferior iliac spine

Greater sciatic notch

Ischial spine

Lesser sciatic notch

Ischial tuberosity

Iliac crest

Anterior superior iliac spine

Anterior inferior iliac spine

Superior pubic ramus

Pubic tubercle

Inferior ramus of pubis

Obturator foramen

Ischial ramus

Figure 2-53. Landmarks of the coxal bones, external view.
From Mathers et al: Clinical anatomy principles, *St Louis, 1996, Mosby.*

Inferior to the ASIS, the next landmark is the **anterior inferior iliac spine** (AIIS); the **posterior inferior iliac spine** (PIIS) is also below the PSIS. Next, a most significant landmark, is the **greater sciatic notch,** which is inferior to the PIIS. The **auricular surface** is located on the posterior, medial portion of ilium and is the articulating surface of the sacrum.

Medially, the wing shape of ilium creates the **iliac fossa,** which supports the inferior portion of the abdominal cavity. Laterally, the ilium provides a broad surface for large hip muscle attachment.

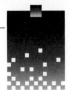

Ischium

The **ischium** is the strongest portion of the coxa and attaches inferior and slightly posterior to the ilium. In addition to forming one third of the acetabulum, the ischium forms the posterior one half of the **obturator foramen,** a large hole in the lower portion of the coxa. Other landmarks include the **ischial spine,** which is the pointed process posterior to the acetabulum, and the **lesser sciatic notch,** which is just below.

The **ischial tuberosity** is the most inferior segment of this bone and is therefore the part of the pelvis on which we sit. The **ischial ramus** is the branch that curves upward to meet the pubis. (Ramus means a branch or part that divides a larger structure.)

Pubis

The **pubis** is the smallest of the three coxal bones, attaching inferior to the ilium. It completes the ring of the pelvis by articulating anteriorly with the pubis of the opposite side. The pubis has a body and two rami (plural). The **body of pubis** is centrally located and lateral to the **pubic symphysis,** where the right and left pubic bones articulate. On the superior edge of the body of pubis, the **pubic tubercle** lies. The **superior pubic ramus** extends laterally from its body, whereas the **inferior pubic ramus** reaches downward toward the ischial tuberosity. The anterior rim of the obturator foramen is formed by both the superior and inferior rami.

Lower extremity

The lower extremity consists of bones of the leg and foot such as the femur, tibia, fibula, tarsals, metatarsals, and phalanges.

Femur

The femur is the longest of all the long bones in the body. Its proximal articulation with the acetabulum creates the hip joint, and its distal articulation with the tibia becomes the knee (Fig. 2-54).

The large round **head of femur** is smooth and symmetrical and has a small indention called the **fovea capitis** at its tip. Just distally is the **neck of femur,** which ends with a trenchlike area before changing its angle and drastically becoming larger. The most superior portion of this broad area is the **greater trochanter of femur,** which is visible from both the anterior and posterior views when oriented lateral to the head and neck. The greater trochanter can be palpated at the point of the hip approximately one-hand length inferior to the crest of ilium.

Descending from the greater trochanter anteriorly, a slightly raised area called the **intertrochanteric line** is located; posteriorly, a larger ridge called the **intertrochanteric crest** is found. Easily visible on the posterior aspect, this intertrochanteric crest leads to the **lesser trochanter of femur.** The

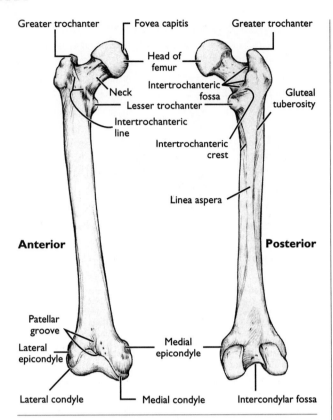

Figure 2-54. Landmarks on the femur.
From Mathers et al: Clinical anatomy principles, *St Louis, 1996, Mosby.*

slight dip between the greater trochanter and the lesser trochanter is the **intertrochanteric fossa.**

A slightly rough area on the posterolateral aspect of the femoral diaphysis is the **gluteal tuberosity.** Continuing down the posterior aspect of the diaphysis, a thin ridge can be palpated running almost the length of the bone. This is the **linea aspera,** an important landmark for muscle attachment. The anterior aspect of the femoral diaphysis is smooth and free of landmarks.

The widest points on the distal epiphysis of femur are the **medial and lateral epicondyles,** which are visible from both anterior and posterior views. The medial epicondyle is on the same side as the head of femur, whereas the lateral epicondyle is on the same side as the greater trochanter. Just distal to these are the larger **medial and lateral condyles of the femur,** which are round, smooth, and facing posteriorly. The condyles of femur articulate with the tibia. The **intercondylar fossa** is the groove between the two condyles. Anteriorly there will be a smooth surface centrally located on the distal epiphysis. This is the articulating surface for the patella, or **patellar groove.**

The distinction between the anterior and posterior surfaces of femur can then be made by locating either the linea aspera (posterior), the dual condyles (also posterior), or the singular patellar surface (anterior). Once the anterior or posterior orientation is made, right or left can be determined by the direction of the head and neck of femur, since these landmarks always point toward the pelvis (medially).

Patella

The **patella** is the largest sesamoid bone in the body, commonly referred to as the *kneecap* (Fig. 2-55). Flattened on its posterior surface and covered with hyaline cartilage, this bone only articulates with the distal epiphysis of femur, acting as a pulley within a large tendinous structure. When the leg is in the straightened position, the patella should feel as though it is *floating* above the femur. The **superior border of patella** is flat, whereas the inferior border, or **apex of patella,** has a slightly rounded point.

Tibia

The **tibia** is the heaviest bone of the lower leg, and it must bear the weight and force of the entire body to and from the foot (Fig. 2-56). Also a long bone, the tibia has a broad flat proximal end that receives the condyles of femur and is referred to as the **tibial plateau.** The **intercondylar eminence** sits midway across the plateau. Below the plateau at the widest point are the **medial and lateral condyles of the tibia,** which are visible from both anterior and posterior views. These tibial condyles differ from those of the femur; they are oriented proximally and are more coarse in surface texture. The proximal end of the fibula will articulate with the tibia just under the lateral tibial condyle and slightly posteriorly. Anteriorly, the raised area between the condyles is the **tibial tuberosity.**

The **soleal line** is the primary landmark on the posterior aspect of tibia; it runs in an oblique direction from the lateral condyle inferiorly. The diaphysis of tibia is slim compared with the large proximal epiphysis. The area of the tibia facing the fibula is called the **interosseous border of tibia.** The distal epiphysis curves abruptly toward the medial side of the lower extremity to form the hooklike **medial malleolus of tibia.** Laterally, the tibia articulates with the fibula again and distally with the talus, a member of the tarsal group.

Fibula

The **fibula** is a rodlike long bone and serves as a surface for muscle attachment but does not contribute to the weight-bearing responsibility of the lower leg (see Fig. 2-56). The proximal **head of fibula** is blunt except for a small **styloid process of fibula** at its superolateral edge. The head articulates with the tibia just inferior and posterior to its lateral condyle. The thin **neck of fibula** precedes the long slender **diaphysis of fibula.** Corresponding with the tibial interosseous border, the **interosseous border of fibula** runs

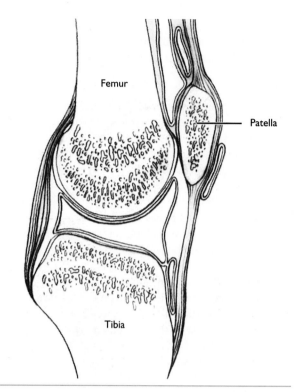

Figure 2-55. Patella.
From Mathers et al: Clinical anatomy principles, St Louis, 1996, Mosby.

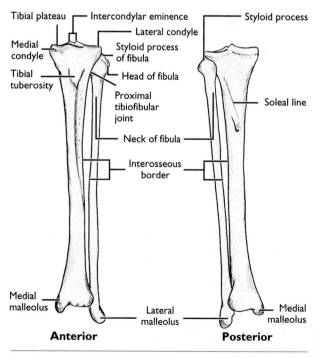

Figure 2-56. Landmarks on the tibia and fibula.
From Mathers et al: Clinical anatomy principles, St Louis, 1996, Mosby.

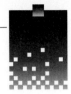

the length of the diaphysis. The entire distal end of fibula is the **lateral malleolus of fibula** and differs from the proximal end by having more of a pointed, tear-drop shape.

Foot

The **foot** is comprised of three groups of bone—the tarsals, metatarsals, and phalanges. Its complex structure accommodates the body's weight-bearing responsibilities, the force of walking, running, and jumping while adjusting to both bipedal and single-leg activity.

Tarsal bones

There are seven **tarsal bones** that form each ankle. Tarsals are short bones that have multiple surfaces, allowing articulation with surrounding bones (Figs. 2-57 and 2-58).

Talus bone

The most superior of the tarsals is the **talus bone,** which articulates with the tibia between the tibial medial and fibular lateral malleoli. This small bone must carry the entire body weight to and from the foot during weight-bearing activities. It articulates distally with the calcaneus bone.

Calcaneus bone

The **calcaneus bone** is the largest of the tarsals and is known as the *heel* of the foot. It is elongated from anterior to poste-

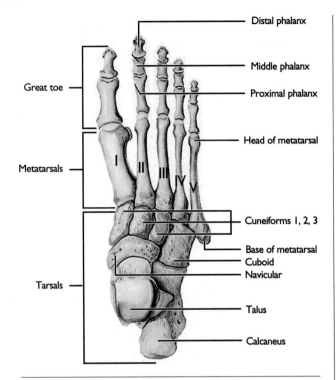

Figure 2-57. Bones of the foot, superior view.
From Thibodeau, Patton: Structure & function of the body, *ed 10 , St Louis, 1996, Mosby.*

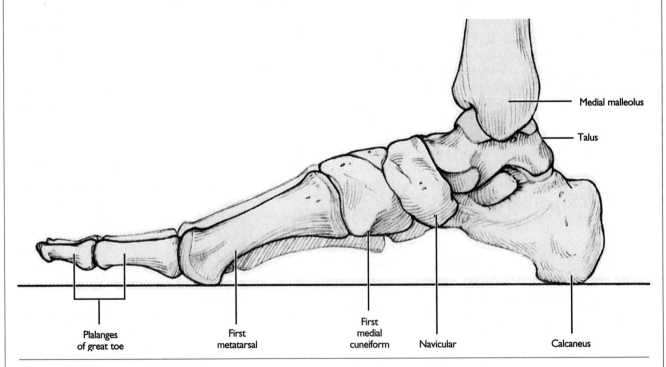

Figure 2-58. Bones of the foot, medial view.
From Mathers et al: Clinical anatomy principles, *St Louis, 1996, Mosby.*

rior, articulating superiorly with the talus and anteriorly with the navicular and cuboid bones.

Navicular bone

The **navicular bone** is a medially oriented tarsal, and it forms the highest portion of the arch of the foot. It articulates posteriorly with the calcaneus bone, laterally with the cuboid bone, and anteriorly with the three cuneiform bones.

Cuboid bone

The laterally oriented **cuboid bone** articulates posteriorly with the calcaneus bone, medially with the navicular bone, and anteriorly with the fourth and fifth metatarsals.

Cuneiform bones

The three **cuneiform bones** are known as *medial, intermediate,* or *lateral* (first, second, or third); the third is the most lateral. In addition to articulating with one another, these tarsals articulate posteriorly with the navicular bone, laterally with the cuboid bone, and anteriorly with the first through fourth metatarsals.

Metatarsal bones

Five **metatarsal bones** are long bones, similar to the metacarpals of the hand. The metatarsals are numbered; the *first* is the most medial and the *fifth* is the most lateral. The proximal epiphysis of each metatarsal is the *base,* and the distal epiphysis is the *head.*

Phalanges

The *digits* of the foot, like the hand, are made up of fourteen tiny long bones. Similarly, the first digit, or the **great toe,** has only two phalanges—the **proximal and distal phalanges.** The remaining four digits each have three phalanges—the **proximal, middle, and distal phalanges.** Like the hand, a *ray* is the full component of a metatarsal and the corresponding phalanges associated with the entire toe. The metatarsals and phalanges make up the **forefoot.**

Exercise 2-23. Pelvic girdle and lower extremity

Provide the bone(s) that best complete(s) the following sentences.

1. The _____, _____, and _____ make up the pelvis.

2. The pelvis articulates proximally to the _____.

3. The pelvis articulates with the _____ at the acetabulum.

4. The _____ is the long bone of the thigh.

5. The _____ of the lower leg lies medially.

Exercise 2-23. Pelvic girdle and lower extremity–cont

6. The _____ of the lower leg lies laterally.

7. The _____, _____,
   _____, _____,
   _____, _____, and
   _____ are individual tarsal bones.

8. The _____ is the most proximal or superior tarsal bone.

9. The _____ and _____ are bones of the foot, distal to the tarsals.

10. There are _____ individual phalanges on one foot.

Exercise 2-24. Landmarks of the pelvic girdle and lower extremity

Provide landmarks of the pelvic girdle and lower extremity.

Ilium: _____ _____
                _____ _____
                _____ _____
                _____ _____
                _____

Ischium: _____ _____
                _____ _____
                _____

Pubis: _____ _____
                _____ _____
                _____

Proximal femur: _____ _____
                _____ _____
                _____ _____
                _____ _____
                _____

Distal femur: _____ _____
                _____ _____
                _____

Patella: _____ _____
                _____

Proximal tibia: _____ _____
                _____ _____
                _____

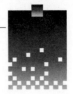

Exercise 2-24. Landmarks of the pelvic girdle and lower extremity–cont

Distal tibia: _____ _____

Fibula: _____ _____
                     _____ _____
                     _____ _____

Foot: _____ _____
                     _____ _____
                     _____ _____
                     _____

Exercise 2-25. Landmarks and directional terms

Complete the following sentences.

1. The ilium is _____ to the ischium.
2. The pubis is _____ to the ischium.
3. The greater trochanter of femur is _____ to the linea aspera of femur.
4. The neck of femur is _____ to the head of humerus.
5. The posterior inferior iliac is _____ to the ischial spine.
6. The acetabulum is _____ to the head of femur.
7. The obturator foramen is _____ to the iliac fossa.
8. The lesser trochanter of femur is _____ to the greater trochanter of femur.
9. The medial condyle of femur is _____ to the medial epicondyle of femur.
10. The patellar surface is _____ to intercondylar notch.
11. The tibial plateau is _____ to the tibial condyles.
12. The tibial tuberosity is _____ to the patella.
13. The head of fibula is _____ to the lateral condyle of tibia.
14. The styloid process of fibula is _____ to the medial malleolus of tibia.
15. The soleal line of tibia is _____ to tibial tuberosity.
16. The neck of fibula is _____ to lateral malleolus of fibula.
17. Calcaneus is _____ to the talus.
18. Navicular is _____ to the calcaneus.
19. Cuboid is _____ to the navicular.

Exercise 2-25. Landmarks and directional terms–cont

20. First cuneiform is _____ to the first metatarsal.
21. Fifth metatarsal is _____ to the cuboid.
22. Second metatarsal is _____ to the third metatarsal.
23. Head of a metatarsal is _____ to the base of the metatarsals.
24. The proximal phalanx is _____ to the head of the metatarsals.
25. The second cuneiform is _____ to the first cuneiform.

Exercise 2-26. Pelvic girdle and lower extremity

Identify the bones and landmarks of the pelvic girdle and lower extremity on Figures 2-59 through 2-65 on pages 50 through 52.

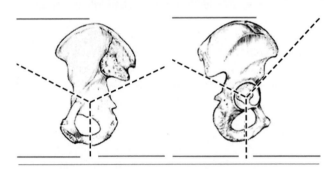

Figure 2-59. Coxal bones, internal and external views.
From Mathers et al: Clinical anatomy principles, *St Louis, 1996, Mosby.*

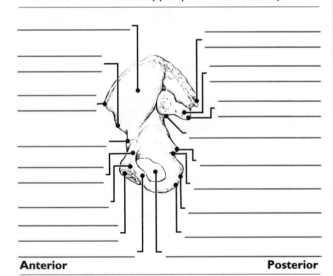

Anterior   **Posterior**

Figure 2-60. Landmarks on the coxal bones, internal view.
From Mathers et al: Clinical anatomy principles, *St Louis, 1996, Mosby.*

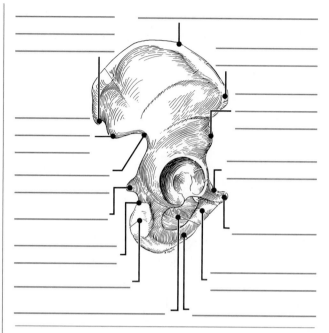

Figure 2-61. Landmarks on the coxal bones, external view.
From Mathers et al: Clinical anatomy principles, *St Louis, 1996, Mosby.*

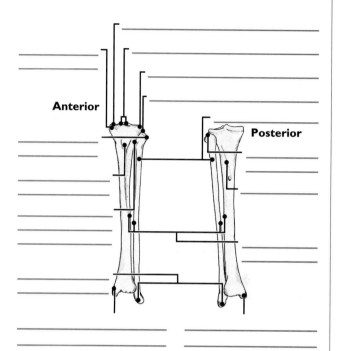

Anterior

Posterior

Figure 2-63. Landmarks on the tibia and fibula.
From Mathers et al: Clinical anatomy principles, *St Louis, 1996, Mosby.*

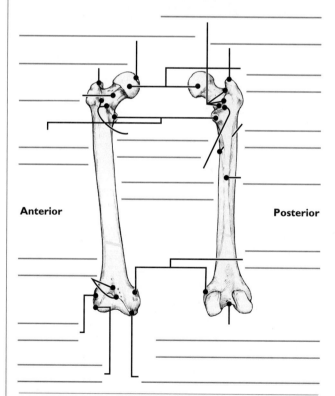

Anterior

Posterior

Figure 2-62. Landmarks on the femur.
From Mathers et al: Clinical anatomy principles, *St Louis, 1996, Mosby.*

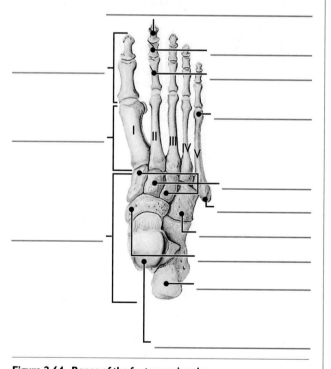

Figure 2-64. Bones of the foot, superior view.
From Thibodeau, Patton: Structure & function of the body, *ed 10, St Louis, 1996, Mosby.*

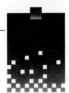

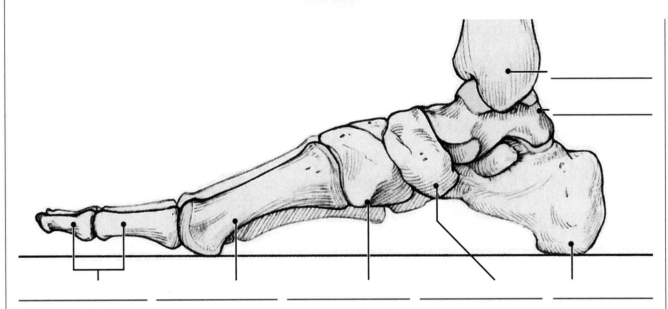

Figure 2-65. Bones of the foot, medial view.
From Mathers et al: Clinical anatomy principles, St Louis, 1996, Mosby.

Bony landmarks will feel differently on every individual. Practice your palpation skills on your study partner, and identify each bony landmark. Compare the locations of landmarks on the right side against the left. With washable color markers or tape, label the following palpable sketetal landmarks on the body of your study partner.

- ■ Iliac crest

- ■ Anterior superior iliac spine

- ■ Posterior superior iliac spine

- ■ Greater trochanter of femur

- ■ Medial and lateral epicondyles of femur

- ■ Patella

- ■ Medial and lateral condyles of tibia

- ■ Head of fibula

- ■ Tibial tuberosity

- ■ Medial malleolus of tibia

- ■ Lateral malleolus of fibula

- ■ Calcaneus

- ■ Head of metatarsals

Provide the location and definition for each landmark term.

Condyle   Location _____
    Definition: _____
Crest   Location _____
    Definition: _____
Epicondyle Location _____
    Definition: _____
Facet   Location _____
    Definition: _____
Foramen   Location _____
    Definition: _____
Fossa   Location _____
    Definition: _____
Groove   Location _____
    Definition: _____
Head   Location _____
    Definition: _____
Ramus   Location _____
    Definition: _____
Sinus   Location _____
    Definition: _____
Tubercle   Location _____
    Definition: _____
Tuberosity Location _____
    Definition: _____

Summary

Concise familiarity with the bones and bony landmarks of the skeleton is essential to the successful study of musculoskeletal anatomy. Strict attention to detail must be maintained when discussing or documenting this material because of the occasional duplication of terminology and landmark names in multiple areas of the body. Accurate spelling is also essential since the incorrect substitution of one or more letters may cause a word to represent an entirely different body part or landmark.

Study Note

It is best to develop the habit of naming a landmark in conjunction with the bone on which it is associated! For example, we have identified the following:
- Greater trochanter *of femur*
- Greater tuberosity *of humerus*
- Styloid process *of fibula*
- Head *of femur*

Key Words

acetabulum
acromial end
acromion process of scapula
ala of ilium
ala of sacrum
anatomic neck
angle of mandible
anterior arch
anterior inferior iliac spine
anterior superior iliac spine
anterior tubercle
apex of patella
appendicular skeleton
articulate
Atlas
auricular surface
axial skeleton
axillary (lateral) border of
    scapula
Axis
bicipital groove
bifid
body of mandible
body of pubis
body of sternum
bone marrow
calcaneus bone
calcium salts
canaliculus
cancellous bone
capitate
capitulum of humerus

carpals
cervical section
clavicle
coccyx
collagen fibers
compact bone
compressive forces
concave curve
condyle
convex curve
coracoid process of scapula
coronal suture
coronoid fossa of humerus
coronoid process of mandible
coronoid process of ulna
cortical bone
costal cartilage
costal facet
coxal bone
cranium
crest
cuboid bone
cuneiform bones
deltoid tuberosity
diaphysis
diaphysis of fibula
digits
dorsal tubercle
endochondral bone
endosteum
epicondyle
epiphyseal plate

epiphysis
ethmoid bone
external auditory meatus
facet
false ribs
femur
fibula
flat bone
floating ribs
foot
foramen
foramen magnum
forefoot
fossa
fovea capitis
frontal bone
glenoid fossa
gluteal tuberosity
great toe
greater sciatic notch
greater trochanter of femur
greater tubercle of humerus
groove
hamate
hand
hard palate
haversian canal
haversian system
head
head of femur
head of fibula
head of humerus

head of radius
head of ulna
hematopoiesis
hook of hamate
humerus
hyaline cartilage
hyoid bone
iliac crest
iliac fossa
ilium
inferior angles of scapulae
inferior articulating facets
inferior nasal conchae
inferior pubic ramus
infraglenoid tubercle
infraspinous fossa of scapula
innominate bones
intercondylar eminence
intercondylar fossa
interosseous border of fibula
interosseous border of radius
interosseous border of tibia
interosseous border of ulna
intertrochanteric crest
intertrochanteric fossa
intertrochanteric line
intervertebral disks
intervertebral foramen
irregular bone
ischial ramus
ischial spine
ischial tuberosity

53

Continued

Key Words—*cont*

ischium
lacrimal bones
lacuna
lambdoidal suture
lamellae
lamina
lateral malleolus of fibula
lesser sciatic notch
lesser trochanter of femur
lesser tubercle of humerus
linea aspera
long bone
lumbar section
lumbar vertebrae
lunate
mandible
mandibular condyle
mandibular fossa
mandibular ramus
manubrium
mastoid process
maxillary bones
medial and lateral condyles
    of femur
medial and lateral condyles
    of tibia
medial and lateral epicondyles
    of femur
medial and lateral epicondyles
    of humerus
medial and lateral malleoli
medial and lateral supra-
    condylar ridges
medial malleolus of tibia
medullary cavity
metacarpal bones
metatarsal bones
nasal bones
navicular bone
neck of femur
neck of fibula
neck of radius
obturator foramen
occipital bone
occipital condyles
occipital protuberance
odontoid facet
odontoid process
olecranon fossa of humerus

olecranon process of ulna
orbit
organic matrix
os coxae
ossification
osteoblasts
osteocytes
osteon structure
palatine bones
parietal bones
patella
patellar groove
pedicle
periosteum
phalanges
pisiform
posterior inferior iliac spine
posterior superior iliac spine
posterior tubercle
proximal, middle, and distal
    phalanges
pubic symphysis
pubic tubercle
pubis
radial fossa of humerus
radial notch of ulna
radial tuberosity
radius
ramus
ray
remodeling
resorption
ribs
root of spine of scapula
sacral canal
sacral section
sacral foramen
sacral hiatus
sacral promontory
sacroiliac facets
sacroiliac joint
sacrum
sagittal suture
scaphoid
scapulae
scapular notch
sesamoid bone
short bone
sinus

soleal line
sphenoid bone
spine of scapula
spinous process
spongy bone
squamosal suture
sternal end
sternum
styloid process of fibula
styloid process of radius
styloid process of temporal
    bones
styloid process of ulna
subscapular fossa
superior angles of scapulae
superior articulating facets
superior border of patella
superior portions of the right
    and left orbits
superior pubic ramus
supinator crest
supraglenoid tubercle
supraorbital foramen
supraspinous fossa
surgical neck
suture
talus bone
tarsal bones
temporal bones
temporal process
tendon
tensile strength
thoracic section
tibia
tibial plateau
tibial tuberosity
trabeculae
transverse foramen
transverse processes
trapezium
trapezoid
triquetrum
trochlea of humerus
trochlear notch
true ribs
tubercle
tuberosity
ulna
ulna notch of radius

ulnar tuberosity
vertebrae
vertebral artery
vertebral body
vertebral (medial) border
    of scapula
vertebral canal
vertebral column
Volkmann's canal
vomer bone
xiphoid process
zygomatic arch
zygomatic bones
zygomatic process

3

Joints

❝ *It is the goal of this chapter to enable the student to identify primary types and structures of joints as they relate to human movement.* ❞

Chapter objectives

To enable the student to:

1. Identify joints in terms of structure and available movement.

2. Define movement terminology.

3. Discuss principal joints and their structure and movement.

Structure and Movement of Joints

A joint is identified as an articulation or an area where bones attach or move against one another. Some joints involve large bony surfaces and others involve only small areas. Some joints (shoulder, hip, knee) allow a great deal of movement, whereas other joints (articulating cranial and facial bones) allow no movement at all. The degree of movement in a particular joint can also differ depending on the age of the individual and his or her physical condition.

The types of tissue that make up a joint can greatly affect the amount of movement that occurs between articulated bones. Some tissues in the body are designed to hold firm and resist outside forces, whereas others have a great deal of elasticity and flexibility; still other tissues that are present in quantity allow only restricted movement. Therefore through examination of the tissues involved, a joint can be classified into one of three specific structural categories—fibrous, cartilaginous, and synovial.

The degree of stability and movement available in a joint makes functional activity possible, allowing an individual to perform common tasks and activities. The three categories of joint movement are synarthrotic, amphiarthrotic, and diarthrotic.

Fibrous joints

A fibrous joint is composed of articulating bones that are joined by dense collagen fibers that have little elasticity and allow no empty spaces between the surfaces (Fig. 3-1). The union of irregular bones by this **fibrous connective tissue** often occurs along their entire common borders. Such structural attachment allows *no movement* to occur between the bones, a category of movement known as **synarthrosis.** There are three types of fibrous joints found in the body— suture, syndesmosis, and gomphosis.

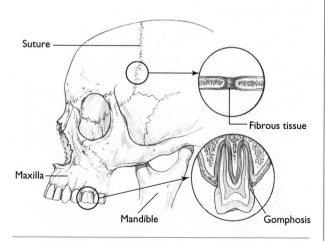

Figure 3-1. Examples of fibrous joints.
From Mathers et al: Clinical anatomy principles, *St Louis, 1996, Mosby.*

Sutures

A **suture** is an area where two flat bones meet side to side. Specific sutures are identified in Chapter 2 wherein the bones of the cranium are discussed and several articulating unions of bone are labeled. Movement is not intended between these bones, at least not in the fully developed adult. As the cranial bones of a young child grow closer together, they attach by way of an extensive fibrous connective tissue network, which still allows growth but holds the bones in place. In adulthood these areas begin to absorb increasing amounts of calcium and the areas *ossify,* becoming more rigid and *immovable.*

Syndesmoses

A **syndesmosis** is an area where bones are joined by a long fibrous connective tissue, which may allow for a small amount of movement because of the tissue's length. A **ligament** is an example of a long fibrous connective tissue that connects bone to bone at specific locations, holding each in relative proximity to one another. A broad surface of bone may be covered by an **interosseous ligament,** as occurs at the landmarks of the interosseous borders between the radius and ulna and between the tibia and fibula. The shafts of these paired long bones are held alongside one another by the interosseous ligaments. A syndesmosis allows attached bones to be *slightly movable.*

Gomphoses

A **gomphosis** is an area where the root of a tooth attaches to either the maxilla or mandible. This very tight union resists intense pressure during chewing and biting. The ligaments in this specialized area are strong and cause this joint to be *immovable.*

Cartilaginous joints

Cartilage is a tissue that is also made of collagen; it is similar to bone and fibrous tissue but has a gel-like quality and lacks calcium. As with fibrous tissue, there is no blood or nutrient supply to cartilage. It is both flexible and strong, making it an effective shock absorber. There are three types of cartilage— hyaline, elastic, and fibrocartilage, and there are two types of cartilaginous joints—synchondrosis and symphysis. It is important to remember that there are no empty spaces between the surfaces of cartilaginous joints.

Synchondroses

A **synchondrosis** is a cartilaginous joint during the youthful years, but it absorbs calcium in adulthood and loses its flexibility. The epiphyseal plate, or growth plate, in a long bone is made of cartilage that later ossifies when growth is complete (see Fig. 2-3). Other synchondroses are between the first rib and sternum and between the manubrium and body of sternum. Once the development of this joint is complete, it is *immovable* or synarthrotic.

Symphyses

A **symphysis** is also primarily made of cartilage, yet this cartilaginous joint has greater elasticity and flexibility than a synchondrosis. An obvious example of this joint is the pubic symphysis at the point where the two pubic bones meet (Fig. 3-2). The articulation of one vertebral body with the one above or below is a second example of a symphysis. The flexible nature of the cartilage between vertebrae allows the vertebral column to move. The strength of the cartilage, however, keeps each vertebra from slipping out of alignment. At the point where the individual bones come into close contact with one another and are joined by pads of fibrocartilage, a *slight degree of movement* is allowed between the bones; this type of movement is called *amphiarthrosis* or **amphiarthrotic joint movement.**

Synovial joints

The most common type of joint in the body is the **synovial joint,** the only one that is *freely movable* (Fig. 3-3). Common synovial joints include the shoulder, hip, knee, wrist, and fingers. These freely movable joints allow a high degree of movement that is necessary for all functional activity; this category of movement is called *diarthrosis* or **diarthrotic joint movement.** Synovial or diarthrotic joints differ from one another in terms of the specific degrees of movement allowed between the bony surfaces. There are six types of synovial or diarthrotic joints, each responsible for specific functional movement. Table 3-1 lists each joint and its movement and includes anatomic examples.

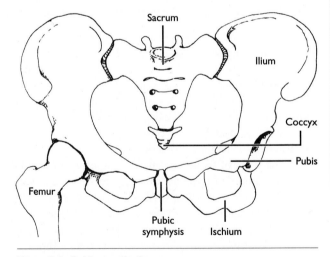

Figure 3-2. Pubic symphysis.
From Edmond: Manipulation and mobilization: extremity and spinal techniques, *St Louis, 1995, Mosby.*

Movement is described as occurring within one of the three planes that divide the body—the sagittal, frontal, and transverse planes. Each plane is described by the two portions of the body that it separates. For instance, the sagittal plane separates right from left; however, moving anterior to posterior would also be along or within the sagittal plane. The frontal plane separates anterior from posterior, but moving from right to left would be movement within the frontal plane. The transverse plane separates superior from inferior, and moving from medial to lateral would be within the transverse plane.

Table 3-1. Six types of synovial (diarthrotic) joints

Joint	Description	Examples	Degrees and planes of motion
Hinge	Concave surface on a convex surface	Elbow–humerus on ulna Knee–femur on tibia	Uniplanar–sagittal
Pivot	One bone rotates on a fixed landmark	Atlas (C_1) on Axis (C_2) Proximal radius on ulna	Uniplanar–transverse
Condyloid	Oval condyle fits into an elliptical groove (biconcave into biconvex)	Mandibular condyle on temporal bone Metacarpal on proximal phalanx	Biplanar–sagittal and frontal
Saddle	Each bone concave in one direction and convex in the other direction	First metacarpal on trapezium	Biplanar–sagittal and frontal
Ball and socket (spheroid)	Round sphere fits into a cup	Humerus on glenoid fossa of scapula Head of femur on acetabulum	Multiplanar–sagittal, frontal, transverse
Gliding	Two semiflat surfaces facing one another	Articular facets of the vertebrae	Multiplanar–sagittal, frontal, transverse oblique

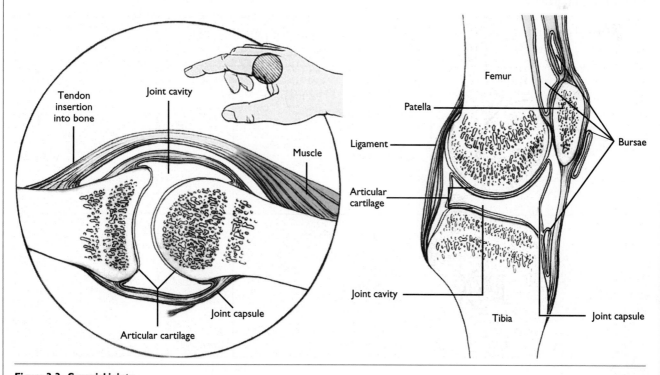

Figure 3-3. Synovial joints.
From Mathers et al: Clinical anatomy principles, *St Louis, 1996, Mosby.*

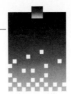

It is possible for a joint movement to occur within just one plane—**uniplanar,** within two planes—**biplanar,** or within all three planes—**multiplanar**. The number of planes in which a movement occurs is also referred to as the **degree of movement.**

Beginning from the anatomic position, several common synovial or diarthrotic joints can be observed. Though the elbow is freely movable, it is limited in the motions it is capable of performing. Bending and straightening the elbow causes movement to occur only in an anterior to posterior direction. This direction of movement occurs within the sagittal plane. Thus this joint movement is uniplanar; it has one degree of motion.

Consider the joints of the fingers between the metacarpal bones and the proximal phalanges. These joints can bend in an anterior to posterior direction when observed in the anatomic position, and the digits can move closer together or farther apart. This direction of movement is in the sagittal plane and then in the frontal plane. Thus this joint movement is biplanar; it has two degrees of motion.

From the anatomic position, the mobile shoulder or glenohumeral joint can move anterior to posterior, right to left, *and* rotate around an internal axis. This direction of movement is multiplanar; it has three degrees of motion.

Carefully consider the six different types of synovial or diarthrotic joints in terms of their structural shape, as well as the planes or degrees of motion that are possible (Fig. 3-4).

Synovial or diarthrotic joints have a complex structure with many essential elements that allow movement and simultaneous joint integrity and stability. These elements include articular cartilage, synovial cavity, joint capsule, synovial membrane, synovial fluid, and ligaments.

The **articular cartilage** in a synovial joint is hyaline cartilage, which covers the ends of the bones, creating a smooth, slick surface. Hyaline cartilage is a good shock absorber and protects the bone tissue from repeated pounding and joint movements.

The **joint cavity** is the empty space between two bones. This gap allows the bones to move back and forth without binding together.

A **joint capsule** is an enclosed sac that surrounds all other structures of the joint. It is made of fibrous connective tissue and attaches to the **periosteum** or covering of the bone. The joint capsule must have the flexibility to allow the joint to move, but it must also help hold the joint together.

The **synovial membrane** is a thin inner lining of the joint capsule. It covers everything except the areas of articular cartilage and is made of loose connective tissue. This tissue has a blood supply that provides nutrients and oxygen, and it secretes **synovial fluid** into the joint cavity. This fluid lubricates the articular surfaces inside the cavity and indirectly provides nutrients and oxygen to the tissues to aid healing.

Though the joint capsule is composed of fibrous connective tissue, it alone does not hold the joint together. Ligaments withstand force and are formed in bundles, which

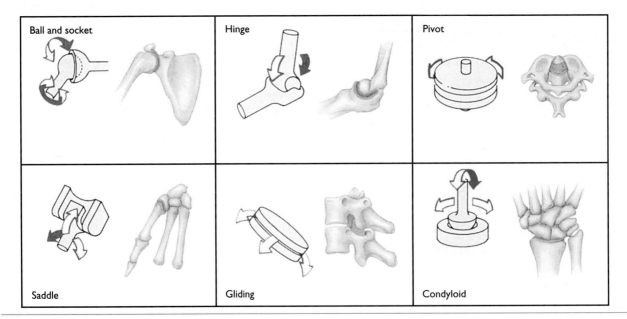

Figure 3-4. Six types of synovial (diarthrotic) joints.
From Thibodeau, Patton: Structure and function of the body, ed 10, St Louis, 1997, Mosby.

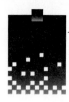

increase their strength. Some ligaments are located inside the joint capsule, whereas others are observed outside. They have virtually no blood supply and, therefore, offer poor healing potential. The various lengths of ligaments allow movements to occur within a limited range.

Other elements not found in all synovial joints include meniscus, bursa, tendon sheaths, labrum, and muscle. These terms are defined in Box 3-1.

Box 3-1. Structures found in synovial joints

Meniscus (pl. *menisci*). Cushion made of fibrocartilage that is generally circular and found in the knee; improves the mobility of the articulating bones while keeping them properly aligned. (Example: the medial and lateral menisci of the knee)

Bursa (pl. *bursae*). Small fluid-filled sac that provides padding for tendons near a joint. (Example: the subacromial bursae of the shoulder)

Tendon sheaths. Long, thin cylinder, whose fluid helps reduce friction on tendon, which frequently pulls back and forth.

Labrum (pl. *labra*). Fibrocartilage located at a ball-and-socket joint, which helps make the socket deeper by creating an additional lip not provided by the bone. (Example: glenoid labrum at the glenoid cavity and acetabular labrum in the hip)

Muscle. Often attaches to the skeleton outside the joint capsule and helps reinforce the stability of the joint

Exercise 3-1. Joints—structure and movement

Answer each question as it pertains to the structure and movement of joints.

1. Which category of joint movement is described as slight?

_____

2. The two pubic bones are held together by what type of joint structure?

_____

3. What type of tissue holds together the sutures of the cranium?

_____

4. Which type of fibrous joint describes the attachment between tibia and fibula?

_____

5. Which type of synovial joint best describes the movement of C_1 and C_2 vertebrae?

_____

6. Which type of joint has an enclosed capsule filled with fluid?

_____

7. What tissue covers the ends of long bones in synovial joints?

_____

8. Amphiarthrosis best describes what degree of joint movement?

_____

9. An interosseous ligament is the primary structure in which type of joint?

_____

10. A temporary joint formed by an epiphyseal plate in a long bone, which allows growth to take place, refers to which type of joint?

_____

11. A freely movable joint is also referred to as what type of joint?

_____

12. The base of the thumb at trapezium and the first metacarpal is an example of what type of joint?

_____

13. The head of femur joins the acetabulum to form which type of joint?

_____

14. How many degrees of motion are possible in a condyloid joint?

_____

15. What is an anatomic example of a hinge joint?

_____

16. A gomphosis is an example of which structural type of joint?

_____

17. A symphysis is an example of which type of joint movement?

_____

18. A fluid-filled sac that provides padding near a joint is which structure?

_____

19. Which synovial joint allows the greatest amount of movement?

_____

20. Which synovial joint allows the least amount of movement?

_____

CHAPTER 3

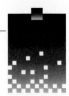

■■■ ■ Exercise 3-2. Joint structures

Complete the following table.

Joint structure	Structures involved	Examples of joints	Mobility
Fibrous	_____	1. _____	1. _____
	_____	2. _____	2. _____
		3. _____	3. _____
Cartilaginous	_____	1. _____	1. _____
	_____	2. _____	2. _____
Synovial	_____	1. _____	1. _____
	_____	2. _____	
	_____	3. _____	
	_____	4. _____	

■■■ ■ Exercise 3-3. Joint movements

Complete the following table.

Joint type	Structure	Motion
Synarthrotic	_____	_____
Amphiarthrotic	_____	_____
Diarthrotic	_____	_____

■■■ ■ Exercise 3-4. Components of joint structures

Identify the components of a joint structure on Figures 3-5, 3-6, and 3-7 below and on page 61.

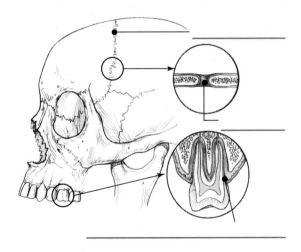

Figure 3-5. Types of joints.
From Mathers et al: Clinical anatomy principles, *St Louis, 1996, Mosby.*

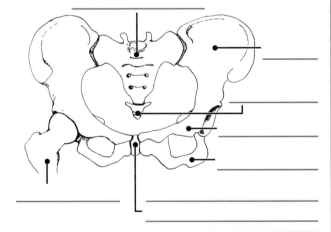

Figure 3-6. Pubic symphysis.
From Edmond: Manipulation and mobilization: extremity and spinal techniques, *St Louis, 1993, Mosby.*

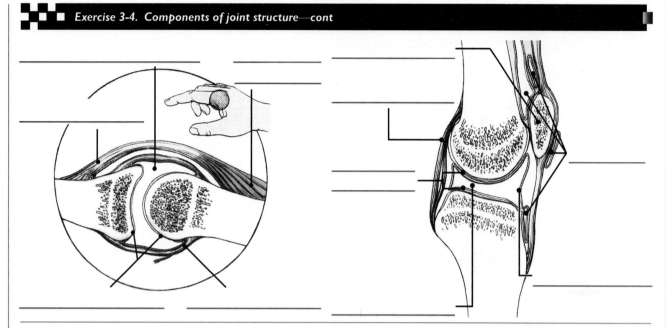

Figure 3-7. Types of joints.
From Mathers et al: Clinical anatomy principles, *St Louis, 1996, Mosby.*

■■ ■ ■   *Exercise 3-5. Synovial (diarthrotic) joints*

Give examples of the following synovial joints.

Joint	Description	Examples	Degrees and planes of motion
Ball and socket			
Hinge			
Pivot			
Saddle			
Gliding			
Condyloid			

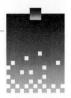

◼ ◼ ◼ **Exercise 3-6. Types of synovial (diarthrotic) joints**

Label Figure 3-8 with the types of synovial (diarthrotic) joints represented.

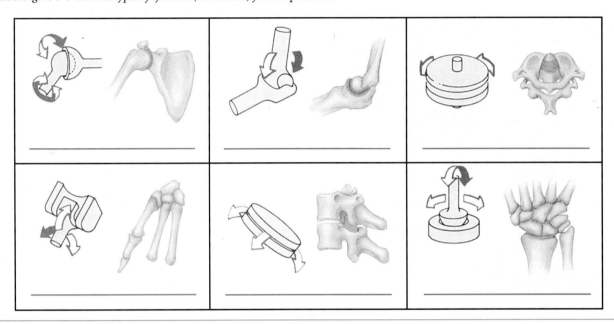

Figure 3-8. Types of synovial (diarthrotic) joints.
From Thibodeau, Patton: Structure and function of the body, *ed 10, St Louis, 1997, Mosby.*

Terminology of Movement

Since the primary purpose in studying anatomy is to understand human movement, it must be realized that the structure of a joint enables an individual to perform actions with direction and control. The physical anatomy of a joint maintains stability at fixed locations, while allowing bones to freely move in response to skeletal muscle.

Activities such as rising from a chair and walking across a room or reaching to pick up an object are actually combinations of individual movements that can be described with respect to specific joints. Each movement, like the landmarks of a bone, can be given a name to make the discussion pertaining to it universal.

Beginning from the anatomic position, all movement occurs at one or more joints. Box 3-2 gives common movement terminology and their definitions (Figs. 3-9 through 3-20).

Box 3-2. Common movement terminology

Flexion Angle between two body parts decreases
Extension Angle between two body parts increases
Hyperextension Excessive increase in angle between two body parts

Box 3-2. Common movement terminology—cont

Lateral flexion To bend vertebral column to the right or left of midline
Abduction To move away from midline of body or body part
Adduction To move toward midline of body or body part
Internal rotation To pivot around an internal axis toward midline
External rotation To pivot around an internal axis away from midline
Dorsiflexion To flex ankle until toes point skyward
Plantar flexion To extend ankle until toes point downward
Ulnar deviation To laterally flex wrist until fifth digit moves toward ulna
Radial deviation To laterally flex wrist until thumb moves toward radius
Pronation To turn hand palm down; to turn foot until lateral edge is raised
Supination To turn hand palm up; to turn foot until medial edge is raised
Inversion To turn sole of foot until it faces inward
Eversion To turn sole of foot until it faces outward
Elevation To move body part superiorly (i.e., shrugging shoulders)

Box 3-2. *Common movement terminology—cont*

Depression To move body part inferiorly (i.e., pressing shoulders downward)

Protraction To move body part anteriorly (i.e., jaw or head pushes forward)

Retraction To move body part posteriorly (i.e., jaw or head pulls backward)

Opposition To rotate metacarpal combined with flexion and abduction—unique to the thumb (necessary movement for thumb to reach toward the little finger in grasping motion)

Reposition Reverse of opposition (i.e., act of returning to anatomic position)

Circumduction Combination of many individual movements; involves flexion followed by abduction, external rotation, extension, adduction, and internal rotation (i.e., extremity moves in a large circle)

Though the illustrations of many of these motions occur in the upper extremity, it is possible to perform abduction, adduction, and internal and external rotation with the lower extremity. Individually, motions occur within one plane. Single plane movements are referred to as *cardinal* or *traditional plane* movements. If an activity is performed in a cardinal plane, it will appear robotic. Normal movement patterns, however, incorporate several individual motions at one time and cross through several planes, moving diagonally. Diagonal movements almost always combine at least one type of flexion or extension with a simultaneous rotational component from coordinated multiple muscle activity. A body part is almost never isolated as one single motion or a single muscle during normal activity.

Movements such as flexion, extension, hyperextension, dorsiflexion, and plantar flexion occur in the sagittal plane. The movements toward and away from midline (abduction, adduction) occur in the frontal plane. Additional movements in this plane include ulnar and radial deviation, lateral trunk flexion, and inversion and eversion of the ankle. Rotational movements (pronation and supination) occur within the transverse or horizontal plane.

To study human movements accurately, attention must be focused on the movements that occur at each joint. The complex activity must be broken down into small segments of

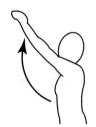

Figure 3-9. Flexion.

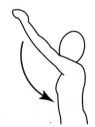

Figure 3-10. Extension.

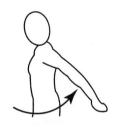

Figure 3-11. Hypertension.

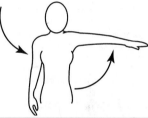

Figure 3-12. Adduction/abduction.

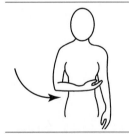

Figure 3-13. Internal rotation.

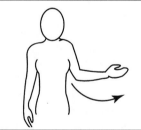

Figure 3-14. External rotation.

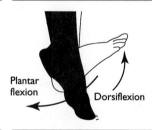

Figure 3-15. Dorsiflexion and plantar flexion.

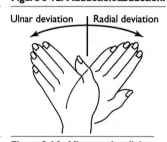

Figure 3-16. Ulnar and radial deviation.

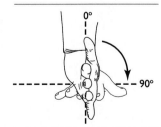

Figure 3-17. Pronation.

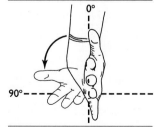

Figure 3-18. Supination.

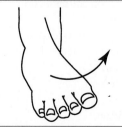

Figure 3-19. Ankle inversion.

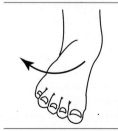

Figure 3-20. Ankle eversion.

From Brister: Mosby's comprehensive physical therapist assistant boards review, *St Louis, 1996, Mosby.*

motion that can be specifically described. For example, when rising from a chair and taking a step, at least twenty gross motor movements at the large joints of the trunk and extremities can be described; these movements do not require as much rotation as most activities (combing hair, eating a meal, or dressing).

With slow, tedious practice and a keen eye, one can develop an accurate sense of the movements that are required to perform the functional activities of everyday life. Many movements become easier to identify once the muscles that are responsible for each movement are labeled. Remember, circumduction and diagonal or multiplanar movements are combinations of sequential and simultaneous single plane motions.

Exercise 3-7. Movement definitions

Match the following terms to the correct definition.

____	1. Flexion	____	13. Pronation
____	2. Extension	____	14. Supination
____	3. Hyperextension	____	15. Inversion
____	4. Lateral flexion	____	16. Eversion
____	5. Abduction	____	17. Elevation
____	6. Adduction	____	18. Depression
____	7. Internal rotation	____	19. Protraction
____	8. External rotation	____	20. Retraction
____	9. Dorsiflexion	____	21. Opposition
____	10. Plantar flexion	____	22. Reposition
____	11. Ulnar deviation	____	23. Circumduction
____	12. Radial deviation		

a. To move away from midline of body or body part
b. To move body part posteriorly
c. To pivot around an internal axis away from midline
d. To laterally flex wrist until fifth digit moves toward ulna
e. Angle between body parts increases
f. To turn palm upward; to turn foot until medial edge of foot is raised
g. To move body part anteriorly
h. To rotate thumb combined with flexion and abduction
i. To extend ankle until toes point downward
j. To laterally flex wrist until thumb moves toward radius
k. To bend vertebral column to the right or left of midline
l. To flex ankle until toes point skyward
m. To turn sole of foot until it faces outward
n. Angle between body parts decreases
o. To return thumb to anatomic position
p. Combination of movements including flexion, abduction, external rotation, extension, adduction, internal rotation
q. Excessive increase in angle between two body parts

Exercise 3-7. Movement definitions—cont

r. To turn sole of foot until it faces inward
s. To move body part inferiorly
t. To pivot around an internal axis toward midline
u. To turn palm down; to turn foot until lateral edge is raised
v. To move body part superiorly
w. To move toward midline of body or body part

Exercise 3-8. Movements

Identify movements on Figures 3-21 through 3-32.

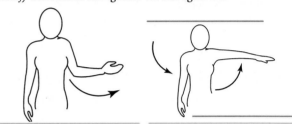

Figure 3-21. _____   **Figure 3-22.** _____

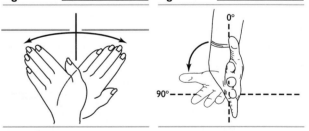

Figure 3-23. _____   **Figure 3-24.** _____

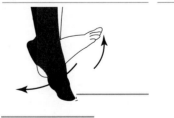

Figure 3-25. _____   **Figure 3-26.** _____

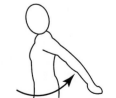

Figure 3-27. _____   **Figure 3-28.** _____

From Brister: Mosby's comprehensive physical therapist assistant boards review, St Louis, 1996, Mosby.

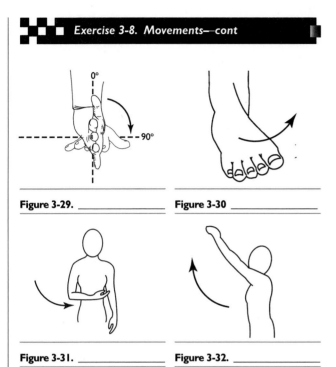

Figure 3-29. _____   Figure 3-30 _____

Figure 3-31. _____   Figure 3-32. _____

From Brister: Mosby's comprehensive physical therapist assistant board review, *St Louis, 1996, Mosby.*

Principle Joints of the Pectoral Girdle and Upper Extremity

The principle joints of the upper extremity are the shoulder, elbow, and wrist. The bones that make up the shoulder are the clavicle, scapula, and humerus. The bones of the elbow are the humerus, ulna, and radius. The bones of the wrist are the radius, ulna, carpals, and metacarpals. For an upper extremity to be fully functional, all the joint structures must allow full range of motion at each joint.

The pectoral girdle is located where the axial skeleton connects with the upper extremity via three bones—the clavicle, scapula, and humerus. Thus the pectoral girdle has four joints—sternoclavicular, acromioclavicular, glenohumeral, and scapulothoracic. The name of a joint and its structures often correspond to the bones and landmarks involved.

Sternoclavicular joint

The **sternoclavicular joint** is a synovial (diarthrotic) joint composed of a synovial capsule, articular cartilage, and several very strong **sternoclavicular ligaments** (Fig. 3-33). Only a slight amount of movement occurs at this joint; thus it is classified as a **gliding joint**. There is also a short **costoclavicular ligament,** which binds the proximal end of the clavicle to the first rib for added stabilization.

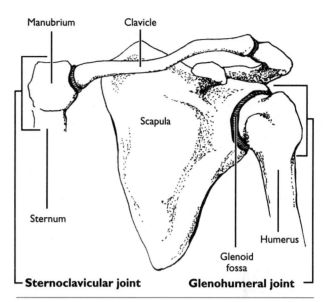

Figure 3-33. Shoulder and sternoclavicular and glenohumeral joints without ligaments.
From Edmond: Manipulation and mobilization: extremity and spinal techniques, *St Louis, 1993, Mosby.*

Acromioclavicular joint

The distal end of the clavicle forms the **acromioclavicular joint,** a gliding diarthrotic joint with a flat butter-knife shape that attaches to the acromion and coracoid processes of scapula. The joint capsule and articular cartilage are located at the acromion process, and stability is maintained by the **acromioclavicular ligaments.** Somewhat proximal to this joint is the **coracoclavicular ligament,** which assists in holding the clavicle in place. The **coracoacromial ligament** attaches the coracoid process to the acromion process (Fig. 3-34).

Glenohumeral joint

The **glenohumeral joint** is also diarthroidal and is classified as a **ball-and-socket (spheroid) joint,** which allows a wide range of mobility. At this joint the glenoid fossa of scapula articulates to the head of humerus (see Fig. 3-33).

Since the humerus is suspended against gravity, the glenohumeral joint depends on connective tissue to keep the scapula and humerus in proper alignment. The shallow fossa of the joint enables it to have a high degree of mobility. The rim of the fossa is reinforced and deepened by a cartilage ring known as the **glenoid labrum.** The synovial capsule encloses the glenoid fossa and the head of humerus by attaching at the rim of the fossa and extending distally over the anatomic neck of humerus to the periosteum.

Three strong ligaments hold this joint intact, they are the **coracohumeral, glenohumeral,** and **transverse humeral ligaments.** The coracohumeral ligaments attach from the coracoid

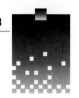

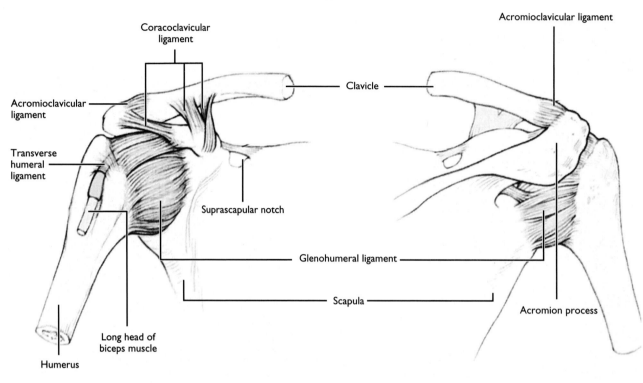

Figure 3-34. Ligaments of the shoulder.
From Mathers et al: Clinical anatomy principles, St. Louis, 1996, Mosby.

process of scapula to the greater tubercle of humerus. The glenohumeral ligament is actually made of three ligaments, which envelop the anterior portion of the joint and reinforce the synovial capsule. The transverse humeral ligament attaches to the greater and lesser tubercles of humerus. This ligament does not actually cross the glenohumeral joint but serves to hold a tendon of the biceps brachii muscle in place.

Further reinforcement of this joint comes from the surrounding muscles and their tendons. The four muscles of the **rotator cuff group** serve this purpose and are discussed at length in Chapter 5, Muscles and Movement of the Shoulder and Upper Extremity.

The shoulder is capable of a wide variety of motions and is perhaps one of the most flexible joints in the body. These motions include flexion, extension, hyperextension, rotation, abduction, adduction, horizontal abduction and adduction, and the combination movement of circumduction.

Scapulothoracic joint

Though there is no synovial joint between the scapula and thorax, there is a great deal of mobility in this region. Aside from the clavicular articulation, the scapula is bound to the trunk by several muscles that allow this bone to glide over the ribs.

Scapular movements include abduction, adduction, elevation, depression, rotation, and anterior tilt. Scapular rotation is labeled according to the specific reference landmark of each rotational direction. Medial rotation refers to the inferior angle of scapula moving toward midline, whereas lateral rotation refers to movement away from midline. Downward rotation is the same motion as medial rotation, however, the reference landmark of downward rotation becomes the acromion process of scapula, which is moving in a downward oblique direction. Upward rotation is synonymous with lateral rotation; however, the reference landmark of upward rotation is also the acromion process, but moving in an upward oblique direction. Anterior tilt occurs when the coracoid process of scapula is pulled in an anterior direction, which "tips" the superior portion of this bone forward (Fig. 3-35).

There exists a relationship between the movements of the scapula and the movements of the humerus. To perform normal shoulder flexion and abduction, the gliding movement of scapula must be present. This movement is known as **scapulohumeral rhythm** and is described as a two-to-one (2:1) ratio of humeral motion to scapular glide. This event is

best demonstrated and observed on a partner by palpating the inferior angle and medial border of scapula while the partner slowly performs shoulder flexion or abduction. A large arc of motion occurs at the glenohumeral joint, while a smaller arc of motion simultaneously occurs as the scapula glides over the thorax.

Elbow

The **elbow** is seemingly simple when observing its obvious movements, but it is complex in its construction. The articulation of the humerus and ulna create a hinge joint for elbow flexion and extension, whereas the proximal articulation of ulna and radius creates a pivot joint for supination and pronation of the forearm (Fig. 3-36).

The trochlea of humerus fits into the trochlear notch of ulna; the capitulum of humerus corresponds to the head of radius; and the olecranon process of ulna fits into the olecranon fossa of humerus. These landmarks are then enclosed in the synovial capsule.

The elbow is reinforced by **ulnar (medial) collateral** and **radial (lateral) collateral ligaments,** which run from the medial epicondyle of humerus to the medial side of ulna and from the lateral epicondyle of humerus to the lateral side of ulna, respectively. Neither collateral ligament attaches to the radius, leaving the radius free to pivot on the ulna. The **annular ligament** runs from the lateral epicondyle of humerus to the medial side of ulna, across the joint over the head of radius, and attaches to the coronoid process of ulna. Note,

this ligament does not attach to the radius, but it forms a sling that holds the radius in place, while it pivots on the ulna during supination and pronation. Also, it is not necessary to flex the elbow in order to perform the rotational components, only to rotate the extremity around an internal axis.

The **radioulnar diaphysis** of both the radius and ulna are held in parallel position by the interosseous ligament, which begins just distal to the radial and ulnar tuberosities (Fig. 3-37). Distally, the articulation between the ulna and radius is a diarthrotic joint with articular cartilage and synovial capsule, allowing a pivot motion to occur during supination and pronation.

Wrist

The **wrist** is a complex joint with many articular surfaces (Fig. 3-38). The distal ends of the radius and ulna are in contact with the proximal row of carpal bones, and the distal carpal row articulates with the bases of the five metacarpals. The various articulations between these fifteen bones make possible the motions of wrist flexion, extension, hyperextension, and ulnar and radial deviation.

The primary stability of this joint comes from the **ulnar and radial collateral ligaments** that run along their respective sides of the wrist, stabilizing the alignment of the carpals. Other ligaments include the **dorsal radiocarpal, palmar radiocarpal, palmar ulnocarpal,** and **intercarpal ligaments,** which criss-cross the carpal region, stabilizing the bony alignment of the radius, ulna, and carpals. Larger liga-

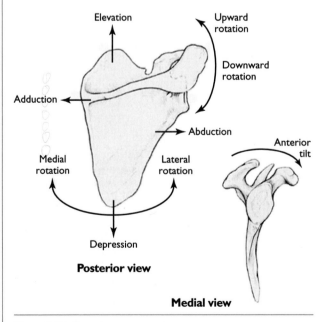

Figure 3-35. Scapular movement.
Edmond: Manipulation & mobilization: extremity & spiral techniquies, *St Louis, 1993, Mosby.*

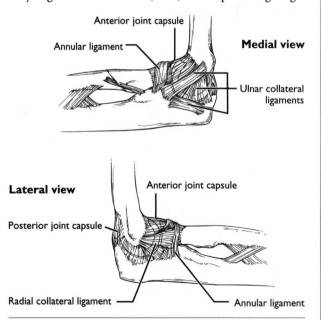

Figure 3-36. Ligaments of the elbow.
From Greenstein: Clinical assessment of neuromusculoskeletal disorders, *St Louis, 1997, Mosby.*

mentous structures unique to this area of the upper extremity are the **flexor and extensor retinacula**. A retinaculum runs transversely across the joint assisting with stability.

Hand

The **hand** is composed of the **carpometacarpal, intermetacarpal, metacarpophalangeal**, and **interphalangeal joints**. Ligaments connecting the bones of these joints are simply named for the joint and its respective location. These include the dorsal and palmar carpometacarpal ligament, the intermetacarpal ligament, and the palmar and collateral ligaments of the hand and digits.

Though there is little or no movement between the carpometacarpal joints, there is slight movement at the intermetacarpal joint that enables the hand to curve anteriorly. Metacarpophalangeal joints are of the condyloid variety, allowing flexion, extention, abduction, and adduction of the digit. Interphalangeal joints are hinge joints that display only flexion and extension.

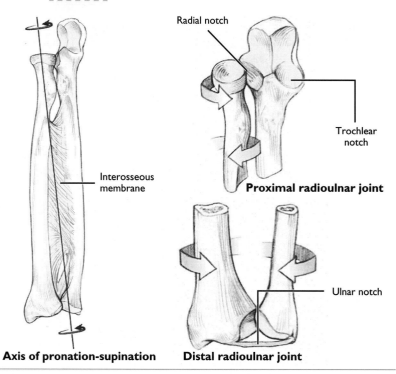

Figure 3-37. Radioulnar joints (axis of pronation and supination).
From Mathers et al: Clinical anatomy principles, *St. Louis, 1996, Mosby.*

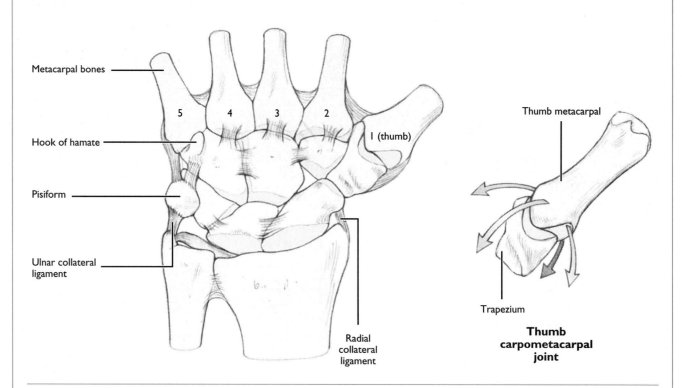

Figure 3-38. Ligaments of the wrist.
From Mathers et al: Clinical anatomy principles, *St. Louis, 1996, Mosby.*

■■■ ■ *Exercise 3-9. Joint structures of the shoulder and upper extremity*

Complete the following table.

Joint	Bones and landmarks	Type of joint	Ligaments and soft tissues	Movements
Sternoclavicular	_____ _____ _____	_____	_____ _____	_____
Acromioclavicular	_____ _____	_____	_____ _____ _____	_____
Glenohumeral	_____ _____	_____	_____ _____ _____ _____ _____ _____ _____ _____	_____ _____ _____ _____ _____ _____
Scapulothoracic	_____ _____	_____	_____	_____ _____ _____ _____ _____ _____
Elbow	_____ _____ _____ _____	_____	_____ _____ _____	_____
Radioulnar	_____ _____ _____ _____ _____	_____	_____	_____ _____
Wrist	_____ _____ _____ _____	_____ _____	_____ _____ _____ _____	_____ _____
Hand	_____ _____ _____ _____	_____	_____ _____ _____	_____

Identify the structures of the pectoral girdle and upper extremity on Figures 3-39 though 3-42 below and on page 71.

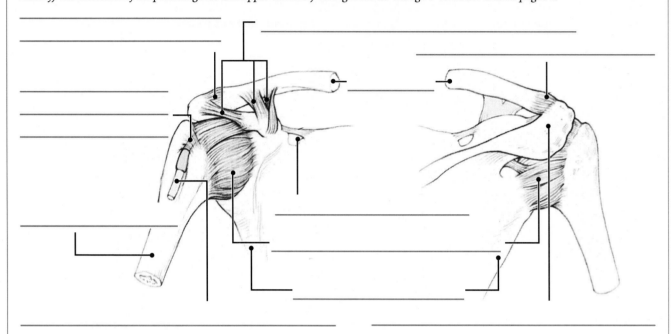

Figure 3-39. Ligaments of the shoulder.
From Mathers et al: Clinical anatomy principles, *St. Louis, 1996, Mosby.*

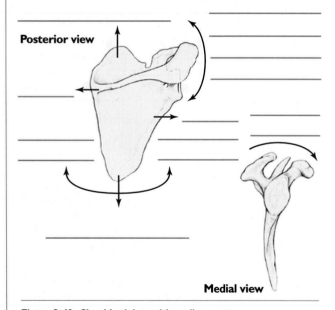

Posterior view

Medial view

Figure 3-40. Shoulder joints without ligaments.
From Edmond: Manipulation and mobilization: extremity and spinal
techniques, *St Louis, 1993, Mosby.*

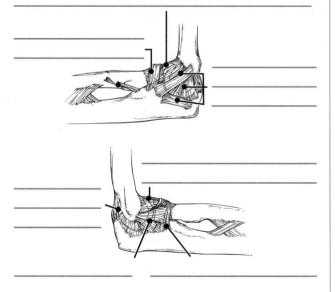

Figure 3-41. Ligaments of the elbow.
From Greenstein: Clinical assessment of neuromusculoskeletal disorders,
St Louis, 1997, Mosby.

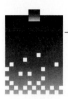

■ ■ **Exercise 3-10. Structures of the pectoral girdle and upper extremity—cont**

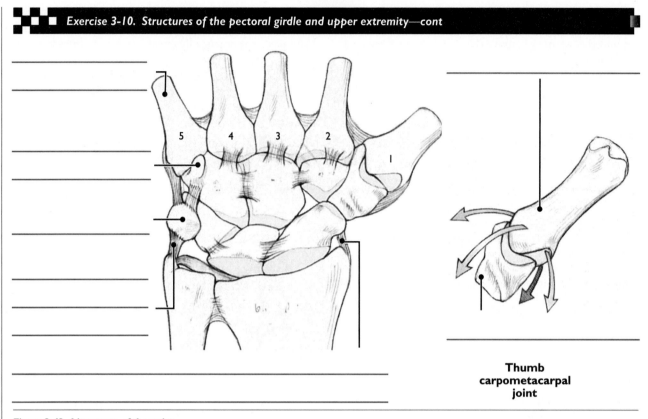

**Thumb
carpometacarpal
joint**

Figure 3-42. Ligaments of the wrist.
From Mathers et al: Clinical anatomy principles, *St. Louis, 1996, Mosby.*

■ ■ **Exercise 3-11. Ligaments of the pectoral
girdle and upper extremity**

*Match the following ligaments to the correct joint. Each joint
may match more than one ligament.*

_____ 1. Interosseous	a. Sternoclavicular
_____ 2. Coracohumeral	b. Acromioclavicular
_____ 3. Glenohumeral	c. Glenohumeral
_____ 4. Transverse humerus	d. Elbow
_____ 5. Ulnar collateral	e. Radioulnar
_____ 6. Radial collateral	f. Wrist
_____ 7. Annular	g. Hand
_____ 8. Radiocarpal	
_____ 9. Palmar intercarpal	
_____ 10. Interphalangeal collateral	
_____ 11. Sternoclavicular	
_____ 12. Flexor retinaculum	
_____ 13. Costoclavicular	
_____ 14. Acromioclavicular	
_____ 15. Coracoclavicular	
_____ 16. Coracoacromial	

Pelvic Girdle and Lower Extremity

The principle joints of the lower extremity are the hip, knee, and ankle. The bones that make up the hip are the coxal bones and femur. The bones of the knee are the femur, tibia, and fibula. The ankle is made up of the tibia, fibula, tarsals, and metatarsals.

Hip

The second pair of ball-and-socket (spheroid) joints is the **hip,** which allows a wide range of movement but not as much as the shoulder (Fig. 3-43). The cuplike acetabulum of the coxal bone is much deeper than the glenoid fossa of the scapula, and the head of femur is more deeply seated than the head of humerus. The acetabulum, like the glenoid fossa, is surrounded by an **acetabular labrum,** which increases the stability of the socket. Therefore the available degree of motion in the hip joint is lessened compared with the shoulder, but the individual movements are the same. These motions are flexion, extension, abduction, adduction, hyperextension, rotation, and the combination movement of circumduction.

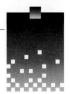

The ligaments of the hip include the **iliofemoral, ischiofemoral,** and **pubofemoral,** which together surround the underlying synovial capsule (Fig. 3-44). A small ligament, called the **ligamentum teres,** runs from the center of the head of femur at an indention called the fovea capitis to the lower part of the acetabulum, protecting a small artery inside. The ligamentum teres keeps the head of femur from slipping upward in the joint space, but its small size does not contribute significantly to the stability of the joint.

Knee

The largest and single-most complicated synovial joint of the body is the knee. Here, the distal femur articulates with the tibia and patella (Fig. 3-45). This tibiofemoral joint is somewhat precarious because the femur and entire body weight rest directly on top of the tibia's flat proximal surface. There are no bony blocks or calcified structures to assist in maintaining proper alignment of the two larger bones. This responsibility lies solely with the connective tissues. The knee is capable of flexion, extension, and slight rotation when in the flexed position.

There are eight significant ligaments that hold this synovial joint together (Fig. 3-46). The deepest are the **anterior and posterior cruciate ligaments,** which are **intracapsular;** that is, they lie inside the joint capsule. *Cruciate* refers to a structure that crosses another; therefore, these ligaments cross one another at their midpoint and lie in opposing directions within the knee. Each is named for its distal attachment. The anterior cruciate ligament attaches to the anterior portion of the tibial plateau and then onto the posterior surface of the epiphysis of femur. The posterior cruciate ligament attaches

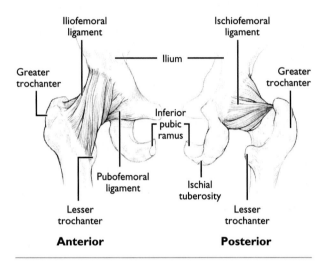

Figure 3-44. Ligaments of the hip joint.
From Mathers et al: Clinical anatomy principles, St. Louis, 1996, Mosby.

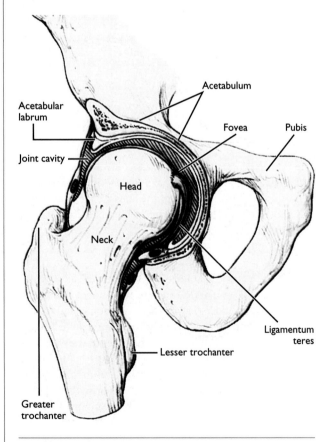

Figure 3-43. Head of femur in the acetabulum.
From Mathers et al: Clinical anatomy principles, St. Louis, 1996, Mosby.

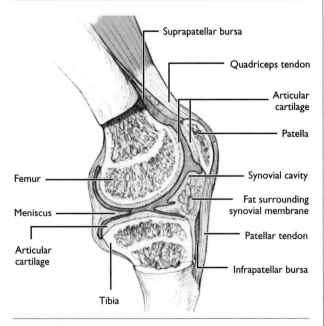

Figure 3-45. Sagittal section, knee joint.
From Mathers et al: Clinical anatomy principles, St. Louis, 1996, Mosby.

distally to the posterior surface of the tibial plateau and reaches forward to attach to the anterior portion of the epiphysis of femur. With these attachments, the two ligaments prevent the femur from slipping off the tibial plateau anteriorly or posteriorly.

Medial and lateral stability come from the collateral ligaments, named for their location. These two ligaments are also known by their distal attachments, **tibial (medial) collateral** and **fibular (lateral) collateral.** The collateral ligaments of the knee are **extracapsular;** that is, they are found outside the joint capsule. Other ligaments of the knee are the **oblique popliteal** and **transverse ligaments.** The oblique popliteal ligament is on the posterior side of the knee and prevents hyperextension. The transverse ligament binds two menisci and anchors them to the anterior side of the tibial plateau (Fig. 3-47).

The medial and lateral menisci are semicircular rings serving a purpose similar to the labra of the ball-and-socket joints by deepening the joint rim and assisting in holding the bones in proper alignment. Both menisci are intracapsular.

The articulation of the patella on the femur is vital to the overall function of the knee in that the patella is responsible for maintaining the alignment of the large **quadriceps tendon,** the attachment for the four muscles of the anterior thigh. The articulating surface of the patella is covered by hyaline cartilage, whereas the rest of this bone is encased with-

in the fibrous tissue of the quadriceps tendon and patellar tendon. The patella must be mobile in its articulation with the femur to accommodate the changing positions of the femur and absorb the tension on the quadriceps tendon. The patellar tendon attaches the patella to the tibial tuberosity.

Ankle

The **ankle joint** possesses precarious mobility and is built on a cluster of irregular surfaces (Figs. 3-48 and 3-49). The proximal articulations are those of the tibia, fibula, talus, and most proximal of the tarsal bones. The tibia and fibula are attached via a fibrous syndesmotic ligament, forming a joint that is classified as synarthrotic—allowing almost no movement. These two bones form a type of trough between which the talus fits. The talotibial joint is a hinge joint, which permits flexion and extension, better known in the ankle as dorsiflexion and plantar flexion.

The articulation of the seven tarsal bones is accomplished by gliding joints on multiple irregular surfaces. Like the carpals, the tarsals are bound by many ligamentous structures, the most complex of which lies medial to the knee joint and is known as the **deltoid ligament.** It has many branches, each named for its distal attachment. Laterally, the **fibulocalcaneal ligament** maintains ankle alignment and stability.

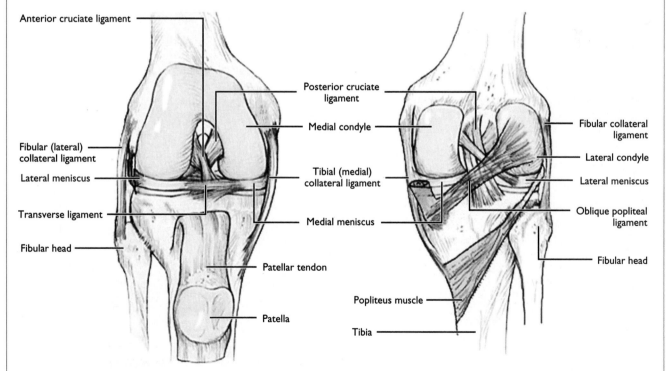

Figure 3-46. Knee joint opened, anterior and posterior views.
From Mathers et al: Clinical anatomy principles, *St. Louis, 1996, Mosby.*

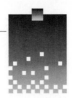

Exercise 3-12. Joint structures of the hip and lower extremity

Complete the following table. Refer to Chapter 2, Human Skeleton, for the landmarks and bones of the lower extremity. It is important to include previously discussed material in your study because of the comprehensive nature of anatomy.

Joint	Bones and landmarks	Type of joint	Ligaments and soft tissues	Movements
Hip				
Knee				
Ankle				

Exercise 3-13. Ligaments of the hip and lower extremity

Match the following ligaments or tendons to the correct joint.

_____ 1. Cruciate ligaments   a. Hip

_____ 2. Acetabular labrum   b. Knee

_____ 3. Collateral ligaments   c. Ankle

_____ 4. Iliofemoral ligament

_____ 5. Deltoid ligament

_____ 6. Oblique popliteal ligament

_____ 7. Patellar tendon

_____ 8. Ischiofemoral ligament

_____ 9. Transverse ligament

_____ 10. Fibulocalcaneal ligament

_____ 11. Pubofemoral ligament

_____ 12. Menisci

_____ 13. Quadriceps tendon

_____ 14. Ligamentum teres

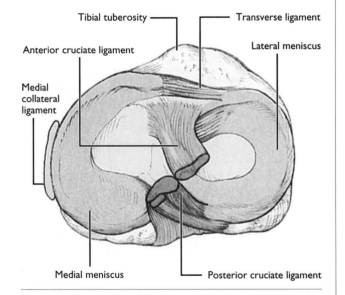

Tibial tuberosity — Transverse ligament

Anterior cruciate ligament — Lateral meniscus

Medial collateral ligament

Medial meniscus — Posterior cruciate ligament

Figure 3-47. Knee joint opened, superior view of tibia.
From Mathers et al: Clinical anatomy principles, St. Louis, 1996, Mosby.

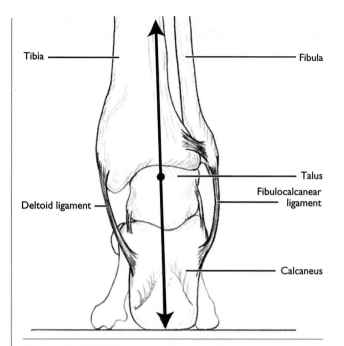

Tibia ———————   ——————— Fibula

                                        ——————— Talus
                                        Fibulocalcanear
                                                ligament
Deltoid ligament ——————

                                        ——————— Calcaneus

Figure 3-48. Weight bearing at the ankle joint.
From Mathers et al: Clinical anatomy principles, St. Louis, 1996, Mosby.

Medial malleolus ——————   ——— Anterior
                                                 tibiotalar
                                            ——— Tibionavicular
                                            ——— Tibiocalcaneal
                                            ——— Posterior
                                                 tibiotalar

Medial cuneiform   Navicular   Calcaneus

Figure 3-49. Deltoid ligament.
From Mathers et al: Clinical anatomy principles, St. Louis, 1996, Mosby.

Exercise 3-14. Identify structures of the hip and lower extremity

Identify the structures of the hip and lower extremity on Figures 3-50 through 3-55 below and on pages 76 and 77.

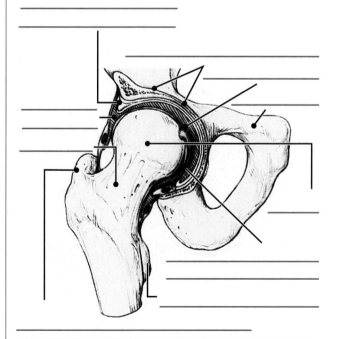

Figure 3-50. Head of femur in the acetabulum.
From Mathers et al: Clinical anatomy principles, St. Louis, 1996, Mosby.

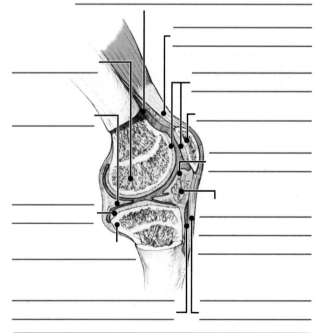

Figure 3-51. Sagittal section, knee joint.
From Mathers et al: Clinical anatomy principles, St. Louis, 1996, Mosby.

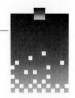

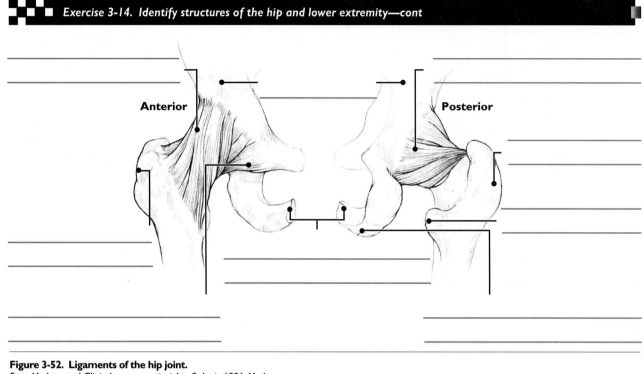

Figure 3-52. Ligaments of the hip joint.
From Mathers et al: Clinical anatomy principles, *St. Louis, 1996, Mosby.*

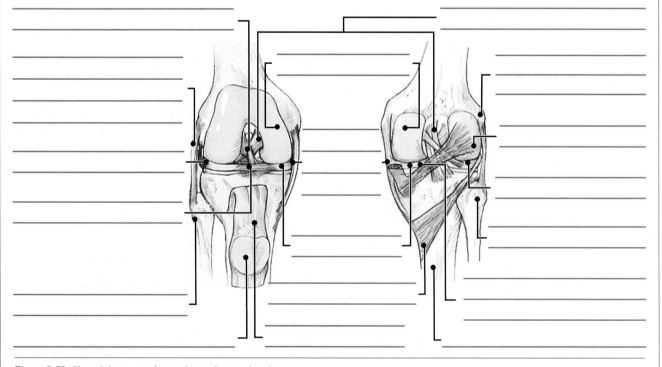

Figure 3-53. Knee joint opened, anterior and posterior views.
From Mathers et al: Clinical anatomy principles, *St. Louis, 1996, Mosby.*

Exercise 3-14. Identify structures of the hip and lower extremity—cont

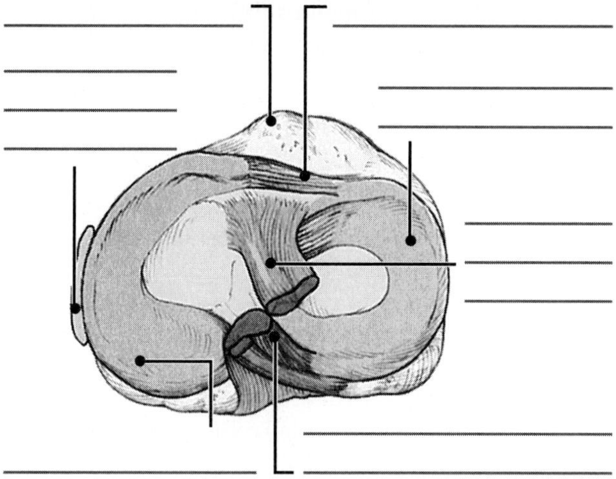

Figure 3-54. Knee joint opened, superior view of tibia.
From Mathers et al: Clinical anatomy principles, *St. Louis, 1996, Mosby.*

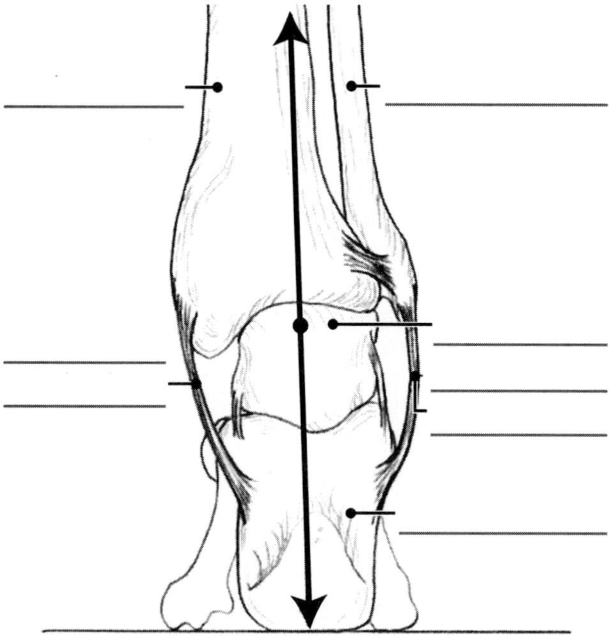

Figure 3-55. Weight bearing at the ankle joint.
From Mathers et al: Clinical anatomy principles, *St. Louis, 1996, Mosby.*

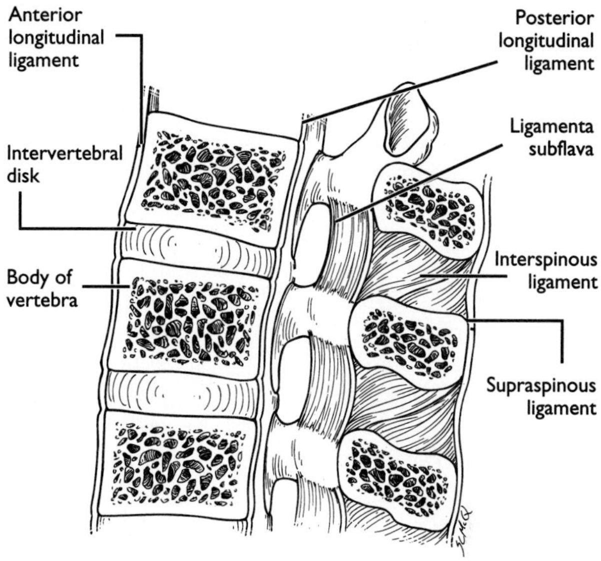

Figure 3-56. Ligaments of vertebrae.
From Greenstein: Clinical assessment of neuromusculoskeletal disorders, *St Louis, 1997, Mosby.*

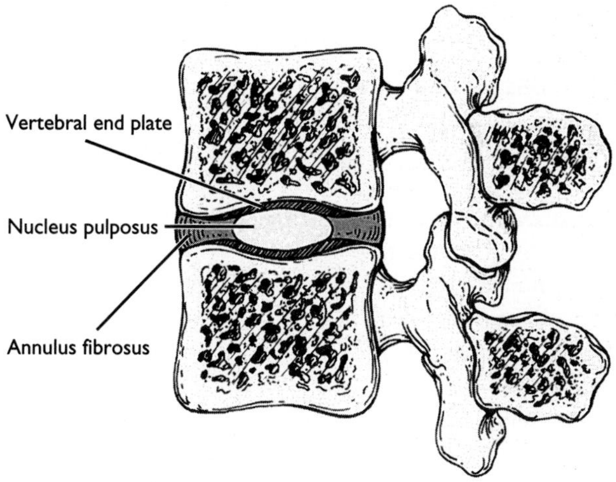

Figure 3-57. Intervertebral disk.
From Cramer, Darby: Basic & clinical anatomy of the spine, spinal cord, and ANS, *St Louis, 1995, Mosby.*

Intervertebral Joints

Two types of joints between vertebrae combine to provide stability and cushion between the vertebral bodies, as well as provide mobility between the articulating facets (Figs. 3-56 and 3-57). Between the bodies of the vertebrae are the **intervertebral disks,** which are constructed of strong fibrocartilage pillow known as the **annulus fibrosus**. Inside this pillow is a soft, elastic **nucleus pulposus** surrounded by clear serous fluid. The annulus fibrosus attachment to the vertebral bodies forms a type of symphysis cartilaginous joint, allowing slight movement between the two bones.

Between the articulating facets of the vertebrae, there can be found articular cartilage, synovial capsules, synovial fluid, and ligaments that hold the joints in alignment. These

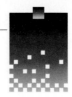

small synovial joints are gliding, allowing movement to occur in between the facets.

The vertebrae are held together collectively by **anterior longitudinal ligaments,** which run between vertebral bodies, and **posterior longitudinal ligaments,** which run between vertebral bodies inside the spinal canal. Other ligaments along the vertebral column attach like structures to one another, such as the tips of the spinous processes (**supraspinous ligaments),** the bases of the spinous processes (**interspinous ligaments),** lamina (**ligamenta subflava),** and transverse processes (**intertransverse ligaments).**

Key Words

abduction
acetabular labrum
acromioclavicular joint
acromioclavicular ligaments
adduction
amphiarthrotic joint movement
ankle joint
annular ligament
annulus fibrosus
anterior cruciate ligament
anterior longitudinal ligaments
anterior tilt
articular cartilage
ball-and-socket joint
biplanar joint movement
bursa
carpometacarpal joint
cartilaginous joint
circumduction
condyloid
coracoacromial ligament
coracoclavicular ligament
coracohumeral ligament
costoclavicular ligament
degree of movement
deltoid ligament
depression
diarthrotic joint movement
dorsal radiocarpal ligament
dorsiflexion
elbow joint
elevation
eversion
extension
extensor retinaculum
external rotation
extracapsular
fibrous connective tissue
fibrous joint
fibula (lateral) collateral ligament
fibulocalcaneal ligament
flexion

flexor retinaculum
glenohumeral joint
glenohumeral ligament
glenoid labrum
gliding joint
gomphosis
hand
hinge
hip
hyperextension
iliofemoral ligament
intercarpal ligament
intermetacarpal joint
internal rotation
interosseous ligament
interphalangeal joint
interspinous ligaments
intertransverse ligaments
intervertebral disks
intracapsular
inversion
ischiofemoral ligament
joint capsule
joint cavity
labrum
lateral flexion
ligament
ligamenta subflava
ligamentum teres
meniscus
metacarpophalangeal joint
multiplanar joint movement
muscle
nucleus pulposus
oblique popliteal ligament
opposition
palmar radiocarpal ligament
palmar ulnocarpal ligaments
patellar ligament
periosteum
pivot
plantar flexion

posterior cruciate ligament
posterior longitudinal ligaments
pronation
protraction
pubofemoral ligament
quadriceps tendon
radial deviation
radial (lateral) collateral ligament
radioulnar diaphysis
reposition
retraction
rotator cuff group
saddle
scapulohumeral rhythm
scapulothoracic joint
spheroid joint
sternoclavicular joint
sternoclavicular ligaments
supination
supraspinous ligaments
suture
symphysis
synarthrotic joint movement
synchondrosis
syndesmosis
synovial capsule
synovial fluid
synovial joint
synovial membrane
tendon sheaths
tibial (medial) collateral ligament
transverse humeral ligament
transverse ligament (collateral ligament
    of the knee)
ulnar deviation
ulnar (medial) collateral ligament
uniplanar joint movement
wrist

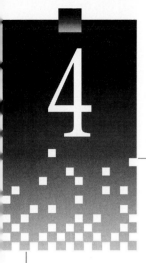

4

Skeletal Muscle Contraction

❝This chapter will enable you to understand the principles of skeletal muscle contraction.❞

Chapter objectives

The student will be able to:

1. Recognize the three different types of muscle tissue.

2. Identify the connective tissues associated with skeletal muscle.

3. Describe the elements of skeletal muscle contraction.

4. Identify types of levers created by the musculoskeletal system.

5. Identify the various roles played by skeletal muscles involved with movement.

6. Describe methods of skeletal muscle contraction as it relates to the movement and stability of the skeleton.

Movement

Movement is defined in this context as a change in the position of a body part or substance from one location to another, occurring inside or around the body as a direct result of contracting muscle tissue. In this chapter, muscle tissue is discussed in depth, and the elements responsible for the movement of the skeleton are identified.

Types of Muscle Tissue

There are three types of muscle tissue—skeletal, cardiac, and smooth. All three types perform contractile duties to move the structures to which they are attached.

The contraction of **skeletal muscle** results in the movement or change in position of the skeleton (Fig. 4-1). This contraction is called voluntary muscle movement, since the contraction and relaxation of most skeletal muscles can be initiated on demand through conscious thought and planning. Voluntary movement also includes skeletal movement that occurs *without* direct conscious thought but through habit and skill. For example, voluntary muscle movements hold vertebrae in place while the body stands upright. Through trial and error, infants learn and develop the skill to control such voluntary muscles, enabling them to effectively control body position in space.

Cardiac muscle is very specialized. When it contracts, it does so in a rhythmic and sequential pattern relative to similar tissue that surrounds it, thus squeezing and relaxing alternately (Fig. 4-2). This coordinated effort results in the forceful propulsion of blood from one heart chamber to another, through the lungs, then out of the heart into the arteries. Human life depends on a constant pressure applied to the volume of blood in our hearts to deliver oxygen to the entire body. Cardiac mus-

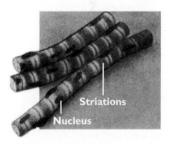

Figure 4-1. Skeletal muscle tissue.

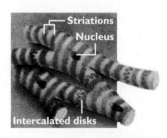

Figure 4-2. Cardiac muscle tissue.
Figs. 4-1 and 4-2 from Thibodeau and Patton: Structure & function of the body, ed 10, St. Louis, 1997, Mosby.

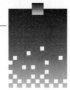

cle contraction is sustained by a constant internal electrical system, and specialized physiology allows for its consistent work without rest, involuntarily, of course.

The third type, **smooth muscle,** is responsible for involuntary contraction, the movement of substances through the arteries, veins, stomach, and intestines (Fig 4-3). In the digestive system, contraction is initiated in the stomach, and signals travel along the intestines in slow repeating waves, carrying along the substances contained inside. These muscle fibers are activated by the part of the nervous system that is not controlled by conscious, voluntary thought. Smooth muscle tissue in the arteries and veins responds to the needs of the body, which go unnoticed by the conscious mind. The mechanism of contraction within smooth muscle is similar to cardiac and skeletal muscle in a most basic sense, but the physiology and nervous system regulation is very different.

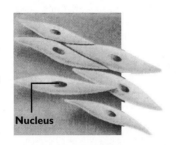

Figure 4-3. Smooth muscle tissue.
From Thibodeau and Patton: Structure & function of the body, ed 10, St. Louis, 1997, Mosby.

Components of Muscle Tissue

With the hands, the muscle belly can be palpated or felt even though it lies deep to the skin, adipose, and layers of connective tissue. To further examine the muscle belly, it must be divided into three levels, each one progressively smaller. These three levels are the **fascicle, muscle fiber, and myofibril,** which are each separated by a different layer of connective tissue.

A muscle fiber is made up of many myofibrils, which are tiny threadlike structures. A single muscle fiber is wrapped by a thin connective tissue layer called the endomysium. Many muscle fibers are bundled together by another layer of connective tissue, called the perimysium, to form a fascicle. Most skeletal muscles are made up of at least several fascicles. Finally, a group of fascicles is wrapped together by the epimysium to form what is known as a single muscle (Fig. 4-4).

For a muscle to make its attachment onto the skeleton, the epimysium may fuse with the periosteum, or bone covering. More common, however, is the development of the epimysium beyond the length of the muscle tissue where it thickens and becomes **tendon.** The tendon then attaches to a periosteum or to the connective tissue of other muscles.

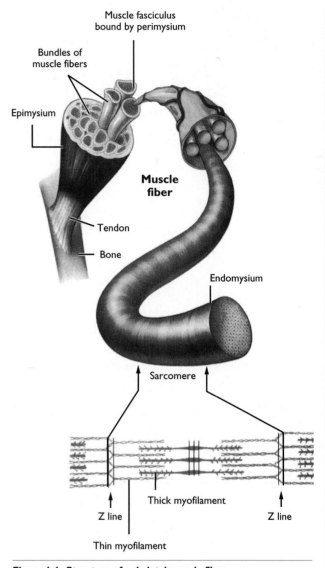

Figure 4-4. Structure of a skeletal muscle fiber.
From Thibodeau: The human body in health & disease, ed 2, St Louis, 1996, Mosby.

Tendons add to the length of the muscle attachment and can resist very strong pulling and friction forces that may occur around joints (Fig. 4-5).

Skeletal Muscle Fiber Contraction

Skeletal muscle fiber contraction occurs at the microscopic level within many myofibrils of a single muscle fiber. According to the commonly held theory, the mechanism within the muscle tissue that performs a contraction is made up of two different microscopic **protein filaments.** These two rodlike filaments (**myofilaments**) are called **actin** and

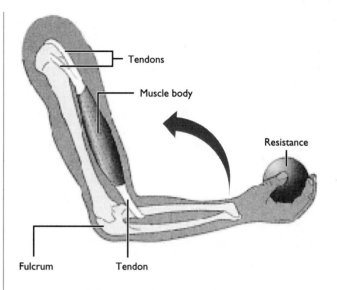

Figure 4-5. **Attachments of a skeletal muscle on a third class lever.**
From Thibodeau and Patton: Structure & function of the body, ed 10, St. Louis, 1997, Mosby.

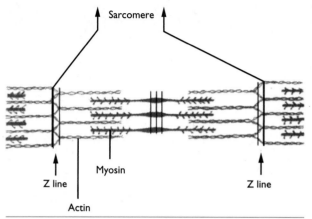

Figure 4-6. **Components of a muscle fiber.**
From Thibodeau: The human body in health & disease, ed 2, St Louis, 1996, Mosby.

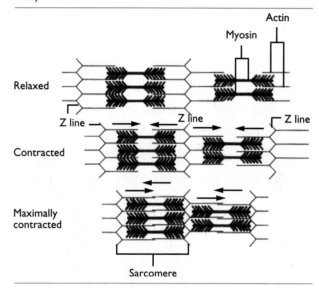

Figure 4-7. **Myofibrils composed of actin and myosin myofilaments.**
From Thibodeau: The human body in health & disease, ed 2, St Louis, 1996, Mosby.

myosin. Actin filaments are thin and form two halves of a rectangular frame around the thicker myosin filaments. Myosin filaments are thick and have tiny budlike projections, and these filaments form bridges between the two halves of the actin frame (Figs. 4-6 and 4-7). Together, these two myofilaments form the protein framework of the muscle fiber called the **sarcomere.**

Through sensitive chemical reactions that occur around the filaments, changes are caused in the surface structures on both the actin and myosin filaments. During stimulation, the myosin buds reach out and attach to specialized locations on the actin filaments. This is followed by a slight wavelike motion of the buds, which pulls the actin filament along a parallel path to the myosin. Thus the two halves of the actin frame are pulled toward one another along a set of myosin filaments, causing the gap between the opposing actin frames to close. A contraction occurs without any shortening of the filaments themselves.

When the chemical changes surrounding the myofilaments subside, the contraction is stopped by the myosin buds that are released from the actin; all the filaments then return to their original positions.

The sarcomere is the smallest single component of muscle tissue contraction, and it is enveloped by a cell membrane called the **sarcolemma.** Sarcomere align end to end and form a myofibril. Each sarcomere is separated by a **Z line** (see Figs. 4-6 and 4-7). Groups of myofibrils are clustered together to form a single muscle fiber. Since a myofibril is enclosed, all the sarcomeres in the myofibril will contract simultaneously when the chemical conditions are right to cause a muscle fiber contraction. Thus there is an **"all-or-none" response** within a single muscle fiber resulting in an instant shortening of its entire length.

Exercise 4-1. Types of muscle tissue

Complete the following table.

Muscle tissue	Voluntary or involuntary	Resulting activity
Skeletal	_____	_____
Cardiac	_____	_____
Smooth	_____	_____

Muscle Fiber Innervation

The ability of muscle tissue to contract is dependent upon its quality of **excitability,** that is the ability of the muscle fiber to be stimulated and then to respond. Skeletal muscles receive impulses from motor neurons, which are branches of larger nerves that lie outside the spinal cord. This is called the **innervation** of the muscle. These nerves are part of the **peripheral nervous system,** whereas the nerves within the brain and spinal cord are part of the **central nervous system.** Each peripheral nerve has its own name, which often corresponds to its body region. The nerve can be further identified by the level of the spinal cord to which it attaches. For example, the axillary nerve is responsible for innervating the triceps brachii muscle in the brachial region. It travels through the axillary region of the body and has roots within the brachial plexus that correspond to the C_5 through T_1 level of the spinal cord.

When a muscle fiber is at rest, the sarcolemma carries a natural voltage of negative polarity; in other words, it is **polarized.** When a muscle fiber is stimulated, it becomes positively charged, or **depolarized.** Inside each muscle fiber is an extensive network of channels called the **sarcoplasmic reticulum;** this network contains high concentrations of positively charged **calcium ions** (see Fig. 4-6). Depolarization of the sarcolemma releases calcium into the sarcomere and triggers the myosin and actin to respond to one another by sliding together in a contraction. This response occurs instantly throughout the entire muscle fiber, thus triggering the "all-or-none" response of every myofibril within the entire muscle fiber. Later, calcium is removed from the sarcomere, the actin and myosin return to their original positions.

Slow Twitch and Fast Twitch Muscle Fibers

Not all muscle fibers are alike in terms of their cellular structure and physiology. **Slow twitch muscle fibers** are designed to perform best during aerobic activity. They have the ability to store oxygen and, as a result, are better suited to withstand prolonged activity. These fibers actually contract at a slow rate, and they can resist fatigue. **Fast twitch muscle fibers** are larger in diameter but do not store oxygen as efficiently. These fibers are designed to perform quick, forceful contractions.

Although all muscles of the body possess both types of muscle fibers, the ratio of slow-to-fast twitch fibers depend on the function performed by each muscle. For instance, the delicate muscles of the face and eyes have a greater number of fast twitch fibers, since these muscles perform quick movements followed by periods of inactivity and are not expected to constantly contract over long periods of time. In contrast, the muscles of the lower

---

Exercise 4-2. Principles of skeletal muscle contraction

Match the following items.

_____	1.	Skeletal muscle
_____	2.	Cardiac muscle
_____	3.	Smooth muscle
_____	4.	Epimysium
_____	5.	Perimysium
_____	6.	Endomysium
_____	7.	Actin
_____	8.	Sarcomere
_____	9.	"All-or-none" response
_____	10.	Myosin
_____	11.	Myofilaments
_____	12.	Z line

a. Protein framework
b. Thin myofilament
c. Smallest component of contraction
d. Contraction of entire motor fiber
e. Voluntary muscle
f. Thick myofilament
g. Divides one sarcomere from another
h. Connective tissue that wraps a group of fascicles
i. Is sustained by electrical system
j. Connective tissue that wraps a single muscle fiber
k. Connective tissue that bundles muscle fibers
l. Involuntary muscle

Exercise 4-3. Components of muscle contraction

Identify the components of muscle contraction in Figure 4-8.

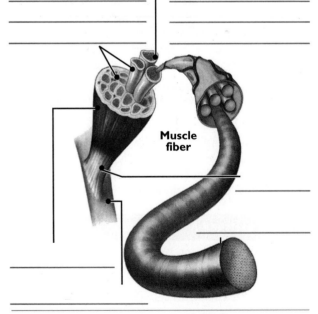

Muscle fiber

Figure 4-8. Structure of a skeletal muscle fiber.
From Thibodeau: The human body in health & disease, *ed 2, St Louis, 1996, Mosby.*

extremity resist fatigue by having larger numbers of slow twitch fibers that allow the muscles to perform under an extended workload.

Musculoskeletal Line of Pull

Skeletal muscle tissue attaches to bone either directly or indirectly by tendon or connective tissue. The attachments are labeled according to which is **fixed** and which is **movable.** The fixed, or immovable, attachment is called the **origin** and is often the most proximal attachment; however, this is not always the case. The movable attachment is called the **insertion.**

The origin and insertion are described according to specific skeletal landmarks to which they attach. The specific location significantly impacts the line of pull that is produced by the muscle contraction. Muscles whose origin and insertion lie within a single plane will more likely have very simple movement patterns, such as only flexion and extension or only abduction and adduction. However, if a muscle belly and its tendon run in an oblique direction or wrap around a shaft or joint, there may be several different motions available through the joint as a direct result of a single muscle's contraction.

Rotational movement is often possible as a result of indirect paths. In every day activities, rotation is performed quite consistently in combination with flexion and extension or abduction and adduction. It is difficult to identify any simple task that does not include some rotational movement of the trunk or an extremity.

Musculoskeletal Lever System

Joints have been well-defined as areas where bones attach and often move. For functional movement to occur, however, there must be the components of both fixed and mobile portions of the bone. For example, a broom is a useful tool for sweeping, but when lying on the floor, it accomplishes nothing. To function, the broom handle must be rigid and stabilized at one end and then grasped at midshaft to provide pull, resulting in the desired motion at the opposite end. Neither flexible handles nor grasping the broom with one hand and pulling are efficient ways to sweep a floor. The effective combination of stability and applied force results in accomplishing work.

Bones provide rigid **levers** that can be both stabilized and moved to accomplish work. Joints are the areas where both stabilization and mobility meet. In all functional movement, one portion of a joint is fixed while the opposite portion becomes mobile in response to pull from skeletal muscle. The location where the stability becomes mobile is the **fulcrum** of the lever. The skeletal attachment is the **force**

applied to the lever, and the object being moved is the **resistance** (see Fig. 4-5).

These components—the fulcrum, force, and resistance—can exist in three different orders. Changing the position of each component changes the type of work accomplished and, more importantly, the efficiency of work accomplished compared with the effort exerted. For example, it takes a great deal of effort to move a heavy object if a short lever arm is used; when the arm is lengthened, the effort required is much less. By the same token, moving the fulcrum to either end or to the middle of the lever can greatly affect the effort required and the work accomplished. Therefore three different classes of levers are discussed.

First class levers

The **first class lever** is the most common form of lever used in simple mechanical machines. The fulcrum is located between the force and the resistance. Common mechanical examples are the seesaw, crowbar, and scissors. The distance between the three components can be changed to effect the force required and the resistance overcome or the work result.

An anatomic example of a first class lever is where the muscles of the neck pull the cranium posteriorly, causing the face to lift upward. The *fulcrum* is located where the cervical spine articulates with the cranium at Atlas (C_1) and the occipital condyles, allowing the cranium to pivot. The *force* is the muscle attachment on the occipital bone, and the *resistance* is actually the weight of the entire head.

Another anatomic example is the posterior brachial region where the triceps brachii muscle attaches to the olecranon process of ulna (Fig. 4-9). The fulcrum is the elbow joint where the capitulum and trochlea of humerus meet the ulna and radius, and the resistance is the hand. The distance between the force and the fulcrum is very short, whereas the distance between the fulcrum and resistance is longer.

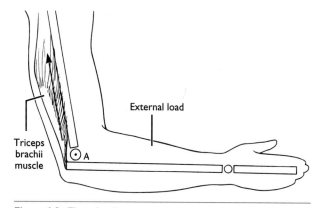

Figure 4-9. First class lever.
From Greenstein: Clinical assessment of neuromusculoskeletal disorders, *St. Louis, 1997, Mosby.*

Second class levers

The components exist in a different order in the **second class lever.** The fulcrum and force are at opposite ends of the lever, and the resistance is in the middle. The most common mechanical example is the wheelbarrow, when force is applied to the handle in an upward direction. This lever pivots on its fulcrum at the wheel, and the resistance is the load to be lifted. This type of lever is ideal for lifting heavy weight.

The anatomic example of a second class lever is lifting the body's weight on the tips of the toes (Fig. 4-10). The fulcrum is the ball of the foot or metatarsal head, the force is applied by muscle attachment on calcaneus, and the resistance is the body weight carried by the lower leg into the ankle.

Third class levers

The most common type of lever found in the human body is the **third class lever.** The resistance and fulcrum are always at opposite ends of the lever, and the force is applied from the middle (Fig. 4-11). The use of a broom with both upper extremities is a good mechanical example of a third class lever. Once again, the broom handle is stabilized at one end by one hand; the work is accomplished at the opposite end, and the force is applied by the other hand along the middle portion of the broom handle.

Anatomically, most skeletal movement is accomplished via third class levers. For instance, with the elbow joint as the fulcrum, the biceps brachii muscle attaches onto the radius just distal to the elbow providing the force, and the weight of the hand is the resistance.

Most other skeletal muscle attachments are similar. The knee joint is a large fulcrum that provides stability and mobility. The muscles of the quadriceps group attach just distal to the knee and pull the weight of the lower leg and foot (Fig. 4-12).

To summarize, the synovial (diarthrotic) joint is a critical structure that allows movement to occur between adjacent bones while stabilizing the bones in their proper alignment. Without healthy synovial joint structures, functional movement can become restricted and even painful.

Methods of Skeletal Muscle Contraction

For work to be accomplished by the skeletal muscles acting on the lever system, there must be coordination between muscle fibers, fascicles, and muscles. If every component were to contract at the same time, the body would become rigid and no activity would result. Therefore, there must be some coordination of stimuli to ensure that movements occur in systematic and controlled patterns.

Muscles receive the stimuli needed for contraction from nerves that carry signals from the brain. Skeletal muscle fibers receive individual impulses from **motor neurons,** and a motor neuron and its specific skeletal muscle fiber make up a motor unit. If the work to be accomplished by a particular muscle is not a large task, few motor neurons will send impulses to the

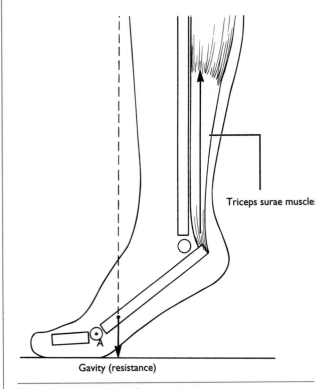

Triceps surae muscle

Gavity (resistance)

Figure 4-10. Second class lever.
From Greenstein: Clinical assessment of neuromusculoskeletal disorders, *St. Louis, 1997, Mosby.*

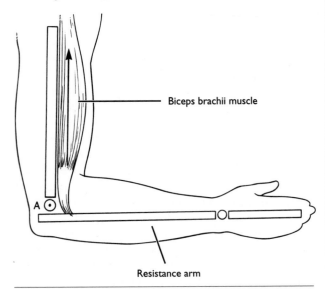

Biceps brachii muscle

A

Resistance arm

Figure 4-11. Third class lever.
From Greenstein: Clinical assessment of neuromusculoskeletal disorders, *St. Louis, 1997, Mosby.*

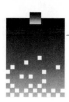

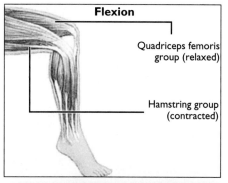

Flexion

Quadriceps femoris group (relaxed)

Hamstring group (contracted)

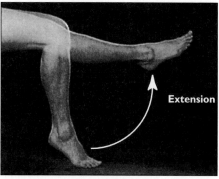

Extension

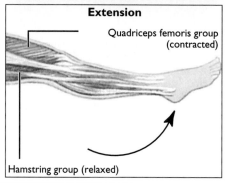

Extension

Quadriceps femoris group (contracted)

Hamstring group (relaxed)

Figure 4-12. Flexion and extension of the lower leg.
From Thibodeau & Patton: Structure & function of the body, ed 10, St. Louis, *1997, Mosby.*

muscle fibers, and only a handful of fibers will contract. If, however, the task becomes larger, the brain will stimulate additional motor units into action. **Recruitment** is an increase in the quantity of motor units that are stimulated within a muscle to accomplish a task. For example, when a person reaches down to pick up a box of unknown weight, the brain may fire only a small number of muscle fibers at first. Very quickly, however, as the actual weight or resistance from the box is realized, a more appropriate number of motor units are recruited within the muscle to accommodate the task.

Between activities, skeletal muscles are rarely completely at rest. Within most muscles there is always a slight amount of contraction present. This sustained contraction is called **muscle tone.** Posture is dependent upon muscle tone. When motor units are damaged, muscle tone may be absent.

Although muscle fibers contract or shorten on the microscopic level, the entire length of the muscle may or may not respond similarly. In some movements, such as active flexion of the elbow, the skeleton is moved by muscles that shorten in the brachial region where the overall length of the muscle bellies changes as the contraction occurs. In this instance, the tone within the muscle is maintained at a level necessary to accomplish the task, while the length of the muscle changes. This is called an **isotonic contraction** (*iso* means *same; tonic* means *muscle tone*) (Fig. 4-13).

There are two types of isotonic contractions common to functional activities, during which the muscle tone remains constant but the length changes as it crosses one or more joints. The first type of isotonic contraction is the shortening of the muscle belly, as described with elbow flexion. Most flexion movements require skeletal muscle to pull a mobile attachment toward a fixed attachment; this is called a **concentric contraction.**

Other activities require a contracting muscle gradually become longer in a controlled manner. This is an **eccentric contraction** and is demonstrated by the muscles of the anterior femoral region when moving from standing to sitting. To keep from flopping down into the chair, the distance between the two attachments must increase in a slow, gradual manner. Another example of an eccentric contraction occurs when lowering a heavy object away from the body. It is possible to release the contraction, allowing gravity to take over and instantly dropping the object; however, maintaining control over the object requires slower lengthening muscle activity. Thus the object is moved eccentrically.

Not all muscle activity requires a change in muscle length or a consistent level of tone. An **isometric contraction** occurs quite regularly; the muscle length remains the same, while the tone dramatically increases across one or more joints. When a muscle attempts to move its attachment but that attachment is somehow fixed, there is an increase in the muscle tone as the muscle attempts to overcome the resistance, but the attachment will not move (see Fig. 4-13). For example, if a person tries to lift an automobile, the muscle tone will increase, but neither the skeleton nor the automobile is likely to move. Isometric contractions are valuable in stabilizing a body part, such as the trunk or scapula, for movements that occur in the extremities. Isometric contractions frequently occur when opposing muscles contract simultaneously, resulting in no movement of the skeleton.

An **isokinetic contraction** occurs when resistance is applied that opposes a movement yet permits a constant rate of movement. This creates the maximum demand on the muscles that surround the joint throughout the full range of motion.

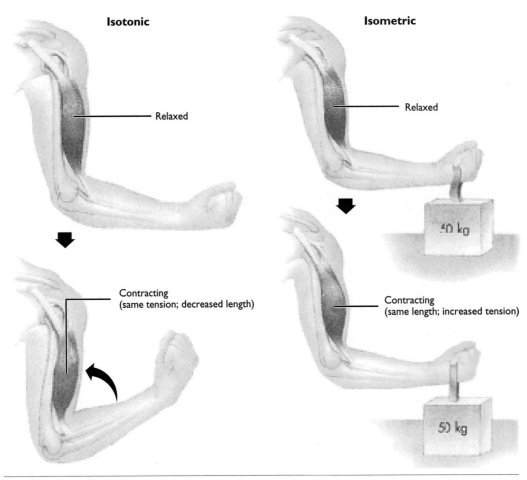

Isotonic

Relaxed

Contracting
(same tension; decreased length)

Isometric

Relaxed

50 kg

Contracting
(same length; increased tension)

50 kg

Figure 4-13. Isotonic and isometric muscle contractions.
From Thibodeau & Patton: Structure & function of the body, ed 10, St. Louis, 1997, Mosby.

Prime Movers, Synergists, Fixators, and Antagonists

For muscle tissue to actually amass enough power to cause movement, especially against resistance, there is an identification of roles that each muscle will play in specific movements. The muscle that carries the greatest responsibility for the work being done and is the primary initiator of the action is called the **prime mover,** or **agonist.** Another muscle that assists the prime mover is said to be in synergy with the prime mover, or a **synergist.**

A muscle that immobilizes or stabilizes the skeleton, not directly causing movement, is called a **fixator.** Muscles performing as fixators often do so in isometric contractions. Most muscles in the body will perform several different roles during different activities. A muscle that opposes a movement is an **antagonist** to the prime mover and its synergists. Antagonists have the ability to reverse, slow, or prevent the movement of prime movers and synergists.

Summary

The coordinated innervation of countless muscle fibers within muscle bellies can create either movement or stability among skeletal components. Understanding the role of muscle tissue will assist in treating patients with movement disorders, as well as the body's overall response to activity demands. In the next chapter the role of individual muscles and their movements of the skeleton are examined.

■ *Exercise 4-4. Types of levers*

Complete the following table.

Class	Mechanical description	Anatomic example
First	_____	_____
Second	_____	_____
Third	_____	_____

■ *Exercise 4-5. Identification of levers*

Identify the correct class of levers in Figure 4-14.

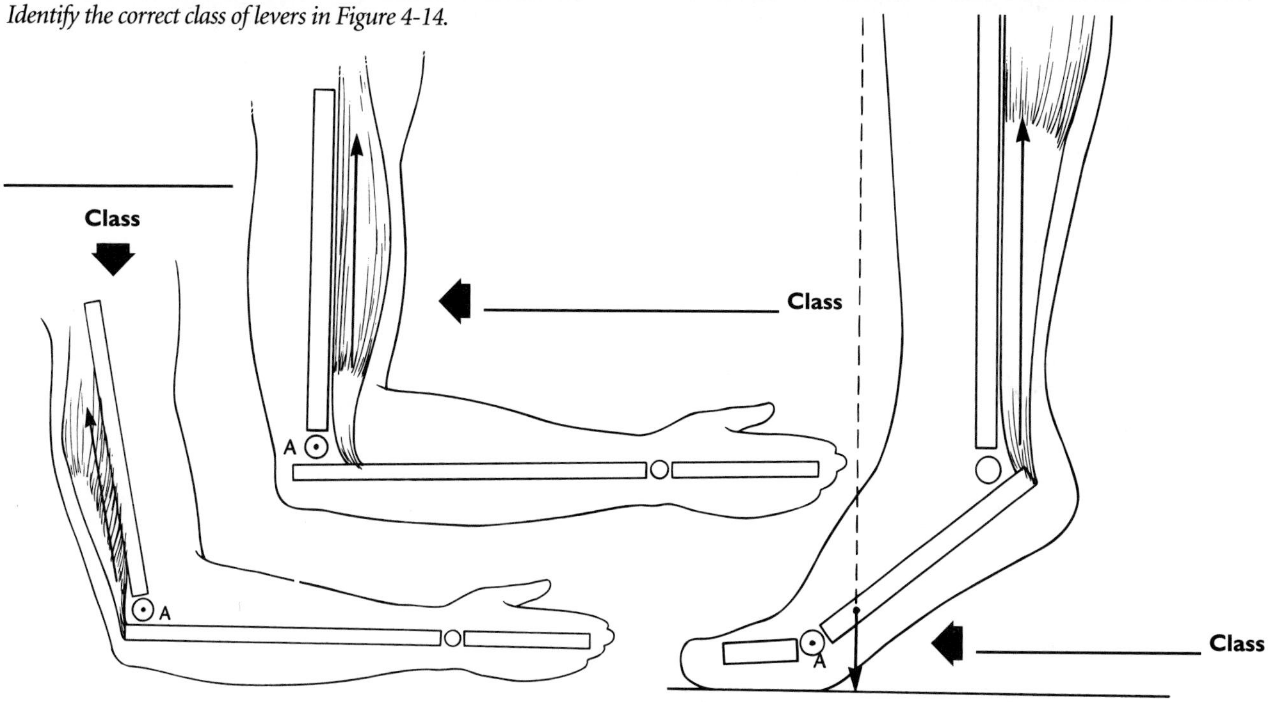

Class _____

Class _____

Class _____

A

A

A

Figure 4-14. The lever systems of the human body.
From Greenstein: Clinical assessment of neuromusculoskeletal disorders, *St. Louis, 1997, Mosby.*

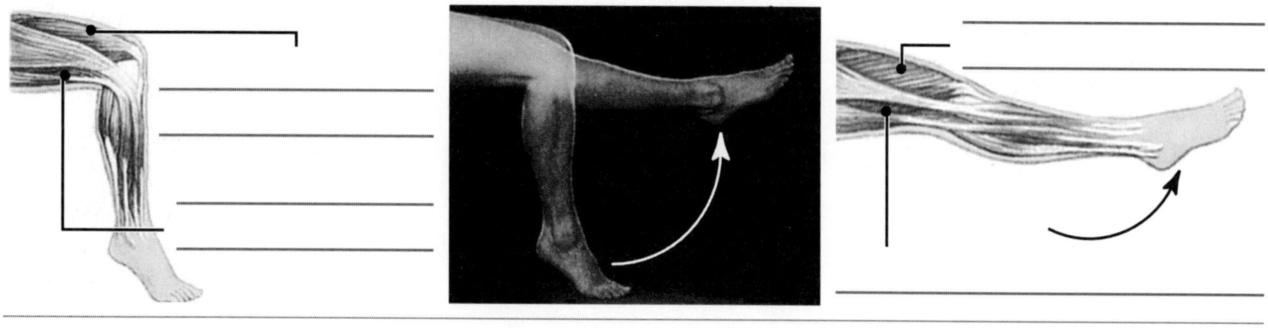

Figure 4-15. _____
From Thibodeau & Patton: Structure & function of the body, ed 10, St. Louis, 1997, Mosby.

Key Words

actin filament	motor neurons
adipose	motor unit
agonist	movable attachment
"all-or-none" response	movement
antagonist	muscle fibers
calcium ions	muscle tone
cardiac muscle	myofibril
central nervous system	myofilaments
cholinesterase	myosin filament
concentric contraction	origin
depolarized	perimysium
eccentric contraction	peripheral nervous system
endomysium	polarized
epimysium	prime mover
excitability	protein filaments
fascicles	recruitment
fast twitch muscle fibers	resistance
first class lever	sarcolemma
fixator	sarcomere
fixed attachment	sarcoplasmic reticulum
force	second class lever
fulcrum	slow twitch muscle fibers
innervation	skeletal muscle
insertion	smooth muscle
involuntary muscle movement	synergist
isokinetic contraction	tendon
isometric contraction	third class lever
isotonic contraction	voluntary muscle movement
levers	Z line

■ ■ Exercise 4-6. *Types of muscle contractions*

Match the following items.

_____ 1. Recruitment   _____ 8. Synergists

_____ 2. Muscle tone   _____ 9. Fixators

_____ 3. Isometric   _____ 10. Antagonists

_____ 4. Isotonic   _____ 11. Isokinetic

_____ 5. Concentric   _____ 12. Eccentric

_____ 6. Fast twitch fibers   _____ 13. Slow twitch fibers

_____ 7. Prime mover

a. Lengthening of muscle belly
b. Opposes movement, permits a constant rate
c. Aerobic, resists fatigue
d. An increase in the number of motor units
e. Forceful contractions
f. Constant firing of few motor units
g. Same muscle length, increased muscle tone
h. Opposes a movement
i. Same muscle tone, change in muscle length
j. Shortening of muscle belly
k. Primary initiator of a movement
l. Holds skeleton in place
m. Assists in a movement

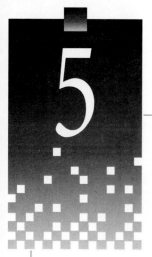

Muscles and Movement of the
Shoulder and Upper Extremity

❝This chapter will enable you to identify individual muscles of the shoulder and upper extremity, their attachments to the skeleton, ensuing skeletal movements, and innervations that affect these movements, as well as enable you to compare and contrast these elements through written exercises.❞

Chapter objectives

The student will be able to:

1. Identify each muscle of the shoulder and upper extremity.

2. Identify the specific skeletal attachment of each muscle.

3. Recognize the innervation of each muscle.

4. Identify the movement created by each muscle as it relates to its skeletal attachment.

5. Discuss the functional significance of each muscle as it relates to the surrounding muscles.

Nomenclature of Skeletal Muscles

Using anatomic terminology as presented in this text, the musculoskeletal system can be discussed as it directly applies to movement. A **nomenclature** is a method that labels or describes a body of information, allowing the information to be categorized into useful sections. The nomenclature of each skeletal muscle discussed in this text includes the **name, origin, insertion, action,** and **innervation** (nerve and root).

Note that the physical size, shape, and direction of the fibers of each muscle greatly contribute to its resulting action. As the details of this system are studied, one must attempt to incorporate a sense of function into normal activities of daily living.

Close examination of normal anatomy is necessary to effectively assist the individual who suffers from trauma or disease. An understanding of the roles of specific structures in a body region will assist in treating the patient who experiences pain or movement dysfunction.

Tissues, such as bone, ligament, tendon, muscle, nerve, and skin each have different rates of repair. Effective treatment may involve protecting a body part, retraining muscle, or preventing disuse or misuse of these structures. Therefore, familiarity with tissues and structures in specific areas of the body is vital to provide patient care with accurate and timely methods.

The human body is not a collection of individual segments that happen to be attached; rather, it is an amazing unit that, in its entirety, is affected by seemingly isolated events. For instance, a slight difference in the length of one lower extremity can, over time, result in abnormal alignment or compensation and pain in the trunk or extremities. An awareness of normal anatomy must be comprehensive, including many movement-related components.

Analysis and Application

Memorizing the nomenclature of musculoskeletal anatomy is, in itself, not useful. However, analyzing and contrasting the similarities and differences between normal movement and that of the individual with pain or movement dysfunction is the first useful step to treatment. This chapter examines individual muscles, groups of muscles that cross a similar joint, and muscles that cross more than one joint, as well as the similarities in action and innervation of each. As the student moves from one group to another, there may be duplication in the muscles discussed. This duplication occurs since the text isolates the muscles that cross individual joints and then discusses the muscles that cross multiple joints. This illustrates the complex nature of human anatomy and movement.

The muscles and movements of the shoulder and upper extremity are divided into five sections and include the

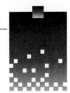

muscles of the scapular stability, shoulder, elbow and forearm, wrist, and those extrinsic and intrinsic to the hand. Each section includes a table arranged according to the nomenclature of skeletal muscle, discussion of significant elements, and exercises that are designed to enhance study and practice.

All skeletal muscles discussed in this text have a right and left component. Unless otherwise noted, the movements result from the contraction of a muscle on one side only, or *unilaterally*. Occasionally, mention is made of actions that require the contraction of both the right and left components, or *bilaterally*.

Muscles of Scapular Stability

The scapular muscle group has the primary function of stabilizing or fixing the scapula on the thorax (Table 5-1). The only bony articulation for the scapula to the axial skeleton is the acromion process on the clavicle to the sternum. The position of the scapula is critical to ensure that the upper extremity is stable and mobile. Though capable of affecting movement, each of these muscles most commonly performs the role of a **fixator**. The innervations of this group originate from the upper cervical nerve roots.

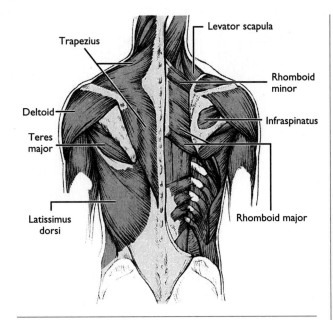

Figure 5-1. Scapular stabilizers.
From Mathers et al: Clinical anatomy principles, St. Louis, 1996, Mosby.

Table 5-1. Muscles of scapular stability

Muscles	Origins	Insertions	Actions	Nerves and root
Trapezius (upper)	External occipital protuberance Crest and superior curved line of occipital bone	Lateral clavicle and acromion process of scapula	*Origin fixed:* scapular elevation and upward rotation *Unilaterally and insertion fixed:* cervical extension, lateral flexion, and rotation to opposite side *Bilaterally and insertion fixed:* cervical extension	Spinal accessory $C_{2,3,4}$
Trapezius (middle)	Spinous process of C_7 to T_{1-5}	Acromion process and spine of scapula	Scapular adduction	Spinal accessory $C_{2,3,4}$
Trapezius (lower)	Spinous processes of T_{6-12}	Root of spine of scapula	Scapular depression and adduction Upward rotation of scapula	Spinal accessory $C_{2,3,4}$
Rhomboids	*Minor:* Spinous processes of C_7 to T_1 *Major:* Spinous processes of T_{2-5}	Vertebral border of scapula from root of spine to inferior angle	Adduction and elevation of scapula Downward rotation of scapula	Dorsal scapular $C_{4,5}$
Levator scapula	Transverse processes of C_{1-4}	Vertebral border of scapula between superior angle and root of spine	Elevates scapula Downward rotation of scapula *Bilaterally and insertion fixed:* cervical extension *Unilaterally and insertion fixed:* rotation and lateral flexion of cervical spine to same side	Dorsal scapular $C_{4,5}$
Serratus anterior	Outer surfaces of upper 8th or 9th ribs and intercostal fascia	Costal surface of vertebral border of scapula	*Origin fixed:* scapular abduction and upward rotation *Insertion fixed:* assists in forced inspiration Stabilizes thorax on a fixed scapula	Long thoracic $C_{5,6,7}$
Pectoralis minor	Outer surfaces of 3rd, 4th, and 5th ribs near costal cartilage	Coracoid process of scapula	Tilts scapula anteriorly *Insertion fixed:* Assists in forced inspiration	Medial pectoral $C_{7,8}$

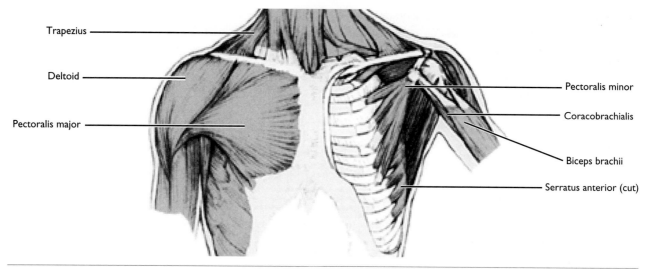

Figure 5-2. Upper trapezius and anterior shoulder muscles.
From Mathers et al: Clinical anatomy principles, *St. Louis, 1996, Mosby.*

The three parts of the **trapezius** are the most superficial muscles of the cervical, thoracic, and posterior shoulder regions (Figs. 5-1 and 5-2). The **upper trapezius,** though effective as a scapular stabilizer, plays a critical role in cervical extension, lateral flexion, and rotation, depending on the unilateral or bilateral activity. Together the **upper and lower trapezius** are capable of opposing one another in scapular elevation and depression, but they compliment each other by participating in upward (lateral) rotation of the scapula. The **middle trapezius** has a simple line of pull that is limited to the transverse plane for scapular adduction.

The **rhomboids,** named for their oblique geometric shape, are a pair of muscles that lies deep to the trapezius group (see Fig. 5-1). Their angular line of pull results in various scapular motions. A muscle that is rather simple in origin and insertion is **levator scapula** (see Fig. 5-1). The actions of this muscle is dependent on the contraction of only one side or the simultaneous contraction of both right and left sides. Differences can also occur with respect to which attachment remains fixed. Though most commonly known for performing scapular movements, **levator scapulae** can affect cervical extension and rotation.

Serratus anterior is hidden by several more superficial muscles and by the scapula with its origin on the anterior thorax and its insertion on the posterior thorax (see Fig. 5-2). This muscle is antagonistic to the trapezius in scapular abduction but works with the trapezius in upward rotation of the scapula. In the event that the scapula is stabilized, serratus anterior is capable of mobilizing its attachment on the ribs, assisting in inspiration.

Another scapular stabilizer is **pectoralis minor;** its origin is on the ribs, and it is a synergist in inspiration (see

Fig. 5-2). This very small muscle tilts the scapula anteriorly by pulling the coracoid process of scapula over the shoulder in a sense, lifting the inferior angle of scapula away from the thorax.

Trapezius, rhomboids, and levator scapulae each originate from the vertebral column, whereas serratus anterior and pectoralis minor both originate from the rib cage. Though the muscles of this group do not cross the glenohumeral joint, their activity has a direct effect on the movement at the shoulder by setting the stage or base to which the proximal humerus is attached. Improper function in the scapular stabilizers results in poor quality movement or the absence of all movement normally performed by the glenohumeral joint.

Functional significance

The muscles of the scapular group are vital to proper postural alignment of the pectoral girdle, upper extremity, and cervical spine. Trapezius, rhomboids, and levator scapulae retract the scapula and pull the shoulders, cervical spine, and head posteriorly. Aside from fixing the scapula for movement of the upper extremity, these muscles open the chest area, helping improve inspiration while keeping the head upright and enabling a full view of the environment. Upper trapezius and levator scapulae lend to cervical rotation to the right or left sides. Serratus anterior and pectoralis minor draw the scapula forward during an upper extremity reach. The scapula is the staging platform on which the humerus moves. This forward posture is necessary to facilitate arm length and shoulder position before performing grasping, pulling, or pushing movements common in activities of daily living. An overview of the muscles of scapular stability is provided in Table 5-1.

■ ■ ■ **Exercise 5-1. Movement analysis: scapular stabilizers**

Indicate the movement(s) that can be performed by each muscle by marking an "X" under each correct action.

Movement	Trapezius upper	Trapezius middle	Trapezius lower	Rhomboids	Levator scapulae	Serratus anterior	Pectoralis minor
Scapular elevation							
Scapular depression							
Scapular rotation—upward							
Scapular rotation—downward							
Scapular adduction							
Scapular abduction							
Scapular tilt—anterior							
Cervical extension							
Cervical rotation							
Cervical lateral flexion							
Assists inspiration							

■ ■ ■ **Exercise 5-2. Innervation analysis: scapular stabilizers**

Indicate the innervation for each muscle by marking an "X" under the correct columns.

Movement	Trapezius upper	Trapezius middle	Trapezius lower	Rhomboids	Levator scapulae	Serratus anterior	Pectoralis minor
Spinal accessory							
Dorsal scapular							
Long thoracic							
Medial pectoral							

Muscles of the Shoulder

The muscles of the shoulder originate from various landmarks on the scapula, clavicle, sternum, and ribs (Table 5-2). The common function of each is movement of the humerus as it pivots within the glenoid fossa of scapula. **Pectoralis major** (Figs. 5-3 and 5-4) is the prominent superficial muscle of the anterior pectoral region. A broad origin allows the differences in the line of pull to its comparatively small insertion, resulting in a variety of shoulder movements. Its larger size also lends to the range of nerve roots that are responsible for the innervation of this muscle. **Coracobrachialis** (Figs. 5-2, 5-4, and 5-5) lies deep to pectoralis major and is a strong shoulder flexor.

Biceps brachii (see Figs. 5-2, 5-3, 5-4, and 5-5) has as its origin two separate tendons that are attached at individual landmarks, allowing some variation in the line of pull.

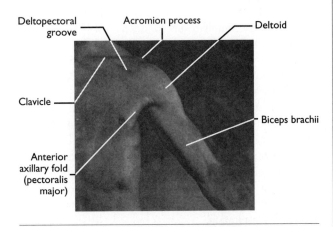

Figure 5-3. Surface anatomy of upper limb, anterior view.
From Mathers et al: Clinical anatomy principles, St. Louis, 1996, Mosby.

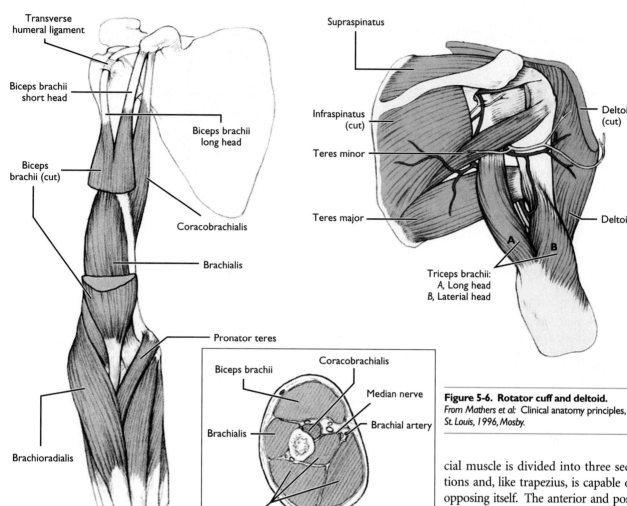

Figure 5-4. Anterior shoulder and elbow.
From Mathers et al: Clinical anatomy principles,
St. Louis, 1996, Mosby.

Figure 5-5. Cross-section of brachial region.
From Mathers et al: Clinical anatomy principles, *St. Louis,
1996, Mosby.*

Figure 5-6. Rotator cuff and deltoid.
From Mathers et al: Clinical anatomy principles,
St. Louis, 1996, Mosby.

The attachment of the long head allows biceps brachii to be a two-joint muscle that crosses the glenohumeral joint and the elbow. Though the biceps brachii can cause simultaneous movements at both the glenohumeral joint and elbow, it is often responsible for movements at only one joint if the other is stabilized by surrounding muscles. A reversal of the line of pull results in moving the humerus and shoulder toward the radius; this can only occur if the forearm and hand are fixed while the rest of the body is mobile as occurs when performing a chin up. The belly of this muscle is easily palpable running anteromedial to humerus.

Deltoid (Figs. 5-1, 5-2, 5-3, 5-6, and 5-7) is also a multi-origin muscle, resulting in a variety of actions. This superfi-cial muscle is divided into three sections and, like trapezius, is capable of opposing itself. The anterior and posterior divisions are antagonistic in action, whereas the middle fibers perform as the primary abductor of the shoulder joint.

The next shoulder muscle has a complex origin and affects movements not only at the shoulder but at the lower portion of the vertebral column, as well as pelvic alignment. **Latissimus dorsi** (Figs. 5-1 and 5-7) has a broad, superficial origin on the posterior trunk. Its insertion, however, lies on the anterior portion of humerus, thus the muscle belly wraps laterally around the trunk and crosses the axillary region under the shoulder before attaching at the bicipital groove of humerus. This muscle effectively pulls the upper extremity into extension, particularly when the humerus begins in the overhead or flexed position, which is common when propelling forward in a wheelchair or when performing a chin up. Similarly, the pull phase of the "butterfly" swimming stroke makes primary use of bilateral latissimus dorsi muscles.

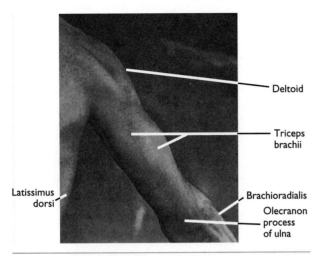

Figure 5-7. Surface anatomy of upper limb, posterior view.
From Mathers et al: Clinical anatomy principles, *St. Louis, 1996, Mosby.*

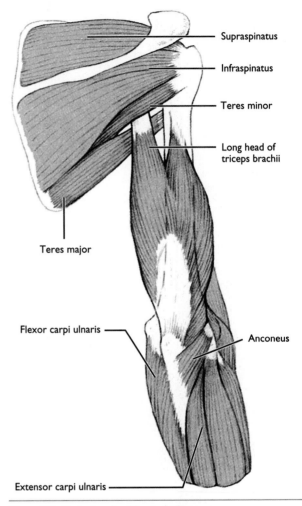

Figure 5-8. Posterior shoulder and elbow.
From Mathers et al: Clinical anatomy principles, *St. Louis, 1996, Mosby.*

Following a similar path along the axillary region as latissimus dorsi, **teres major** (Figs. 5-1 and 5-8) also runs from the posterior trunk to the anterior aspect of humerus. As a result of a similar line of pull, this muscle performs the same actions at the glenohumeral joint as latissimus dorsi. Teres major is sometimes referred to as *little latissimus.*

Another multihead, two-joint muscle is the **triceps brachii** (see Figs. 5-5, 5-7, and 5-8). With its singular inner-vation at the olecranon process of ulna, it is the largest of the two-elbow extensor muscles; the other is **anconeus.** This muscle is able to perform duties of shoulder adduction and extension via the long head of triceps brachii.

The four muscles of the **rotator cuff** have the primary responsibility for holding the head of humerus in alignment with the glenoid fossa of scapula under the weight of the upper extremity and the forces of gravity that act on it. Though other muscles crossing the glenohumeral joint contribute to the integrity of the joint, the rotator cuff is the most efficient stabilizer because of the strategic position of the four muscles around the head of humerus and their relatively short length. Each of the four has its origin on the scapula and insertion on the proximal humerus near the greater tubercle. The line of pull of each muscle directly correlates to its resulting effect on the movement of the head of humerus. The rotator cuff mus-cles are the deepest of all muscles of the shoulder.

The first rotator cuff muscle is **supraspinatus** (see Fig. 5-6), named for its origin. This muscle passes superi-orly over the head of humerus and is responsible for initiat-ing the movement of shoulder abduction. After supraspinatus contracts, the middle portion of the deltoid then continues to move the joint through its full available range in abduction.

During full abduction of humerus (excluding any rotation of the bone), it is common that the tendon of supraspinatus can become trapped between the greater tubercle of humerus and the acromion process of scapula. This common injury requires treatment of the inflamed or torn soft tissue, as well as modifications in the movement at the glenohumeral joint.

Infraspinatus and **teres minor** (see Figs 5-6 and 5-8) both approach the greater tubercle of humerus posteriorly and thus pull in the direction of lateral or external rotation. **Subscapularis** is one of only two muscles of the body with an origin on the ventral or anterior aspect of the scapula. The other is serratus anterior, which is also named for the landmark of origin. As the only medial rotator of humerus in this muscle group, subscapularis joins latissimus dorsi and teres major in the axillary region inferior to the gleno-humeral joint. An overview of the muscles of the shoulder is provided in Table 5-2.

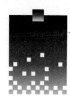

Table 5-2. Muscles of the shoulder and rotator cuff

Muscles	Origins	Insertions	Actions	Nerves and root
Pectoralis major	Medial one half of clavicle Lateral margin of sternum Cartilage of ribs 1 to 6	Lateral lip of bicipital groove just distal to greater tubercle of humerus	*Glenohumeral joint:* Flexion (upper fibers), adduction, medial rotation, and horizontal adduction of humerus (transverse plane)	Medial and lateral pectoral $C_{5,6,7,8}$ to T_1
Coracobrachialis	Coracoid process of scapula	Anteromedial surface of middle of shaft of humerus, anterior to deltoid tuberosity	*Glenohumeral joint:* Flexion, adduction	Musculocutaneous $C_{6,7}$
Biceps brachii	*Short head:* coracoid process of scapula *Long head:* Supraglenoid tubercle of scapula by a tendon that lies along bicipital groove of humerus	Tuberosity of radius	*Glenohumeral joint:* Flexion Long head may assist with abduction if humerus is laterally rotated *At the elbow:* Flexion and supination *Insertion fixed:* humerus toward forearm, "chin-up"	Musculocutaneous $C_{5,6}$
Deltoid	*Anterior fibers:* anterolateral one third of clavicle *Middle fibers:* acromion process of scapula *Posterior fibers:* spine of scapula	Deltoid tuberosity of humerus	*Glenohumeral joint: whole:* abduction *Anterior:* assists in flexion, medial rotation of humerus *Posterior:* assists in extension, lateral rotation of humerus	Axillary $C_{5,6}$
Latissimus dorsi	Spinous processes distal to last six thoracic vertebrae Last three or four ribs Fascia from lumbar and sacral regions Posterior external rim of iliac crest Inferior angle of scapula	Bicipital groove of humerus	*Glenohumeral joint:* adduction, extension, medial rotation of humerus *Insertion fixed and unilateral:* assists in tilting pelvis anteriorly and laterally *Bilaterally:* hyperextension of vertebral column	Thoracodorsal $C_{7,8}$
Teres major	Dorsolateral surface of inferior angle of scapula	Distal to lesser tubercle of humerus	*Glenohumeral joint:* adduction, extension, medial rotation of humerus	Inferior subscapular C_6
Triceps brachii	*Long head:* infraglenoid tubercle of scapula *Lateral head:* proximal posterolateral shaft of humerus *Medial head:* distal posterolateral shaft of humerus	Olecranon process of ulna and deep fascia of forearm	*Glenohumeral joint:* long head performs adduction and extension *At elbow:* extension of humerus	Radial $C_{7,8}$
Supraspinatus	Supraspinous fossa of scapula	Superior to greater tubercle of humerus	*Glenohumeral joint:* initiates abduction Stabilizes head of humerus in glenoid fossa	Suprascapular C_5
Infraspinatus	Infraspinous fossa of scapula	Posterior to greater tubercle of humerus	*Glenohumeral joint:* lateral rotation of humerus Stabilizes head of humerus in glenoid cavity	Suprascapular $C_{5,6}$
Teres minor	Lateral portion of infraspinous fossa of scapula	Posterior to greater tubercle of humerus	*Glenohumeral joint:* lateral rotation of humerus Stabilizes head of humerus in glenoid cavity	Axillary $C_{5,6}$
Subscapularis	Entire subscapular fossa of scapula	Lesser tubercle of humerus	*Glenohumeral joint:* medial rotation of humerus Stabilizes head of humerus in glenoid cavity	Superior and inferior Subscapular $C_{5,6}$

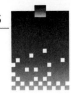

Study Note

A common memory aide when learning new vocabulary is the use of an *acrostic*, a word formed by the first or last letters in a series of words. The acrostic associated with the rotator cuff muscles is **SITS**.

S upraspinatus
I nfraspinatus
T eres minor
S ubscapularis

Be careful not to confuse *teres minor* of this group with teres major (little latissimus).

Functional significance

Pectoralis major and coracobrachialis are powerful in pulling the humerus toward midline. This movement often occurs while grasping either a **fixed** or **movable** object with the hand. Pulling toward midline is necessary when closing a door or turning a steering wheel. Biceps brachii, with its two-joint activity, makes it possible to bring the hand toward the face with palm up for eating, grooming, and upper body dressing.

Shoulder abduction is initiated by supraspinatus and completed with the middle deltoid, which brings the humerus into position so the hand may be placed away from midline. Reaching toward any object above waist level and away from the trunk necessitates some degree of abduction. In contrast, adduction and extension are performed by latissimus dorsi and teres major. This pair of muscles controls forceful rowing movements when the upper extremity opposes resistance in pulling objects toward the trunk or downward from overhead.

While the rotator cuff holds the head of humerus in place on the glenoid fossa of scapula, the contribution to humeral rotation should not be overlooked. External rotation by infraspinatus and teres minor provides the ability to reach away from midline without rotating the entire trunk to do so. This motion is often combined with abduction and flexion when reaching in a diagonal path upward, which occurs when putting on a shirt or coat. Internal rotation by subscapularis provides the ability to reach the hand behind the trunk during bathing, pulling up pants, or reaching into a back pocket.

Exercise 5-3. Movement analysis: shoulder and rotator cuff

Indicate the movement(s) that can be performed by each muscle by marking an "X" under each correct action.

Movement	Flexion	Extension	Abduction	Adduction	Medial rotation	Lateral rotation
Pectoralis major						
Coracobrachialis						
Biceps brachii						
Deltoid						
Latissimus dorsi						
Triceps brachii						
Teres major						
Supraspinatus						
Infraspinatus						
Teres minor						
Subscapularis						

Exercise 5-4. Innervation analysis: shoulder and rotator cuff

Indicate the innervation for each muscle by marking an "X" under the correct columns.

Muscles	Pectoral	Musculocutaneous	Axillary	Thoracodorsal	Radial	Suprascapular	Subscapular
Pectoralis major							
Coracobrachialis							
Biceps brachii							
Deltoid							
Latissimus dorsi							
Triceps brachii							
Teres major							
Supraspinatus							
Infraspinatus							
Teres minor							
Subscapularis							

Exercise 5-5. Scapular stabilizer muscles

Identify the scapular stabilizer muscles in Figure 5-9.

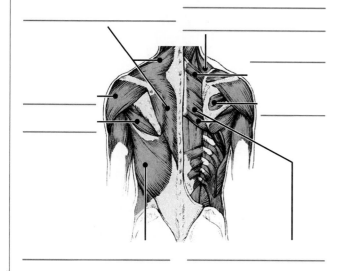

Figure 5-9. Scapular stabilizers.
From Mathers et al: Clinical anatomy principles, *St. Louis, 1996, Mosby.*

Exercise 5-6. Shoulder muscles

Identify the shoulder muscles in Figure 5-10.

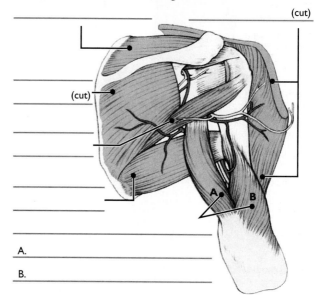

A.

B.

Figure 5-10. Posterior shoulder.
From Mathers et al: Clinical anatomy principles, *St. Louis, 1996, Mosby.*

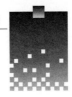

Muscles of the Elbow and Forearm

Since the elbow has only one degree of movement—flexion and extension—the muscles in this area have a relatively direct line of pull. The two-joint muscle, **biceps brachii** (see Figs. 5-2, 5-3, 5-4, and 5-5), is a synergist for elbow flexion, though not the most efficient muscle capable of performing this action. Its single insertion on the radius means this muscle also assists in supination, where the radius pivots around the ulna. The most efficient elbow flexor is **brachialis** (see Figs 5-4 and 5-5), with its short muscle belly and dedicated line of pull from the diaphysis of humerus to the ulna. This muscle shares the same principle innervation as biceps brachii. With sufficient strength, both brachialis and biceps brachii perform well when their distal attachment becomes fixed, allowing the humerus to move toward the forearm, which occurs when performing a *chin-up* or transfer activity when the trunk is pulled toward the hands.

The third elbow flexor, **brachioradialis** (see Figs. 5-4, 5-7, and 5-11), has a similar line of pull to that of biceps brachii from the humerus to the radius. However, the distal location of the insertion does not lend itself to strength in elbow flex-

ion. Though this muscle is not the primary muscle to any one individual movement, it is synergistic to elbow flexion, pronation and supination.

Elbow extension is performed primarily by the two-joint muscle, **triceps brachii** (see Figs. 5-5, 5-6, 5-7, and 5-8), assisted by anconeus, the *little helper*. Both cross the elbow posteriorly over the olecranon process of ulna and are innervated by the radial nerve.

The three muscles of the forearm are dedicated to supination and pronation. **Supinator** (Figs. 5-12 and 5-13) has a line of pull that runs along an oblique plane with its origin on the fixed ulna and inserting on the mobile shaft of radius. Performing this action against resistance, which

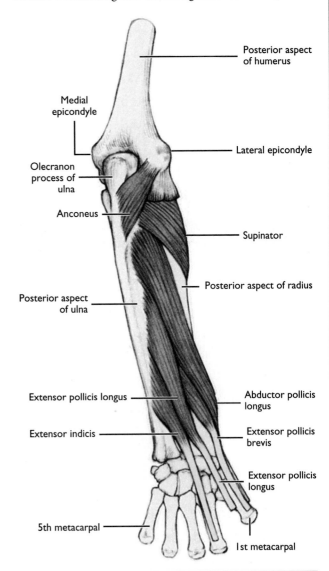

Figure 5-11. Superficial forearm extensor muscles.
From Mathers et al: Clinical anatomy principles, St. Louis, 1996, Mosby.

Figure 5-12. Extensor muscles of digits I and II.
From Mathers et al: Clinical anatomy principles, St. Louis, 1996, Mosby.

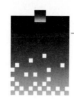

occurs when holding an object in the hand, requires assistance from both biceps brachii and brachioradialis.

Pronator teres (Figs. 5-4, 5-14, and 5-15) and **pronator quadratus** (Figs. 5-14, 5-16, and 5-17) are obvious in their action. Pronator teres runs obliquely from distal humerus, wrapping around the midshaft of the radius, whereas pronator quadratus runs transversely from distal ulna to distal radius. The two have the innervation of the median nerve in common.

Functional significance

The muscles synergistic to elbow flexion obviously serve to pull the hand closer to the face and trunk and also assist in placing the hand on a surface close to the trunk, such as the arm of a chair before standing. When the insertion is fixed, the reverse action is common in activities such as using the upper extremity to pull to standing. This group includes biceps brachii, brachialis, and brachioradialis.

Biceps brachii and supinator are frequently contracted in coordination with brachioradialis, pronator teres, and pronator quadratus when supination and pronation are needed. Turning a door knob or a key in a car ignition, eating, drinking from a cup, and grooming are examples of these motions. An overview of the shoulders of the elbow and forearm is provided in Table 5-3.

Table 5-3. Muscles of the elbow and forearm

Muscles	Origins	Insertions	Actions	Nerves and root
Biceps brachii	*Short head:* coracoid process of scapula *Long Head:* supraglenoid tubercle of scapula	Tuberosity of radius	*Glenohumeral joint:* flexion Long head may assist with abduction if humerus is laterally rotated *At the elbow:* flexion and supination *Insertion fixed:* humerus toward forearm (chin-up)	Musculocutaneous $C_{5,6}$
Brachialis	Anterodistal aspect of humerus	Coronoid process and tuberosity of ulna	Elbow flexion *Insertion fixed:* humerus toward forearm (chin-up)	Musculocutaneous $C_{5,6}$ Small branch from radial
Brachioradialis	Proximal to lateral epicondyle of humerus	Lateral to styloid process of radius	Elbow flexion Assists in pronation to midposition Assists in supination to midposition	Radial $C_{5,6}$
Triceps brachii	*Long head:* infraglenoid tubercle of scapula *Lateral head:* proximal posterolateral shaft of humerus *Medial head:* distal posterolateral shaft of humerus	Olecranon process of ulna and deep fascia of forearm	*Glenohumeral joint:* long head performs adduction and extension *At elbow:* extension of humerus	Radial $C_{7,8}$
Anconeus	Lateral epicondyle of humerus, posterior aspect	Olecranon process of ulna	Elbow extension	Radial $C_{7,8}$
Supinator	Lateral epicondyle of humerus Radial collateral ligament Annular ligament Medial ulna	Proximolateral radius	Supination	Radial C_6
Pronator teres	*Humeral head:* medial epicondyle of humerus Ulnar head: coronoid process of ulna	Lateral midshaft of radius	Pronation Assists in elbow flexion	Median $C_{6,7}$
Pronator quadratus	Anterior surface of distal ulna	Anterolateral aspect of distal radius	Pronation	Median C_8 to T_1

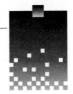

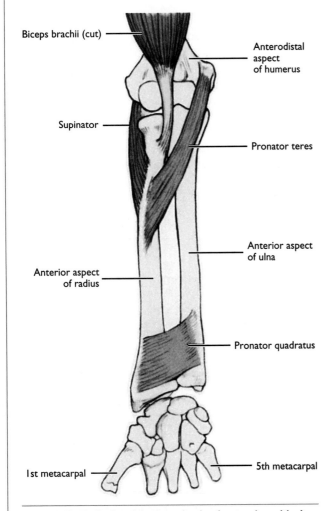

Figure 5-13. Radioulnar joint in supination (anatomic position).
From Mathers et al: Clinical anatomy principles, St. Louis, 1996, Mosby.

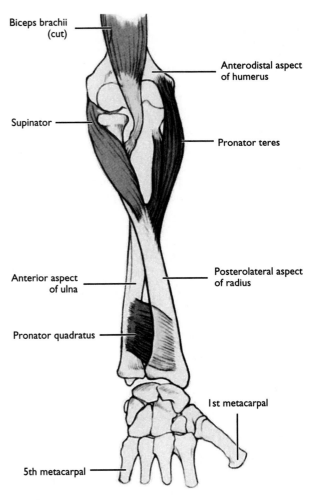

Figure 5-14. Radioulnar joint in pronation.
From Mathers et al: Clinical anatomy principles, St. Louis, 1996, Mosby.

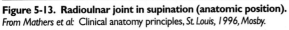

Exercise 5-7. Movement analysis: elbow and forearm

Indicate the movement(s) that can be performed by each muscle by marking an "X" under each correct action.

Muscles that cross the shoulder and elbow	Elbow flexion	Elbow extension	Pronation	Supination
Biceps brachii				
Triceps brachii				

Muscles that cross the elbow only	Elbow flexion	Elbow extension	Pronation	Supination
Brachialis				
Brachioradialis				
Anconeus				
Supinator				
Pronator teres				

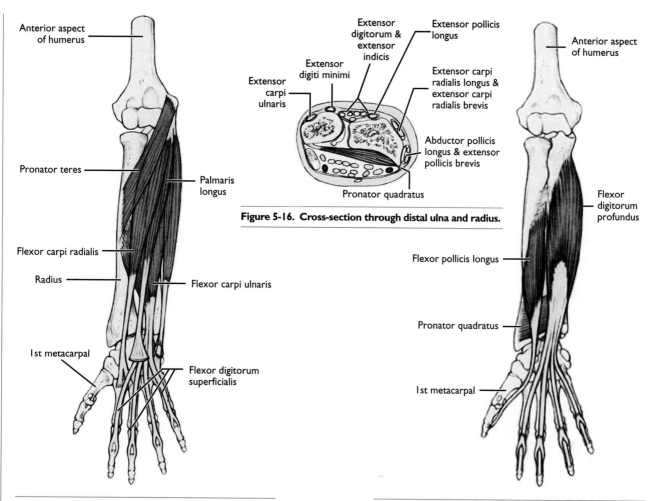

Figure 5-16. **Cross-section through distal ulna and radius.**

Figure 5-15. **Superficial forearm flexor muscles.**

Figure 5-17. **Deep forearm flexor muscles.**

Figures 5-15, 5-16, and 5-17 from Mathers et al: Clinical anatomy principles, St. Louis, 1996, Mosby.

 Exercise 5-8. Innervation analysis: elbow and forearm

Indicate the innervation for each muscle by marking an "X" under the correct columns.

Muscles that cross the shoulder and elbow	Radial	Musculocutaneous	Median
Biceps brachii			
Triceps brachii			

Muscles that cross elbow only	Radial	Musculocutaneous	Median
Brachialis			
Brachioradialis			
Anconeus			
Supinator			
Pronator teres			

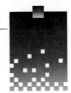

Exercise 5-9. Movement analysis: radio-ulnar joint

Indicate the movement(s) that can be performed by each muscle by marking an "X" under each correct action.

Muscles	Supination	Pronation
Supinator		
Pronator teres		
Pronator quadratus		

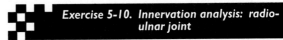

Exercise 5-10. Innervation analysis: radio-ulnar joint

Indicate the innervation for each muscle by marking an "X" under the correct columns.

Muscles	Radial	Median
Supinator		
Pronator teres		
Pronator quadratus		

Exercise 5-11. Muscles of the shoulder and elbow

Identify the muscles of the shoulder and elbow on Figures 5-18 and 5-19.

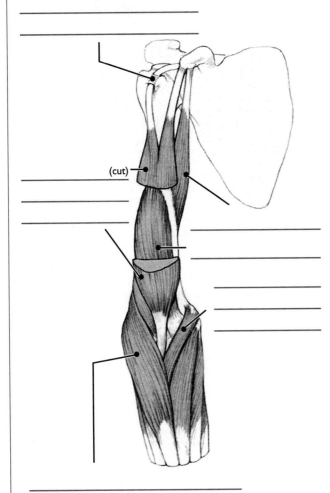

(cut)

Figure 5-18. Anterior brachial region.
From Mathers et al: Clinical anatomy principles, St. Louis, 1996, Mosby.

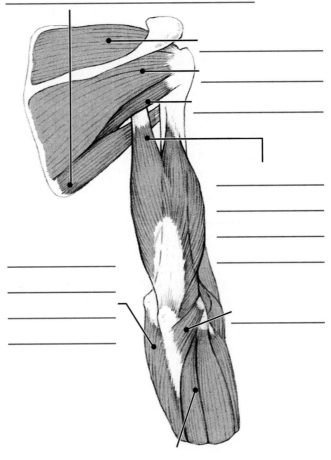

Figure 5-19. Posterior brachial region.
From Mathers et al: Clinical anatomy principles, St. Louis, 1996, Mosby.

Muscles of the Wrist and Muscles Extrinsic to the Hand

The principle muscles that cause flexion of the wrist joint include **flexor carpi radialis** (Figs. 5-15 and 5-20), **flexor carpi ulnaris** (see Figs. 5-11 and 5-15), and **palmaris longus** (see Fig. 5-15). All originate from the medial epicondyle of humerus and, as a group, can be palpated over the ulnar aspect of the forearm. The differences in insertion of these muscles reflect their effect on the deviation of the hand from midline. This deviation movement and the general location of the insertion is reflected in the name of the muscle.

Muscles that affect movement of a body part but whose attachments lie outside the part are called **extrinsic muscles.** These include flexor, abductor, and extensor muscles of the hand and digits that have their origin proximal to the wrist on either the humerus, radius, or ulna.

Muscles that assist in wrist flexion but perform flexion of the phalangeal joints include **flexor digitorum superficialis** (Figs 5-15, 5-20, and 5-21), **flexor digitorum profundus** (Figs. 5-16, 5-20, 5-21, and 5-22), and **flexor pollicis longus** (Figs 5-16 and 5-20). *Digitorum* refers to digits II through V, whereas *pollicis* refers to the thumb, or digit I. Flexor digitorum superficialis inserts via four tendons that are *bifid,* or divided, into two parts that allow the tendon to attach to the sides of the middle phalanges without covering the anterior surfaces. The tendons of flexor digitorum profundus lie deep to the tendon of flexor digitorum superficialis until the latter becomes bifid. At that point the tendon of flexor digitorum profundus runs between the two attachments and inserts at the base of the distal phalanx. Thus the tendon of flexor digitorum superficialis forms a tunnel of sorts through which flexor digitorum profundus can pass. Flexor pollicis longus inserts on the distal phalanx of the thumb.

The tendons of these three muscles pass deep to the **flexor retinaculum** (Figs. 5-20 and 5-21), the ligamentous tissue that runs transverse to the anterior aspect of the carpals. Its function is to hold the tendons of the long flexor muscles in place during contraction, making the line of pull effective between the origin and insertion of these multiple-joint muscles. Tendons of the digits are held in place by **fibrous sheaths.**

Primary extensors of the wrist include **extensor carpi radialis longus** (see Figs. 5-11 and 5-17), **extensor carpi radialis brevis** (see Figs. 5-11, and 5-17), and **extensor carpi ulnaris** (see Figs. 5-8, 5-11, and 5-17). Opposite the wrist flexors, these muscles originate from the lateral epicondyle of humerus and can be easily palpated during their contraction. Similar to other muscles of the wrist and hand, the actions of these muscles are reflected in their names.

Having an origin on the posterior aspect of the forearm, **abductor pollicis longus** (Figs. 5-11, 5-12, 5-17, and 5-23), **extensor pollicis brevis** (see Figs. 5-12, 5-17, and 5-23), and **extensor pollicis longus** (see Figs. 5-11, 5-12, and 5-23) each lend control to the thumb and are innervated by the radial nerve. The tendons of extensor pollicis brevis and extensor pollicis longus can be easily palpated on the posterior aspect of the first metacarpal. During active extension of the thumb with the wrist in the neutral position, a depression forms between the two tendons, known as the *anatomic snuffbox.*

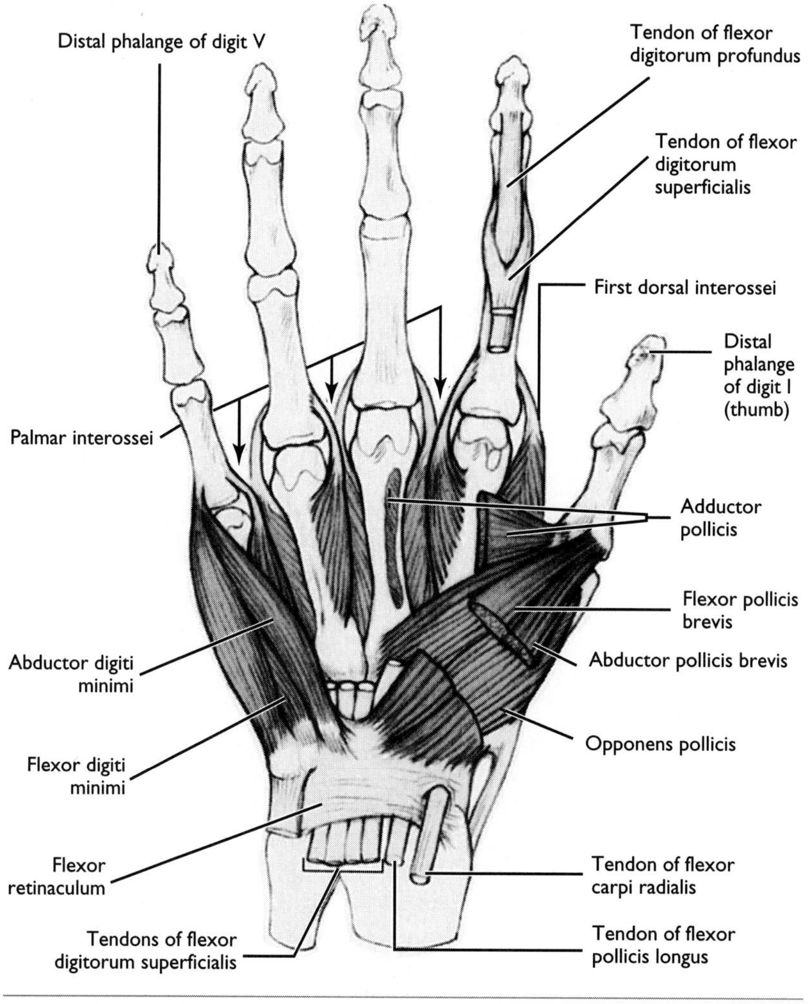

Distal phalange of digit V

Tendon of flexor digitorum profundus

Tendon of flexor digitorum superficialis

First dorsal interossei

Distal phalange of digit I (thumb)

Palmar interossei

Adductor pollicis

Flexor pollicis brevis

Abductor pollicis brevis

Abductor digiti minimi

Opponens pollicis

Flexor digiti minimi

Flexor retinaculum

Tendon of flexor carpi radialis

Tendon of flexor pollicis longus

Tendons of flexor digitorum superficialis

Figure 5-20. Intrinsic muscles of the hand.
From Mathers et al: Clinical anatomy principles, *St. Louis, 1996, Mosby.*

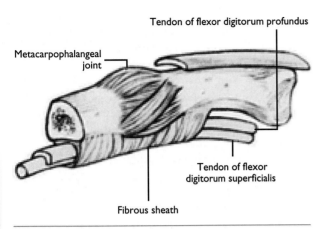

Tendon of flexor digitorum profundus

Metacarpophalangeal joint

Tendon of flexor digitorum superficialis

Fibrous sheath

Figure 5-21. Flexor tendons and assembly.
From Mathers et al: Clinical anatomy principles, *St. Louis, 1996, Mosby.*

Extensor digitorum (see Figs. 5-11 and 5-17), **extensor indicis** (see Figs. 5-11, 5-12, and 5-17), and **extensor digiti minimi** (see Figs. 5-11 and 5-17) each run along the dorsum or posterior aspect of the wrist and hand. Extensor digitorum is the only one of this group that divides into multiple tendons and serves several digits. Extensor indicis is dedicated to digit II, or the index finger, whereas extensor digiti minimi is dedicated to digit V, the little finger.

All extensor wrist and hand muscles are innervated by the radial nerve. As a group, the tendons of these muscles also run deep to the **extensor retinaculum,** (see Fig. 5-23) the ligament that runs transverse to the carpals and metacarpals on the dorsum of the hand. Continuation of this retinaculum into the digits is referred to as the **extensor hood mechanism** or **extensor expansion.** An overview of the muscles of the wrist and those extrinsic to the hand is provided in Table 5-4.

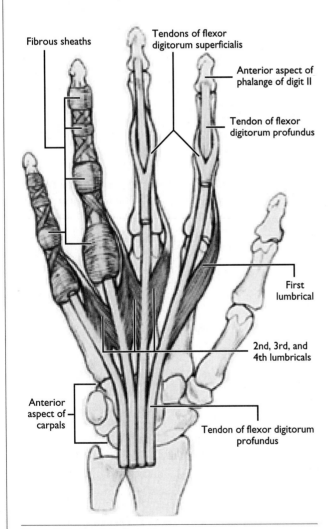

Figure 5-22. Lumbrical muscles.
From Mathers et al: Clinical anatomy principles, *St. Louis, 1996, Mosby.*

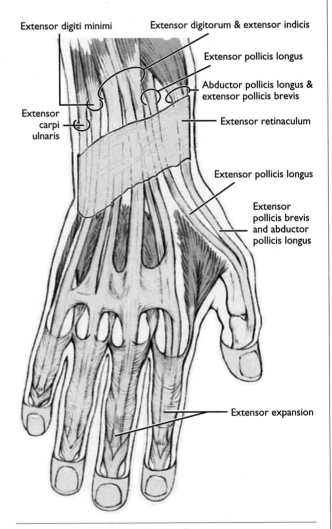

Figure 5-23. Dorsum of hand and wrist.
From Mathers et al: Clinical anatomy principles, *St. Louis, 1996, Mosby.*

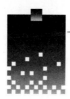

Table 5-4. *Muscles of the wrist and muscles extrinsic to the hand*

Muscles	Origins	Insertions	Actions	Nerves and root
Flexor carpi radialis	Medial epicondyle of humerus	Base of 2nd & 3rd metacarpal on palmar surface	Wrist flexion Radial deviation May assist with elbow flexion	Median $C_{6,7}$
Flexor carpi ulnaris	Medial epicondyle of humerus Olecranon process of ulna	Pisiform, hamate, and base of 5th metacarpal	Wrist flexion Ulnar deviation May assist with elbow flexion	Ulnar C_8
Palmaris longus	Medial epicondyle of humerus	Palmar fascia	Wrist flexion May assist with elbow flexion	Median $C_{6,7}$
Flexor digitorum superficialis	Medial epicondyle of humerus Coronoid process of ulna Anterior radius distal to radial tuberosity	Via four tendons on middle phalanges of digits II to V	Flexes MCP and PIP joints of digits II to V Assists in wrist flexion	Median $C_{7,8}$ to T_1
Flexor digitorum profundus	Anteromedial shaft of ulna interosseous membranes	Via four tendons into bases of distal phalanges on palmar surface	Flexes DIP joints of digits II to V Assists in PIP, MCP, and wrist flexion	Digits II and III: median Digits IV and V: ulnar C_8, T_1
Flexor pollicis longus	Anterior radius distal to tuberosity Interosseous membrane	Distal phalanx of thumb, palmar aspect Flexor retinaculum	IP flexion of thumb Assists in MCP and CMC flexion of thumb May assist in wrist flexion	Median C_8T_1
Extensor carpi radialis longus	Lateral epicondyle of humerus	Base of 2nd metacarpal	Extends wrist Radial deviation May assist in elbow flexion	Radial $C_{6,7}$
Extensor carpi radialis brevis	Common extensor tendon of lateral epicondyle of humerus	Base of 3rd metacarpal	Extends wrist May assist with radial deviation	Radial $C_{6,7}$
Extensor carpi ulnaris	Common extensor tendon of lateral epicondyle of humerus	Base of 5th metacarpal bone, ulnar aspect	Extends wrist Ulnar deviation	Radial $C_{6,7,8}$
Abductor pollicis longus	Posterior aspect of ulna and radius Interosseous membrane	Base of 1st metacarpal, radial aspect	Abduction and extension of CMC of thumb Radial deviation	Radial $C_{6,7}$
Extensor pollicis brevis	Posterior aspect of radius Interosseous membrane	Base of proximal phalanx of thumb, posterior aspect	Extension and abduction of CMC joint of thumb Extension of MCP joint of thumb Assists with radial deviation	Radial $C_{6,7}$
Extensor pollicis longus	Posterior aspect of ulna Interosseous membrane	Base of distal phalanx of thumb, posterior aspect	Extension of IP joint of thumb Assists in extension of MCP and CMC joints of thumb Assists in wrist extension and radial deviation	Radial $C_{6,7,8}$
Extensor digitorum	Common extensor tendon of lateral epicondyle of humerus	Via four tendons into the extensor hood mechanism and bases of middle and distal phalanges of digits II to V Tendons are bound to collateral ligaments	Extend MCP joints Assists in extension of DIP and PIP joints of digits II to V Assists in abduction of index, ring, and little fingers Assists in wrist extension	Radial $C_{6,7,8}$
Extensor indicis	Posterodistal shaft of ulna	Extensor digitorum tendon of digit II by extensor expansion	Extends MCP joint Assists with extension of DIP and PIP joints of index finger Assists in adduction of index finger	Radial $C_{7,8}$
Extensor digiti minimi	Common extensor tendon from lateral epicondyle of humerus	Extensor digitorum tendon of digit V by extensor expansion	Extends MCP joint Assists with extension of DIP and PIP joints of digit V Assists in abduction of digit V	Radial $C_{7,8}$

MCP, Metacarpophalangeal; *CMC*, carpometacarpal; *IP*, interphalangeal; *PIP*, proximal interphalangeal; *DIP*, distal interphalangeal.

■■■ ■ **Exercise 5-12. Movement analysis:** *muscles of the wrist and muscles extrinsic to the hand*

Indicate the movement(s) that can be performed by each muscle by marking an "X" under each correct action.

Muscles that cross the elbow and wrist	Flexion	Extension	Radial deviation	Ulnar deviation
Flexor carpi radialis				
Flexor carpi ulnaris				
Palmaris longus				
Flexor digitorum superficialis				
Extensor carpi radialis longus				
Extensor carpi radialis brevis				
Extensor carpi ulnaris				
Extensor digitorum				

Muscles that cross the wrist	Flexion	Extension	Radial deviation	Ulnar deviation
Flexor digitorum profundus				
Flexor pollicis longus				
Abductor pollicis longus				
Extensor indicis				
Extensor pollicis brevis				
Extensor pollicis longus				

■■■ ■ **Exercise 5-13. Innervation analysis:** *muscles of the wrist and muscles extrinsic to the hand*

Indicate the innervation for each muscle by marking an "X" under the correct columns.

Muscles that cross the elbow and wrist	Median	Radial	Ulnar
Flexor carpi radialis			
Flexor carpi ulnaris			
Palmaris longus			
Flexor digitorum superficialis			
Extensor carpi radialis longus			
Extensor carpi radialis brevis			
Extensor carpi ulnaris			
Extensor digitorum			
Extensor digiti minimi			

Muscles that cross only the wrist	Median	Radial	Ulnar
Flexor digitorum profundus			
Flexor pollicis longus			
Abductor pollicis longus			
Extensor indicis			
Extensor pollicis brevis			
Extensor pollicis longus			

Muscles Intrinsic to the Hand

Muscles that affect movement of a body part and whose attachments lie within that body part are called **intrinsic muscles.** These include muscles of the hand and digits that have their origin distal to the radius and ulna. The innervation of the intrinsic muscles of the hand comes from the median and ulnar nerves.

The primary flexor muscles of digits II through IV are extrinsic to the hand, whereas the intrinsic hand flexors are dedicated to the first and fifth digits only. **Flexor pollicis brevis** (Figs. 5-20 and 5-24) and **flexor digiti minimi** (Figs. 5-20 and 5-24) each originate from the anterior aspect of the carpals and insert on the proximal phalanx of their respective digits. Both assist in the complex motion of opposition, bringing the first and fifth digits into close approximation to one another.

The muscles and soft tissue that make up the raised portion of the palm over the first metacarpal is called the **thenar eminence.** The raised area of the palm over the fifth metacarpal is called the **hypothenar eminence.** The dorsum or posterior surface of the hand lacks significant soft tissue and muscle.

Extension of the interphalangeal joints is facilitated by the **lumbricals** (Fig. 5-22), a group of muscle bellies that have their origin off the tendons of flexor digitorum profundus over the anterior aspect of the metacarpals. The tendons of the lumbricals reach around to the lateral surface of the metacarpophalangeal joint and attach to the extensor expansion. It is this ligamentous insertion that causes the line of pull to become one of extension to the interphalangeal joints while simultaneously performing flexion at the metacarpophalangeal joints.

The **dorsal interossei** (Figs. 5-20 and 5-25) and **palmar interossei** (Figs. 5-20 and 5-26) are responsible for abduction and adduction of digits II through IV. With an ulnar innervation, both originate from the metacarpals and insert into the proximal phalanx of their respective digit. The thumb and little finger abduct via **abductor pollicis brevis** (see Figs. 5-20 and 5-24) and **abductor digiti minimi** (see Figs. 5-20 and 5-24).

Opposition of the hand involves the combination of flexion, abduction, and rotation of the first and fifth metacarpals and is affected by **opponens pollicis** (see Figs. 5-20 and 5-24) and **opponens digiti minimi** (see Figs. 5-20 and 5-24). At their insertion, these muscles wrap around the metacarpal shafts lending to the rotational component of the action.

Finally, the fan-shaped **adductor pollicis** (see Figs. 5-20 and 5-26) stretches across the web-space between the first and second metacarpal, pulling the thumb toward midline during grasp.

Functional significance

The muscles of the wrist, both extrinsic and intrinsic to the hand, are responsible for accurate hand placement for large movements such as a wave or grip, but more importantly, they enable the body to perform fine movements such as writing, typing, or pinching. Muscles that perform flexor and adductor tasks are responsible for a strong grip with opposition of the first and fifth digit, whereas extensors and abductors allow the hand to open and reposition. Pinching movements are more digit specific and include some form of opposition with the thumb. Pointing with the index finger involves simultaneous flexor and extensor differences between the digits and occurs when dialing a telephone, handwriting, and tying shoes. An overview of the muscles intrinsic to the hand is provided in Table 5-5.

Summary

A thorough examination of the muscles of the upper extremity is vital to understand the relationships between the hands, arms, and shoulders and the body's interaction with the environment. The upper extremity has the greatest degree of movement, flexibility, and utility of any portion of the body. Virtually all activities in which the body participates involve the use of the hands, arms, or shoulders.

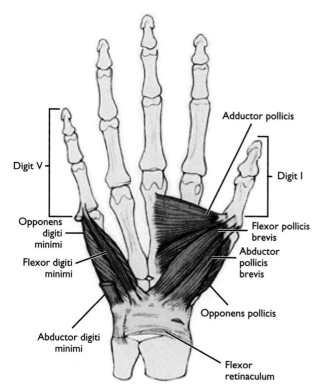

Digit V

Opponens digiti minimi

Flexor digiti minimi

Abductor digiti minimi

Adductor pollicis

Digit I

Flexor pollicis brevis

Abductor pollicis brevis

Opponens pollicis

Flexor retinaculum

Figure 5-24. Palmar intrinsic hand muscles.
From Mathers et al: Clinical anatomy principles, St. Louis, 1996, Mosby.

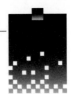

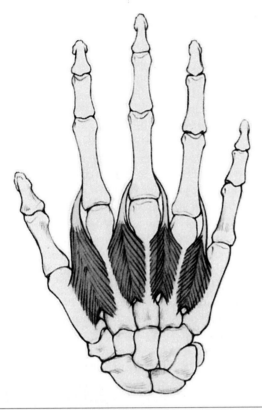

Figure 5-25. Dorsal interossei muscles.
From Mathers et al: Clinical anatomy principles, *St. Louis, 1996, Mosby.*

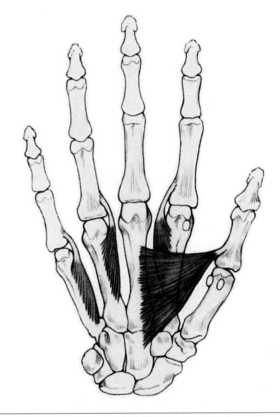

Figure 5-26. Palmar interossei and adductor pollicis muscles.
From Mathers et al: Clinical anatomy principles, *St. Louis, 1996, Mosby.*

Table 5-5. *Muscles of the wrist and muscles intrinsic to the hand*

Muscles	Origins	Insertions	Actions	Nerves and root
Flexor pollicis brevis	Flexor retinaculum and trapezium, trapezoid, and capitate	Base of proximal phalanx of thumb, radial aspect	Flexes MCP and CMC joints of thumb Assists in opposition of thumb	Median and ulnar $C_{6,7,8}$ to T_1
Flexor digiti minimi	Hook of hamate and flexor retinaculum	Base of proximal phalanx of digit V, ulnar aspect	MCP flexion of digit V Assists in opposition	Ulnar C_8, to T_1
Lumbricals	Adjacent portions of tendons of flexor digitorum profundus	Extensor expansion on dorsum of each digit, radial aspect	Extends IP joints and simultaneously flexes MCP joints of the digits II to V Extends the IP joints when MCP joints are extended	Digits I and II: median Digits III and IV: ulnar $C_{6,7,8}$ to T_1
Dorsal interossei	Via two heads from adjacent sides of metacarpal shafts, posterior aspect	*Digits I and II:* base of PIP, radial aspect *Digits III and IV:* base of PIP, ulnar aspect	Abduction of digits II, III, and IV from midline of hand Assists in MCP flexion and IP extension	Ulnar C_8 to T_1
Palmar interossei	Palmar aspect of 2nd, 4th, and 5th metacarpals	Base of PIP of 2nd digit, ulnar aspect Base of PIP of 4th and 5th digits, radial aspect	Adducts digits II, IV, and V Assists in MCP flexion and IP extension	Ulnar $C_8 T_1$

CMC, Carpometacarpal; *IP,* interphalangeal; *MCP,* metacarpophalangeal; *PIP,* proximal interphalangeal.

Table 5-5. Muscles of the wrist and muscles intrinsic to the hand—cont

Muscles	Origins	Insertions	Actions	Nerves and root
Abductor pollicis brevis	Trapezium, scaphoid, and flexor retinaculum	Base of proximal phalanx of thumb, radial aspect Extensor expansion	Abduction of CMC and MCP joints of thumb Assists in opposition	Median $C_{6,7}$
Abductor digiti minimi	Pisiform bone and flexor carpi ulnaris tendon	Base of proximal phalanx of digit V, ulnar aspect	Abducts and assists in flexion of the MCP joint of digit V May assist with extension of IP joints of digit V	Ulnar $C_8 T_1$
Opponens pollicis	Flexor retinaculum, trapezium	Radial aspect of 1st metacarpal	*Opposition of thumb:* flexion and abduction with medial rotation of CMC joint of thumb	Median $C_{6,7}$
Opponens digiti minimi	Hook of hamate bone and flexor retinaculum	Shaft of 5th metacarpal, ulnar aspect	*Opposition of digit V:* flexion and slight lateral rotation of CMC joint of digit V	Ulnar C_8 to T_1
Adductor pollicis	*Oblique head:* capitate, trapezoid, and bases of 2nd and 3rd metacarpals *Transverse head:* palmar surface of 3rd metacarpal	Proximal phalanx of thumb, ulnar aspect	Adduction of CMC joint Flexion of MCP joint Ulnar deviation; assists in opposition	Ulnar C_8 to T_1

CMC, Carpometacarpal; *DIP,* distal interphalangeal; *IP,* interphalangeal; *MCP,* metacarpophalangeal; *PIP,* proximal interphalangeal.

■□■ Exercise 5-14. Movement analysis: intrinsic muscles of the hand

Indicate the movement(s) that can be performed by each muscle by marking an "X" under each correct action.

Muscles	Extension MCPs	Flexion MCPs	Extension IPs	Flexion IPs	Abduction	Adduction
Lumbricals						
Dorsal interossei						
Palmar interossei						
Abductor digiti minimi						
Flexor digiti minimi						
Opponens digiti minimi						
Flexor pollicis brevis						
Abductor pollicis brevis						
Opponens pollicis						
Adductor pollicis						

MCP, Metacarpophalangeal; *IP,* interphalangeal.

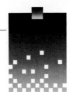

Exercise 5-15. Innervation analysis: intrinsic muscles of the hand

Indicate the innervation for each muscle by marking an "X" under the correct columns.

Muscles	Ulnar	Median
Lumbricals		
Dorsal interossei		
Palmar interossei		
Abductor digiti minimi		
Flexor digiti minimi		
Opponens digiti minimi		
Flexor pollicis brevis		
Abductor pollicis brevis		
Opponens pollicis		
Adductor pollicis		

Exercise 5-16. Extensor muscles of the forearm, wrist, and hand

Identify the muscles of the forearm, wrist, and hand on Figures 5-27, 5-28, 5-29.

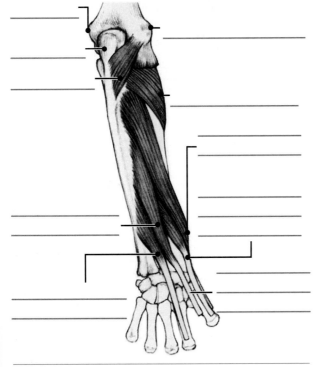

Figure 5-27. Extensor muscles of digits I and II.
From Mathers et al: Clinical anatomy principles, *St. Louis, 1996, Mosby.*

Exercise 5-16. Extensor muscles of the forearm, wrist, and hand—cont

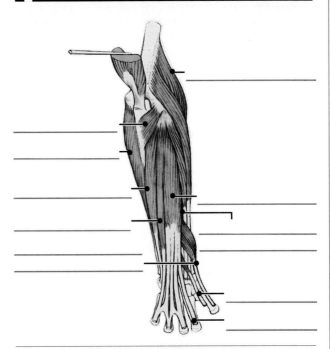

Figure 5-28. Superficial forearm extensor muscles.
From Mathers et al: Clinical anatomy principles, *St. Louis, 1996, Mosby.*

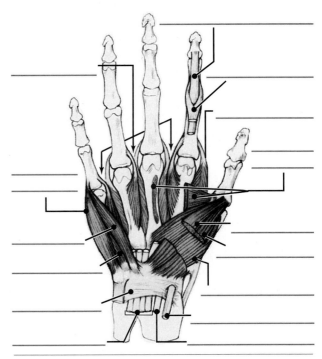

Figure 5-29. Intrinsic muscles of the hand.
From Mathers et al: Clinical anatomy principles, *St. Louis, 1996, Mosby.*

■ *Exercise 5-17. Illustrate muscles of the shoulder and upper extremity*

On the illustrations provided, draw a unilateral view (right or left) of the following muscles of the shoulder and upper extremity with the correct origin and insertion. Be sure to show the direction of the fibers of each muscle.

Posterior view		Anterior view	
Trapezius (upper, middle, lower)	Infraspinatus	Pectoralis major	Flexor carpi ulnaris
Rhomboids	Extensor carpi radialis longus	Biceps brachii	Flexor digitorum superficialis
Levator scapulae	Extensor carpi ulnaris	Brachialis	Flexor pollicis longus
Latissimus dorsi	Extensor digitorum	Pronator teres	Lumbricals
Triceps brachii	Extensor pollicis longus	Lumbricals	Flexor digiti minimi
Supraspinatus	Extensor digiti minimi	Flexor carpi radialis	Adductor pollicis

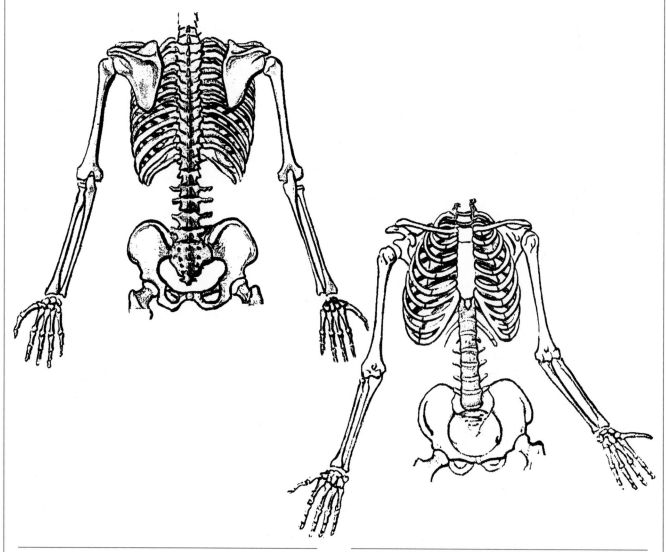

Figure 5-30. Posterior view of skeleton.
From Fritz: Fundamentals of therapeutic massage, *St. Louis, 1996, Mosby.*

Figure 5-31. Anterior view of skeleton.
From Fritz: Fundamentals of therapeutic massage, *St. Louis, 1996, Mosby.*

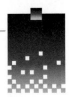

Exercise 5-18. Palpate muscles of the shoulder and upper extremity

With the list of 24 muscles in Exercise 5-17, attempt to palpate each muscle belly on your study partner. With washable markers or adhesive labels, note the location of the muscle belly and its origin and insertion. Be sure to show the direction of the fibers of each muscle. Compare your accuracy with other classmates!

Exercise 5-19. Review muscles of the shoulder and upper extremity

Complete the following based on your familiarity with the muscles of this chapter.

1. Where on the body can the belly of upper trapezius be palpated?

2. What portion of trapezius originates at the spinous processes of T_6 to T_{12}?

3. Is it possible to palpate the insertion of serratus anterior?

4. If the scapula is stabilized inferiorly, what is the bilateral action of levator scapula?

5. The rhomboids lie _____ to trapezius.

6. What single nerve is responsible for innervating muscles that perform strong glenohumeral flexion?

7. What two muscles are responsible for the *rowing* motion?

8. Though latissimus dorsi inserts near the bicipital groove, this landmark is the path of a tendon of what muscle?

Exercise 5-19. Review muscles of the shoulder and upper extremity—cont

9. What muscle is responsible for initiating shoulder abduction?

10. List the muscles of the rotator cuff.

11. What single nerve is responsible for innervating muscles that perform strong elbow flexion?

12. What is the primary innervation for elbow extension?

13. Supinator and both pronator muscles originate from and insert on the same bone. Why is there such a difference in their actions?

14. The medial aspect of distal humerus is the common origin for what muscle group (named by the common action)?

15. Is extensor pollicis brevis extrinsic or intrinsic to the hand?

16. Most extensor muscles of the wrist and hand have what common origin?

17. What is the innervation of the extensor and abductor muscles of the wrist and hand?

■ **Exercise 5-19. Review muscles of the shoulder and upper extremity—cont**

18. What is the innervation that is responsible for ulnar deviation and flexion of digits IV and V?

_____

19. What is the action of palmaris longus?

_____

20. The tendons of what two muscles form the anatomic *snuff box?"*

_____

_____

21. What extrinsic muscle is specific to movements of the second digit?

_____

22. What intrinsic muscle facilitates the *table top* movements of metacarpophalangeal flexion with simultaneous extension of the interphalangeal joints?

_____

23. Flexion, abduction, and opposition of the 5th digit occur via innervation from what nerve?

_____

24. What muscle can be palpated at the web-space between the first and second metacarpals?

_____

25. What muscle performs abduction of digits II, III, and IV?

_____

■ **Exercise 5-20. Muscles of the anterior shoulder**

Identify the muscles of the anterior shoulder on Figure 5-32.

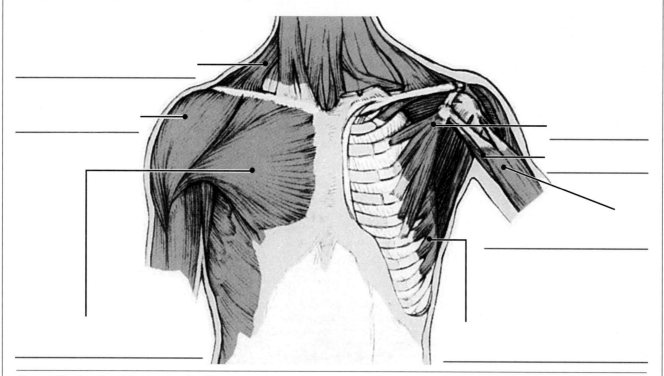

Figure 5-32. Muscles of the anterior shoulder.
From Mathers et al: Clinical anatomy principles, *St. Louis, 1996, Mosby.*

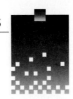

Key Words

abductor digiti minimi
abductor pollicis brevis
abductor pollicis longus
action
adductor pollicis
anconeus
biceps brachii
bilateral
brachialis
brachioradialis
central nervous system
coracobrachialis
deltoid
dorsal interossei
extensor carpi radialis brevis
extensor carpi radialis longus
extensor carpi ulnaris
extensor digiti minimi

extensor digitorum
extensor expansion
extensor hood mechanism
extensor indicis
extensor pollicis brevis
extensor pollicis longus
extensor retinaculum
extrinsic muscles
fixator
fixed
flexor carpi radialis
flexor carpi ulnaris
flexor digiti minimi
flexor digitorum profundus
flexor digitorum superficialis
flexor pollicis brevis
flexor pollicis longus
flexor retinaculum

hypothenar eminence
infraspinatus
innervation
insertion
intrinsic muscles
latissimus dorsi
levator scapula
lumbricals
movable
name
nomenclature
opponens digiti minimi
opponens pollicis
origin
palmar interossei
palmaris longus
pectoralis major
pectoralis minor

pronator quadratus
pronator teres
rhomboids
rotator cuff muscles
serratus anterior
subscapularis
supinator
supraspinatus
synergist
teres major
teres minor
thenar eminence
trapezius (upper, middle, lower)
triceps brachii
unilateral

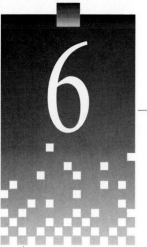

6

Muscles and Movement of the
Hip and Lower Extremity

*❝This chapter will enable you to identify individual muscles
of the hip and lower extremity, their attachments to the
skeleton, ensuing skeletal movements, and innervations that
affect these movements, as well as enable you to compare and
contrast these elements through written exercises.❞*

Chapter objectives

wwThe student will be able to:

1. Identify each muscle of the hip and lower extremity.

2. Identify the specific skeletal attachment of each muscle.

3. Recognize the innervation of each muscle.

4. Identify the movement created by each muscle as it relates
to its skeletal attachment.

5. Discuss the functional significance of each muscle as it
relates to the surrounding muscles.

Muscles of the Hip

The hip and lower extremity are perhaps the most muscular
areas of the body, both having the greatest number of muscles
that surround the skeleton, the largest muscle mass, and the
potential to display the greatest strength through powerful
movement. By observing athletes whose muscles have been
enhanced by extensive training and exercise, the stability and
beauty of mobility in this region is demonstrated.

Muscles of the anterior hip

The first group to be discussed is the anterior portion of the
hip, which involves muscle attachments on the lumbar vertebrae, coxal bones, femur, and tibia. Pulling a **movable** end
toward a **fixed** point, this anterior group is primarily responsible for flexing the hip, or bringing the femur toward the

pelvis. This movement is only possible when the pelvis and
lower trunk are stabilized, usually by having the leg that is
opposite the moving one fixed to the ground. The anterior
hip muscles can operate by moving the femur while the trunk
is stabilized against a chair or the ground, often working both
legs simultaneously, or *bilaterally.*

The first of the hip flexors are **psoas major** and **iliacus.**
These three are often referred to in combination with one
another as **iliopsoas** (Fig. 6-1). With origins on the lumbar
vertebrae and ilium, this muscle group stretches across the
inguinal region, lies deep to the internal organs, and cannot
be easily palpated. Crossing the iliofemoral joint or hip anteriorly, they are the principle muscles for the task of flexion.
Psoas minor blends with psoas major, having its origin on the
vertebral column, but this small, often absent muscle does not
cross the hip.

Three other muscles of this group cross both the hip
and knee, with their origins in the inguinal and coxal regions.
Sartorius, also called the *tailor's strap,* has a long, thin muscle
belly that starts from the anterior superior iliac spine and
wraps around the femur anteriorly to insert on the anteromedial surface of the tibia. A *tailor* is one who sews fabric or
leather, sometimes bracing it between the legs or sitting cross-
legged on the floor; this posture is called a *tailor sit* with hips
flexed, laterally rotated, and knees flexed. Though sartorius is
superficial to other muscles of the lower extremity, its thin,
straplike shape makes it difficult to palpate.

Tensor fasciae latae has its origin just lateral to that of
sartorius (Figs. 6-2 and 6-3). It has a short muscle mass and
inserts into the large tendinous structure of the **iliotibial
band** along the lateral aspect of the tibia and fibula (see Fig. 6-
3). Tensor fasciae latae is an important abductor, pulling the
femur away from midline. It can be palpated near its origin,
especially while contracting.

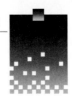

Rectus femoris has its origin inferior to sartorius and tensor fasciae latae; it crosses the hip and knee in a linear fashion directly down the front of the femur to the patella (see Fig. 6-2). The dual role of this muscle is hip flexion and knee extension. The rectus femoris can be best palpated near the proximal end of the femur, since more distally it becomes covered by the well-formed medial and lateral knee extensors. A summary of the anterior muscles of the hip is provided in Table 6-1.

Muscles of the gluteal group

The posterior hip muscles are the **gluteal group** that lies in three layers. **Gluteus maximus** is the largest of the group and the most superficial (see Fig. 6-3). Its fibers run in a lateral, oblique direction to the hip from the sacrum, inserting into the iliotibial band alongside the tensor fasciae latae and at the gluteal tuberosity of femur (Fig. 6-4). Gluteus maximus is a strong hip extensor, considering the relatively short muscle belly compared with its long tendinous insertion.

Gluteus medius lies deep to gluteus maximus but somewhat superficial to and alongside **gluteus minimus** (see Fig. 6-4 and 6-6). Both the gluteus medius and minimus are important in hip abduction but have complex roles with respect to the rotation of the femur. The origin of gluteus medius is fan-shaped, tapering into an insertion over the top of the greater trochanter covering its lateral aspect (Figs. 6-5, and 6-6). Reaching across the joint as it does, the gluteus medius muscle is able to oppose itself, since the anterior fibers pull the greater trochanter into medial rotation, while the posterior fibers pull it into lateral rotation. Simultaneous activity results in a compromise between the two, which is then abduction without rotation.

The origin of gluteus minimus is slightly more lateral and inferior on the ilium that gluteus medius, whereas its insertion is more anterior on the greater trochanter. The line of pull for the insertion toward origin results in medial rotation of the femur. See Table 6-2 for a summary of the muscles of the gluteal group.

Lateral rotator muscles of the hip

Although lateral rotation of the femur is accomplished by muscles in several groups, the six short muscles located deep beneath gluteus maximus are, together, the prime movers. **Piriformis, gemellus superior, obturator internus, gemellus inferior, obturator externus,** and **quadratus femoris** all have their origins on the inferior aspect of the sacrum, ischium, and pubis (see Figs. 6-5 and 6-6). By attaching onto the

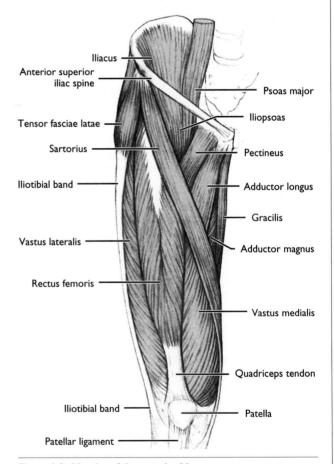

Figure 6-1. Iliopsoas muscle.
From Mathers et al: Clinical anatomy principles, *St. Louis, 1996, Mosby.*

Figure 6-2. Muscles of the anterior hip.
From Mathers et al: Clinical anatomy principles, *St. Louis, 1996, Mosby.*

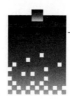

Table 6-1. Muscles of the anterior hip

Muscles	Origins	Insertions	Actions	Nerves and root
Psoas major and psoas minor	Transverse processes of all lumbar vertebrae Bodies of T_{12} and all lumbar vertebrae	Iliac fossa and lesser trochanter of femur	Hip flexion *Reverse action:* flexion of lumbar spine and pelvis on fixed femur	Lumbar plexus $L_{1,2,3,4}$
Iliacus	Anterior iliac fossa and crest Base of sacrum	By tendon of psoas major onto shaft of femur, distal to the lesser trochanter	Hip flexion *Insertion fixed and acting bilaterally:* flexion of trunk on fixed femur	Femoral $L_{2,3}$
Sartorius	Anterior superior iliac spine	Runs posterior to medial epicondyle of femur to attach on anteromedial surface of tibial shaft	Hip flexion, abduction, and lateral rotation of femur Knee flexion Assists in medial rotation of tibia	Femoral $L_{2,3}$
Tensor fasciae latae	Anterolateral iliac crest Anterior superior iliac spine	Iliotibial band, which inserts on lateral condyle of tibia	Hip flexion, abduction, and medial rotation of femur Assists in knee extension	Superior gluteal $L_{4,5}$
Rectus femoris	Anterior inferior iliac spine, just superior to acetabulum	Base of patella via quadriceps tendon to patellar ligament, which attaches to tibial tuberosity	Hip flexion and knee extension	Femoral $L_{2,3,4}$

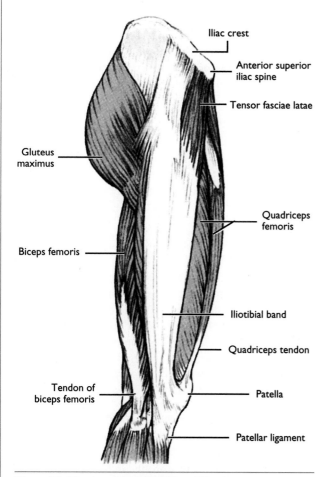

Figure 6-3. Muscles of the lateral hip and knee.
From Mathers et al: Clinical anatomy principles, *St. Louis, 1996, Mosby.*

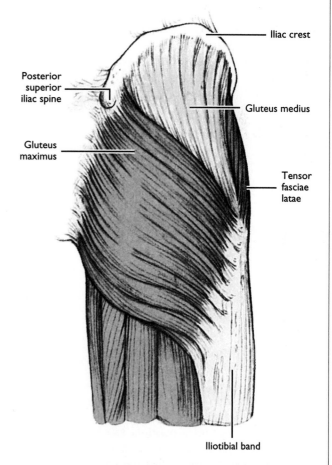

Figure 6-4. Gluteal region, superficial layer.
From Mathers et al: Clinical anatomy principles, *St. Louis, 1996, Mosby.*

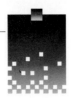

Table 6-2. Muscles of the gluteal group

Muscles	Origins	Insertions	Actions	Nerves and root
Gluteus maximus	Posterior superior iliac spine Posterior surface of sacrum and coccyx Aponeurosis of erector spinae	Iliotibial band over greater trochanter and gluteal tuberosity	Hip extension and lateral rotation of femur *Lower fibers:* assist in hip adduction *Upper fibers:* assist in hip abduction Stabilizes knee in extension	Inferior gluteal $L_5, S_{1,2}$
Gluteus medius	Posterolateral surface of ilium, just inferior to crest From anterior superior iliac spine, across to the posterior superior iliac spine	Lateral aspect of greater trochanter of femur	Hip abduction *Anterior fibers:* assist in hip flexion and medial rotation of femur *Posterior fibers:* assist in hip extension and lateral rotation of femur	Superior gluteal $L_{4,5}, S_1$
Gluteus minimus	Posterolateral surface of ilium, from near anterior superior iliac spine to margin of greater sciatic notch (inferior to origin of gluteus medius)	Anterior aspect of greater trochanter of femur	Hip abduction and medial rotation of femur Assists in hip flexion	Superior gluteal

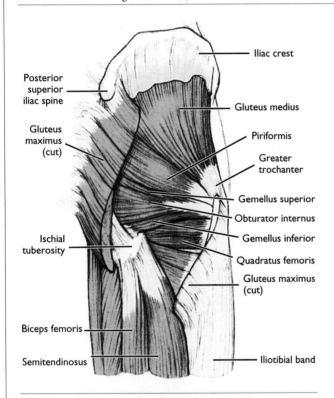

Figure 6-5. Gluteal region, middle layer.
From Mathers et al: Clinical anatomy principles, *St. Louis, 1996, Mosby.*

Labels on figure: Iliac crest · Posterior superior iliac spine · Gluteus medius · Gluteus maximus (cut) · Piriformis · Greater trochanter · Gemellus superior · Obturator internus · Gemellus inferior · Quadratus femoris · Gluteus maximus (cut) · Ischial tuberosity · Biceps femoris · Semitendinosus · Iliotibial band

Study Note

Devise your own acrostic so that you can remember the muscles that perform lateral rotation of the hip. The letters represent names or words in a sentence.

P _____
G _____
O _____
G _____
O _____
Q _____

Adductor muscles of the hip

The five muscles along the medial femoral region make up the **adductor group.** This group is responsible for pulling the femur closer to midline while also enhancing in hip flexion. **Pectineus, adductor longus, adductor brevis, adductor magnus,** and **gracilis** each have their origin on the pubis while the first four insert on the femur (Figs. 6-8 and 6-9). Gracilis is the only two-joint muscle of this group; it reaches across the length of the femur to insert on the tibia.

Hamstring muscles of the posterior hip and knee

Moving again to the posterior side of the femur, the **hamstring group** of muscles contributes to hip extension as a result of their attachment from the ischial tuberosity and insertion along the sides of the tibia. **Biceps femoris—long head, semitendinosus,** and **semimembranosus** are two-joint

greater trochanter from a posterior direction, the line of pull results in rotation away from midline. Piriformis, the most superior of this group, is positioned such that its muscle belly runs through the greater sciatic notch, whereas obturator internus passes through the lesser sciatic notch (Fig. 6-7). See Table 6-3 for a summary of the lateral rotator muscles of the hip.

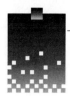

Table 6-3. Lateral rotator muscles of the hip

Muscles	Origins	Insertions	Actions	Nerves and root
Piriformis	Anterior surface of sacrum Medial side of greater sciatic notch	Through greater sciatic notch to superior aspect of greater trochanter of femur	Lateral rotation of hip Assists in abduction when hip is flexed	Sacral plexus $S_{1,2}$
Gemellus superior	Posterolateral aspect of ischial spine	Greater trochanter of femur	Lateral rotation of femur Assists in abduction when hip *is* flexed	Sacral plexus $L_5, S_{1,2}$
Obturator internus	Anteromedial surface of membrane over obturator foramen and surrounding bone	Around rami of ischium through lesser sciatic notch to medial aspect of greater trochanter	Lateral rotation of femur Assists in abduction when hip is flexed	Sacral plexus $L_5, S_{1,2}$
Gemellus inferior	Superior portion of ischial tuberosity	Medial side of greater trochanter of femur	Lateral rotation of femur Assists in abduction when hip is flexed	Sacral plexus $L_{4,5}, S_{1,2}$
Obturator externus	Posterolateral surface of membrane over obturator foramen and surrounding bone	Trochanteric fossa of femur	Lateral rotation of femur Assists in hip adduction	Obturator $L_{3,4}$
Quadratus femoris	Ischial tuberosity	Posterodistal to greater trochanter	Lateral rotation of femur May assist in hip adduction	Sacral plexus $L_{4,5}, S_{1,2}$

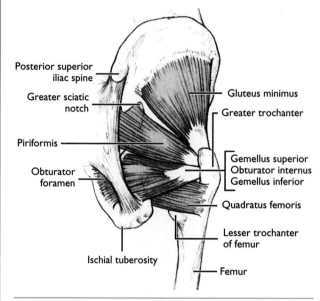

Figure 6-6. Gluteal region, deep layer.
From Mathers et al: Clinical anatomy principles, St. Louis, 1996, Mosby.

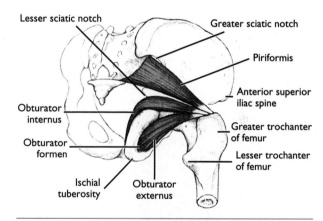

Figure 6-7. Deep rotators of the hip (posterolateral view).
From Mathers et al: Clinical anatomy principles, St. Louis, 1996, Mosby.

muscles that cross the hip and knee (Fig. 6-10). Though they all originate together, biceps femoris—long head lies lateral to the distal femur, whereas semitendinosus and semimembranosus lie medial to distal femur.

Functional significance

For a person to participate in tasks of daily living, there must be a foundation of stability in the trunk and proximal joints, especially in the hip, for accurate movements to occur in the distal extremities. The muscles of the hip are functionally grouped according to the primary actions at the particular joint: flexors, extensors, abductors, lateral rotators, and adductors. These groups are often antagonistic to one another, and from this opposition comes the much needed stability of the joint for posture. Whereas the activities of some of these groups may be more obvious than others, they are all necessary in normal standing posture and bipedal mobility.

Usually thought of as movers of the femur, hip muscles also play an important role in maintaining proper alignment of the pelvis and lower back. Dysfunction in the muscles of the proximal lower extremity often results in malalignment and movement deviations of the trunk, shoulders, cervical spine, and upper extremities during activities such as walking or running. The term commonly used to refer to normal walking is **ambulate.**

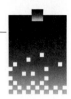

Table 6-4. Adductor muscles of the hip

Muscles	Origins	Insertions	Actions	Nerves and root
Pectineus	Anterior aspect of superior pubic ramus	Between lesser trochanter and linea aspera	Hip adduction Assists in hip flexion	Femoral $L_{2,3}$
Adductor longus	Anterior surface of body of pubis	Midshaft of femur at medial lip of linea aspera	Hip adduction Assists in hip flexion	Obturator $L_{2,3,4}$
Adductor brevis	Anterior aspect of inferior pubic ramus	Medial and just distal to lesser trochanter of femur	Hip adduction Assists in hip flexion	Obturator $L_{2,3,4}$
Adductor magnus	Inferior pubic ramus Ramus of ischium Ischial tuberosity	Length of linea aspera and medial condyle of femur	Hip adduction	Obturator and sciatic $L_{2,3,4}$
Gracilis	Inferior body of pubis	Runs posterior to medial condyle of femur, attaching on antero-medial aspect of tibia	Hip adduction Assists in knee flexion and medial rotation of femur	Obturator $L_{2,3,4}$

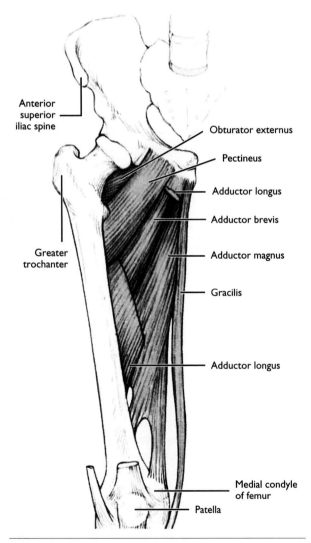

Figure 6-8. Adductor muscles, anterior superficial layer.
From Mathers et al: Clinical anatomy principles, St. Louis, 1996, Mosby.

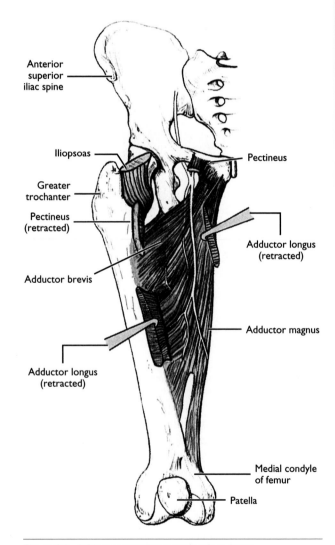

Figure 6-9. Adductor muscles, anterior deep layer.
From Mathers et al: Clinical anatomy principles, St. Louis, 1996, Mosby.

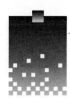

The muscles of the anterior hip perform some degree of flexion during forward ambulation, a motion more exaggerated during stair climbing. When lying in bed, the hips are flexed when the knees are brought toward the head before rolling to one side and a sitting position is achieved. In reverse action, hip flexion is the movement that controls the trunk on fixed bilateral femurs when shifting position in a chair. The pull of the hip flexors from a fixed femur can cause the pelvis to tip anteriorly, resulting in an abnormal alignment of the lumbar vertebrae.

The hip extensors, including both the gluteal and hamstring groups, are perhaps even more critical than the hip flexors to everyday activities. Hip extension must occur to achieve upright posture, not only in standing but while sitting. When rising to stand from a chair, it is the hip extensors that, in a type of reverse action, pull the trunk backward over the extended lower extremities. Without adequate hip extensors, one may be inclined to use the upper extremities to achieve an upright stance. It is hip extension that gives the *push off* during walking, propelling the body forward and away from the last step. To compensate for a lack of hip extension, the hip flexors may *pull* the body forward, a very energy-consuming task.

Abduction of the femur by the sartorius, tensor fasciae latae, and gluteal group helps separate the feet to maintain a wider, stable base of support during standing. In the event that the femur is fixed (standing on one leg), gluteus medius on the stance side pulls the coxal origin toward the femoral insertion. This reverse action keeps the pelvis level when the leg opposite is swinging forward. Without appropriate abductor strength, the hip of the swinging leg will drop and ambulation will become cumbersome and less energy-efficient. This drop of the pelvis opposite the weak abductor muscles is referred to as the "Trendelenburg sign" (Figs. 6-11, *A* and 6-11, *B*).

Lateral rotation is a motion that often accompanies abduction and extension of the hip, providing stability during standing and ambulation. In walking, the movement allows the feet and lower leg to be properly aligned just before striking the ground. A lack of lateral rotation at this point can result in the foot pointing toward midline, adding stress to the knees as force is transferred through the joint upon impact.

Figure 6-10. Muscles of the posterior hip and knee.
From Mathers et al: Clinical anatomy principles, St. Louis, 1996, Mosby.

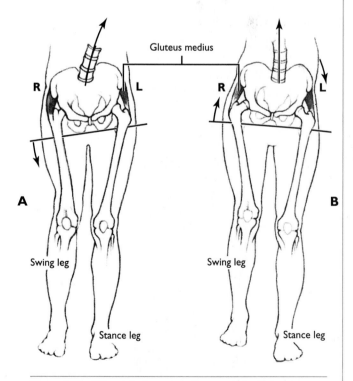

Figure 6-11. A, Trendelenburg sign; B, normal hip alignment.
From Mathers et al: Clinical anatomy principles, St. Louis, 1996, Mosby.

Muscles of the Knee

The knee is the most complex joint of the body because of the precarious stacking of one long bone directly on top of another, the intricate network of ligaments, and the fifteen muscles that surround the joint. This discussion begins by looking again at the two-joint muscles of the hip that cross the knee. Eight of the 15 muscles in this region have their origin proximal to the hip. **Sartorius, tensor fasciae latae, rectus femoris, gluteus maximus, gracilis, biceps femoris—long head, semitendinosus,** and **semimembranosus** each have long muscle bellies with tendons that insert onto the iliotibial band, proximal tibia, and fibula (Fig. 6-12). Each contributes to knee flexion with the exception of rectus femoris, a muscle that is directly responsible for knee extension. All participate in rotation of the tibia on the femur, again with the exception of rectus femoris.

The long tendinous insertions of sartorius, gracilis, and semitendinosus blend together at their attachments on the anteromedial aspect of the tibia. These structures are collectively referred to as the **per anserinus** or *foot of a goose* (Fig. 6-12 and 6-22).

Another muscle that is part of the hamstring group but is not discussed earlier is **biceps femoris—short head.** Having an origin on the shaft of the femur, this portion of biceps femoris crosses only the knee and assists in its flexion. It blends with the long head to insert into the lateral side of the lower leg over the fibular head and lateral condyle of tibia.

Beginning an anterior inspection of the joint, the **quadriceps femoris** muscle group, led by rectus femoris, performs knee extension without a rotational component (Fig. 6-13). **Vastus intermedius, vastus medialis,** and **vastus lateralis** attach proximally onto their respective portions of the

shaft of femur and insert into the base of the patella by a common **quadriceps tendon** (see Fig. 6-13). This sesamoid bone is then attached to the tibial tuberosity via the **patellar ligament,** an extension of the tendon as it surrounds the patella (see Fig. 6-12). With the exception of vastus intermedius, which lies deep to rectus femoris, vastus medialis and vastus lateralis can be palpated on their respective sides of femur.

Study Note

Strict attention to spelling is very important when using anatomic terminology. Provide the action of the following muscles with similar names.

Quadratus femoris: _____

Quadriceps femoris: _____

Quadratus lumborum—lateral flexion of the lumbar vertebrae (see Fig. 6-1).

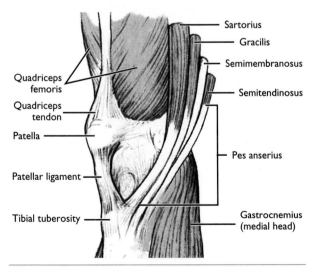

Figure 6-12. Medial knee.
From Mathers et al: Clinical anatomy principles, *St. Louis, 1996, Mosby.*

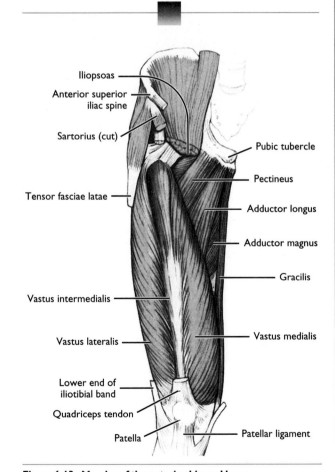

Figure 6-13. Muscles of the anterior hip and knee.
From Mathers et al: Clinical anatomy principles, *St. Louis, 1996, Mosby.*

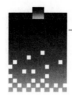

Aside from biceps femoris—short head, the only other single-joint muscle that crosses the posterior aspect of the knee is **popliteus,** a small muscle that runs from the lateral condyle of the femur to the medial portion of the tibia (Fig. 6-14). This muscle only performs rotation between the femur and tibia; the direction of this rotation is dependent on which bone is fixed. When the lower extremity is in a non–weight-bearing position, only the femur is fixed to the pelvis; thus the tibia is able to rotate medially when the insertion of popliteus moves in the direction of the lateral femoral condyle, pointing the foot toward midline.

When the body bears weight through the designated lower extremity, the origin and insertion of the popliteus are then reversed. The mobile femoral condyle is pulled toward the fixed medial tibial surface. This resulting action is lateral rotation of femur on tibia.

Gastrocnemius and **plantaris** are two-joint muscles that cross the knee and ankle, affecting motions at both joints (Fig. 6-15). Gastrocnemius, like biceps femoris, has two heads that originate from each of the condyles of femur posteriorly. This superficial muscle descends down the sural region to insert into the heavy **tendocalcaneus,** commonly called the *Achilles tendon* (see Figs. 6-14 and 6-15). Plantaris lies deep to the belly of gastrocnemius, originating slightly superior to its proximolateral attachment. This muscle has a short belly and a long distal tendon that blends into tendocalcaneus on the medial side. Both muscles assist with knee flexion but are more powerful in their influence on the ankle. As with other muscles of this area, the tibial nerve is the innervation. See Tables 6-5, 6-6, and 6-7 for overviews of the muscles of the knee, hamstring group, and quadriceps femoris.

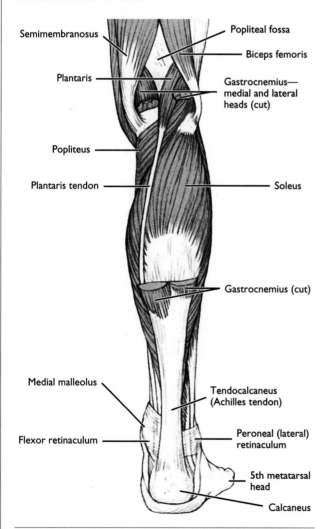

Figure 6-14. Muscles of the posterior lower leg, middle layer.
From Mathers et al: Clinical anatomy principles, St. Louis, 1996, Mosby.

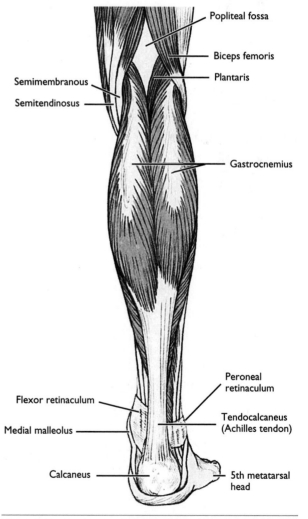

Figure 6-15. Muscles of the posterior lower leg, superficial layer.
From Mathers et al: Clinical anatomy principles, St. Louis, 1996, Mosby.

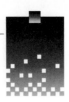

Table 6-5. Muscles of the knee

Muscles	Origins	Insertions	Actions	Nerves and root
Sartorius	Anterior superior iliac spine	Runs posterior to medial epicondyle of femur to attach on anteromedial surface of tibial shaft	Knee flexion Assists in medial rotation of tibia Hip flexion; abduction and lateral rotation of femur	Femoral $L_{2,3}$
Tensor fasciae latae	Anterior iliac crest and anterior superior iliac spine	Iliotibial band that attaches on lateral condyle of tibia	Assists in knee extension Hip flexion; abduction and medial rotation of femur	Superior gluteal $L_{4,5}$
Rectus femoris	Anterior inferior iliac spine just superior to acetabulum	Base of patella via quadriceps tendon to patellar ligament Patellar ligament attaches to tibial tuberosity	Knee extension Hip flexion	Femoral $L_{2,3,4}$
Gluteus maximus	Posterior superior iliac spine Posterior surface of sacrum and coccyx Aponeurosis of erector spinae	Iliotibial band over greater trochanter and gluteal tuberosity	Stabilizes knee in extension Hip extension and lateral rotation of femur *Lower fibers:* assist in hip adduction *Upper fibers:* assist in hip abduction	Inferior gluteal $L_5, S_{1,2}$
Gracilis	Inferior body of pubis	Runs posterior to medial condyle of femur, attaching on antero-medial aspect of tibia	Assists in knee flexion and medial rotation of femur Hip adduction	Obturator $L_{2,3,4}$
Biceps femoris—long head	Ischial tuberosity	Lateral aspect of fibular head and lateral condyle of tibia	Knee flexion Hip extension Lateral rotation of tibia Assists in lateral rotation of femur	
Biceps femoris—short head	Posterior midshaft of femur at linea aspera	Shares insertion with biceps femoris—long head	Knee flexion and lateral rotation of tibia	Sciatic $S_{1,2}$
Semitendinosus	Ischial tuberosity	Medial surface of proximal tibia	Knee flexion and medial rotation of tibia Hip extension Assists in medial rotation of femur	Sciatic $L_5, S_{1,2}$
Semimembranosus	Ischial tuberosity	Medial surface of proximal tibia	Knee flexion and medial rotation of tibia Hip extension Assists in medial rotation of femur	Sciatic $L_5, S_{1,2}$
Popliteus	Posterolateral condyle of femur	Soleal line on posteromedial surface of proximal tibia	*Origin fixed, non–weight-bearing:* medial rotation of tibia *Insertion fixed, weight-bearing:* lateral rotation of femur Assists in knee flexion	Tibial $L_{4,5}, S_1$
Gastrocnemius	Via two heads on the posterior surface of medial and lateral condyles of femur	Tendocalcaneus, which attaches to posterior calcaneus	Assists in knee flexion Plantar flexion of ankle	Tibial L_5, S_1
Plantaris	Lateral supracondylar ridge of femur	Tendon descends medially to blend with tendocalcaneus	Assists in knee flexion Plantar flexion of ankle	Tibial L_5, S_1

Table 6-6. Muscles of the hamstring group

Muscles	Origins	Insertions	Actions	Nerves and root
Biceps femoris— long head	Ischial tuberosity	Lateral aspect of fibular head and lateral condyle of tibia	Knee flexion Hip extension Lateral rotation of tibia Assists in lateral rotation of femur	Sciatic $S_{1,2}$
Biceps femoris— short head	Posterior midshaft of femur at linea aspera	Shares insertion with biceps femoris—long head	Knee flexion and lateral rotation of tibia	Sciatic $S_{1,2}$
Semitendinosus	Ischial tuberosity	Medial surface of proximal tibia	Knee flexion and medial rotation of tibia Hip extension Assists in medial rotation of femur	Sciatic $L_5, S_{1,2}$
Semimembranosus	Ischial tuberosity	Medial surface of proximal tibia	Knee flexion and medial rotation of tibia Hip extension Assists in medial rotation of femur	Sciatic $L_5, S_{1,2}$

Table 6-7. Muscles of the quadriceps femoris group

Muscles	Origins	Insertions	Actions	Nerves and root
Rectus femoris	Anterior inferior iliac spine just superior to the acetabulum	Base of patella via quadriceps tendon to patellar ligament Patellar ligament attaches to tibial tuberosity	Knee extension Hip flexion	Femoral $L_{2,3,4}$
Vastus intermedius	Proximal and anterolateral shaft of femur	Base of patella via quadriceps tendon to patellar ligament Patellar ligament attaches to tibial tuberosity	Knee extension	Femoral $L_{2,3,4}$
Vastus medialis	Anteromedial aspect of shaft of femur	Medial aspect of base of patella via quadriceps tendon to patellar ligament	Knee extension	Femoral $L_{2,3,4}$
Vastus lateralis	Anteromedial aspect of shaft of femur	Lateral aspect of base of patella via quadriceps tendon to patellar ligament	Knee extension	Femoral $L_{2,3,4}$

Functional significance

Since the principle movements at the knee are flexion and extension, the muscles are discussed in these functional groups. The two-joint muscles of the hip that affect the movements at the knee and participate in knee flexion include sartorius, tensor fasciae latae, and gracilis. Active knee flexion occurs during walking to effectively shorten the leg that swings forward. Without adequate flexion at this joint, the body must compensate by exaggerating its hip flexion or swinging the extremity away from midline to prevent the leg from dragging the ground. Other instances of knee flexion occur during common daily tasks such as bathing and dressing and stair climbing.

Knee extension involves the quadriceps femoris muscle group. During ambulation, knee extension prepares the body for the next heel strike of the swinging leg and maintains the position while the body's weight is carried onto and over the foot. Rotation at the knee is not a large arch of motion but is generally an accessory to the medial and lateral rotation that occurs at the hip.

■ *Exercise 6-1. Movement analysis: muscles of the hip*

Indicate the movement(s) that can be performed by each muscle by marking an "X" under each correct action.

Muscles that cross the hip	Flexion	Extension	Abduction	Adduction	Lateral rotation	Medial rotation
Psoas major and minor						
Iliacus						
Gluteus medius						
Gluteus minimus						
Piriformis						
Gemellus superior						
Obturator internus						
Gemellus inferior						
Obturator externus						
Quadratus femoris						
Pectineus						
Adductor longus						
Adductor brevis						
Adductor magnus						
Muscles that cross the hip						
Sartorius						
Tensor fasciae latae						
Rectus femoris						
Gluteus maximus						
Gracilis						
Biceps femoris—long head						
Semitendinosus						
Semimembranosus						

Exercise 6-2. Innervation analysis: muscles of the hip

Indicate the correct innervation for each muscle by marking an "X" under the correct columns.

Muscles that cross the low back and hip	Lumbar Plexus	Femoral	Gluteal	Sacral Plexus	Obturator	Sciatic
Psoas major and minor						
Iliacus						
Gluteus medius						
Gluteus minimus						
Piriformis						
Gemellus superior						
Obturator internus						
Gemellus inferior						
Obturator externus						
Quadratus femoris						
Pectineus						
Adductor longus						
Adductor brevis						
Adductor magnus						

Muscles that cross the hip and knee						
Sartorius						
Tensor fasciae latae						
Rectus femoris						
Gluteus maximus						
Gracilis						
Biceps femoris—long head						
Semitendinosus						
Semimembranosus						

Exercise 6-3. Movement analysis: muscles of the knee

Indicate the movement(s) that can be performed by each muscle by marking an "X" under each correct action

Muscles that cross the knee and hip	Knee flexion	Knee extension	Knee rotation
Sartorius			
Tensor fasciae latae			
Rectus femoris			
Gluteus maximus			
Gracilis			
Biceps femoris—long head			
Semitendinosus			
Semimembranosus			

Muscles that cross the knee only			
Biceps femoris—short head			
Vastus intermedius			
Vastus medialis			
Vastus lateralis			
Popliteus			

Muscles that cross the knee and ankle			
Gastrocnemius			
Plantaris			

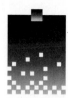

Indicate the correct innervation for each muscle by marking an "X" under the correct columns.

Muscles that cross the knee and hip	Femoral	Gluteal	Obturator	Sciatic	Tibial
Sartorius					
Tensor fasciae latae					
Rectus femoris					
Gluteus maximus					
Gracilis					
Biceps femoris—long head					
Semitendinosus					
Semimembranosus					

Muscles that cross the knee only					
Biceps femoris—short head					
Vastus intermedius					
Vastus medialis					
Vastus lateralis					
Popliteus					

Muscles that cross the knee and ankle					
Gastrocnemius					
Plantaris					

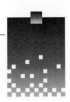

■ ■ ■ □ ■ **Exercise 6-5. Muscles and landmarks of the hip and knee**

Identify the muscles and landmarks of the hip and knee on Figures 6-16, 6-17, 6-18, and 6-19.

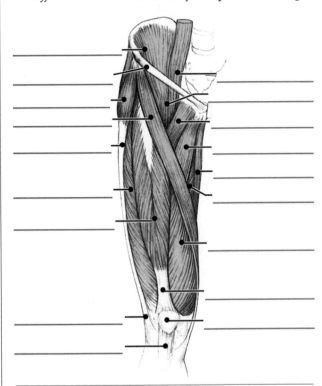

Figure 6-16. Muscles of the anterior hip.
From Mathers et al: Clinical anatomy principles, St. Louis, 1996, Mosby.

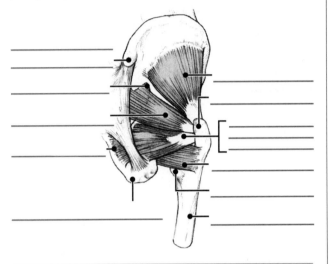

Figure 6-18. Gluteal region, deep layer.
From Mathers et al: Clinical anatomy principles, St. Louis, 1996, Mosby.

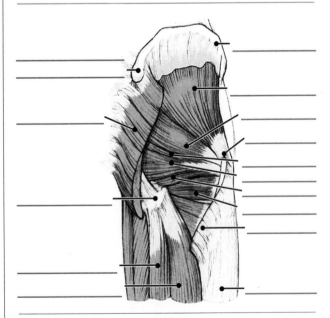

Figure 6-17. Gluteal region, middle layer.
From Mathers et al: Clinical anatomy principles, St. Louis, 1996, Mosby.

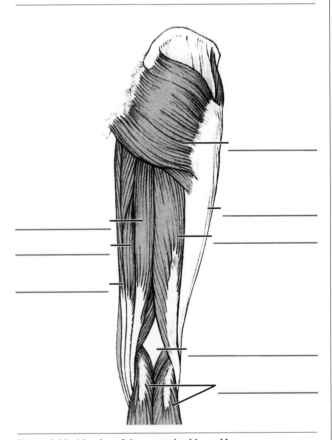

Figure 6-19. Muscles of the posterior hip and knee.
From Mathers et al: Clinical anatomy principles, St. Louis, 1996, Mosby.

Muscles of the Ankle

Though the ankle is bony upon palpation, it is surrounded by the tendons of muscles that have contractile tissue located in the sural and crural regions of the lower leg, commonly known as the *shin* and *calf.* A review of the motions at the ankle includes plantar flexion or pointing the toes inferiorly. Dorsiflexion pulls the toes skyward in an extension movement. Inversion pulls the forefoot (metatarsal heads) toward midline, whereas eversion turns the forefoot away from midline.

Muscles that have an origin proximal to the ankle but insert on the foot are called **extrinsic muscles of the foot,** whereas muscles that have their origin and insertion within the foot are called **intrinsic muscles.** Many extrinsic muscles insert on the bones of the digits and can affect the movements of the metatarophalangeal (MTP) and interphalangeal (IP) joints.

Extrinsic muscles of the foot

Though **gastrocnemius** and **plantaris** have already been discussed as working together to achieve knee flexion, they are more powerful as plantar flexors (see Fig. 6-15). Together, gastrocnemius and **soleus** form the **triceps surae muscle group,** with triceps referring to the total of three heads, whereas *surae* refers to the region of the posterior lower leg. Soleus is deep to its two counterparts, originating at the oblique soleal line on the posteroproximal tibial shaft and blending into tendocalcaneus.

Tibialis posterior, flexor digitorum longus, and **flexor hallucis longus** complete the muscles in the sural region; all originate from the midshaft of the tibia and fibula and the interosseous membrane (Figs. 6-20 and 6-21). (Just as *pollicis* referred to the thumb during the discussion of the hand, *hallucis* refers to the great toe, or digit I, of the foot.) As the deepest muscles in this area, both participate in plantar flexion and inversion of the ankle. Flexors digitorum longus and

hallucis longus have more specific duties according to their distal tendon attachments. Flexor digitorum longus divides into four parts that correspond to the lateral four toes, whereas flexor hallucis longus is dedicated to the great toe. The long tendons of these extrinsic muscles run along the plantar surface, or *sole,* of the foot.

The long tendons of the muscles of the ankle and those extrinsic to the foot are held in place by **flexor retinaculum,** a ligamentous structure that runs transverse to the ankle (see Fig. 6-21). The deep-lying tendons are able to track smoothly, maintaining the proper line of pull between attachments as a result of the strong sleeve that is formed by the flexor retinaculum.

Moving to the anterior aspect of the lower leg, **tibialis anterior, extensor digitorum longus,** and **extensor hallucis longus** perform movements opposite that of the previous muscle group (Figs. 6-20 and 6-22). Tibialis anterior is easily palpated just lateral to the midline of tibia, the area common-

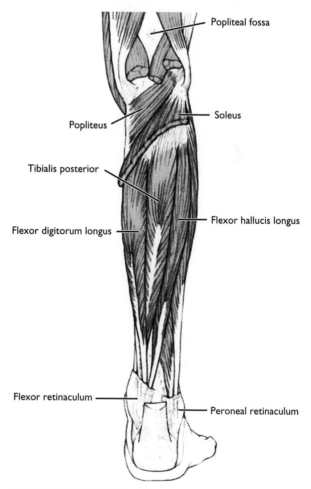

Figure 6-21. Muscles of the posterior lower leg (deep layer).
From Mathers et al: Clinical anatomy principles, St. Louis, 1996, Mosby.

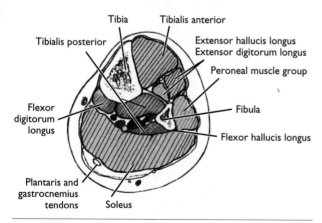

Figure 6-20. Cross-section of lower leg.
From Mathers et al: Clinical anatomy principles, St. Louis, 1996, Mosby.

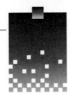

ly called the *shin*. Dorsiflexion is the principle ankle movement, with tibialis anterior contributing to inversion. Extensors digitorum longus and hallucis longus perform as their names describe, extending the digits. The innervation is the deep peroneal nerve.

Similar to the flexor retinaculum, the dorsiflexor and extensor tendons are held in place by several transverse ligaments known as the **extensor retinaculum** (see Fig. 6-22). These ligaments crisscross the ankle superficial to the tendons, ensuring proper tracking and an accurate line of pull.

Lateral to the lower leg are **peroneus tertius, peroneus longus,** and **peroneus brevis** (Fig. 6-23). Peroneus tertius

shares its origin with extensor digitorum longus, inserting onto the fifth metatarsal base. Peroneus longus and peroneus brevis both insert via tendons that pass behind the lateral malleolus, attaching anteriorly onto the metatarsals and tarsals. Particularly unique, the tendon of peroneus longus reaches across the entire width of the foot transversely on the plantar side and attaches onto the first metatarsal. Their lines of pull enable peroneus longus and peroneus brevis to perform eversion of the foot, turning the plantar surface away from the midsagittal plane of the body. The **peroneal retinaculum** holds these tendons in place as they course around the lateral malleolus toward the plantar surface of the foot (see Fig. 6-21). For an overview of the muscles of the ankle and those extrinsic to the foot, see Table 6-8.

Intrinsic muscles of the foot

Intrinsic muscles of the foot are all contained distal to the talus and control the fine movements of the forefoot and dig-

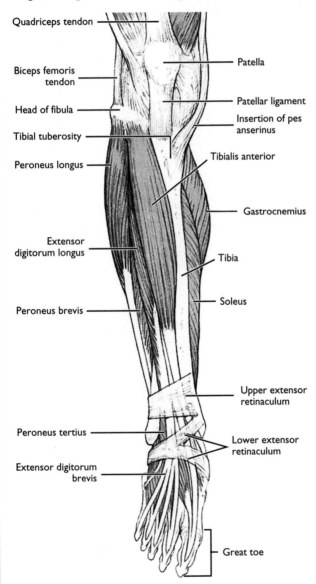

Figure 6-22. Muscles of the anterior lower leg.
From Mathers et al: Clinical anatomy principles, St. Louis, 1996, Mosby.

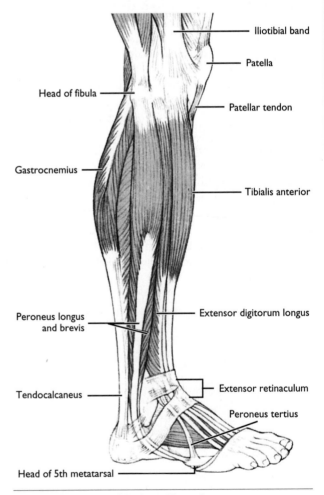

Figure 6-23. Muscles of the lateral lower leg.
From Mathers et al: Clinical anatomy principles, St. Louis, 1996, Mosby.

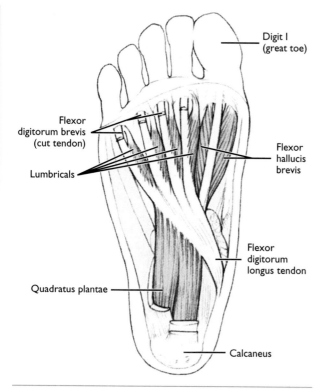

Figure 6-24. Muscles of sole of foot, layer two.
From Mathers et al: Clinical anatomy principles, *St. Louis, 1996, Mosby.*

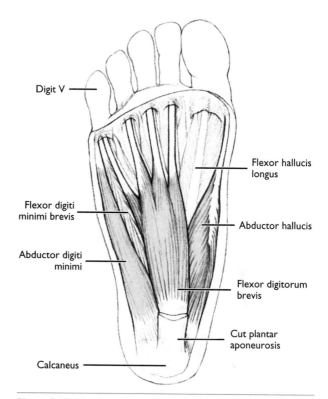

Figure 6-25. Muscles of sole of foot, layer one.
From Mathers et al: Clinical anatomy principles, *St. Louis, 1996, Mosby.*

its. **Flexor digitorum brevis, flexor hallucis brevis,** and **flexor digiti minimi brevis** have their attachments on the plantar surface of the tarsals, metatarsals, and digits (Figs. 6-24, 6-25, and 6-26). Flexor digitorum brevis divides into four tendons, whereas flexor hallucis brevis divides into two before inserting onto its respective digit. Flexor digiti minimi brevis has a single tendon for the fifth digit of the foot.

    Extensor digitorum brevis and **extensor hallucis brevis** are found on the dorsum or superior aspect of the foot (Fig. 6-27). These intrinsic muscles lie deep to the tendons of extensors digitorum longus and hallucis longus and share their common insertions.

    Other foot intrinsic muscles are the **lumbricals,** which like their counterpart in the hand, have an origin from the long flexor tendons (see Fig. 6-24). Again, the lumbricals perform the complex action of flexing the MTP joints while extending the more distal IP joints because of the insertion on the extensor hood. **Abductor hallucis** (see Fig. 6-25) and **adductor hallucis** (see Fig. 6-26) are responsible for the mediolateral alignment of the great toe. **Quadratus plantae** (see Fig. 6-26) is an accessory muscle of flexion that stabilizes the tendon of flexor digitorum longus and assists in maintaining its line of pull for efficient flexion of the digits. For an overview of the muscles of the ankle and those intrinsic to the foot, see Table 6-9.

Functional significance

The weight-bearing activity of ambulation is examined as the muscles of the ankle and those extrinsic to the foot perform plantar flexion, dorsiflexion, inversion, and eversion. Active plantar flexion by the triceps surae muscles and the long toe flexors provide a *push off* action that propels the body forward. Perhaps not so obvious is the use of this functional group during a sit-to-stand movement from a chair. The ankle is usually placed passively into a few degrees of dorsiflexion after scooting forward on the chair. As the body rises in response to trunk, hip, and knee extension, the plantar flexors help push away from the floor. If plantar flexion was exaggerated at this point, the body would stand and continue to rise up on the balls of the feet in a hop. The strength of this muscle group against the entire weight of the body is, in itself, amazing.

    Dorsiflexion is not as noticeable and is a less drastic movement, without which simple walking would be a tedious and tiring task. During the swing portion of ambulation when the hip and knee are flexing, dorsiflexion must occur to sufficiently shorten the leg and prevent it from dragging the ground. Consistently dragging the feet or toes is a sign that dorsiflexion may not be occurring.

    Inversion and eversion both occur during ambulation in an effort to negotiate uneven terrain and to carry the body over a planted foot without undue stress on the ankle, knee, and hip. Non–weight-bearing activities that involve these movements include bathing and dressing of the lower extremities.

During ambulation, flexion and extension of the joints of the digits compliment the plantar flexion and dorsiflexion of the ankle and add to the forceful *push off,* as well as to the necessary limb length changes.

Figure 6-26. Muscles of sole of foot, layers three and four.
From Mathers et al: Clinical anatomy principles, St. Louis, 1996, Mosby.

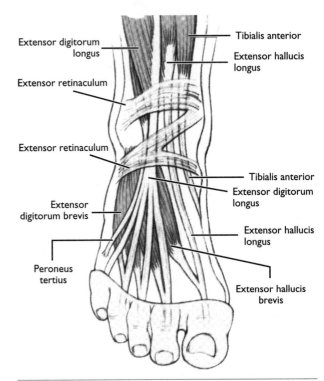

Figure 6-27. Muscles and tendons on dorsum of foot.
From Mathers et al: Clinical anatomy principles, St. Louis, 1996, Mosby.

Table 6-8. Muscles extrinsic to the foot

Muscles	Origins	Insertions	Actions	Nerves and root
Gastrocnemius	Via two heads on the posterior surface of medial and lateral condyles of femur	Tendocalcaneus, which attaches to posterior calcaneus	Plantar flexion of ankle Assists in knee flexion	Tibial L_5, S_1
Plantaris	Lateral supracondylar ridge of femur	Tendon descends medially to blend with tendocalcaneus	Plantar flexion of ankle Assists in knee flexion	Tibial L_5, S_1
Soleus	Posteroproximal fibula and soleal line of tibia	Tendocalcaneus	Plantar flexion of ankle	Tibial $S_{1,2}$
Tibialis posterior	Interosseus membrane and midshaft of tibia and fibula	Plantar surfaces of tarsals and base of metatarsals II-IV	Inversion of foot Assists in plantar flexion of ankle	Tibial $L_{4,5}, S_1$
Flexor digitorum longus	Posterior midshaft of tibia	Plantar surfaces of bases of distal phalanges of digits II-V	Flexion of MTP and IP joints of digits II-V Assists in plantar flexion and inversion	Tibial L_5, S_1
Flexor hallucis longus	Distal shaft of fibula and interosseous membrane	Plantar surfaces of base of distal phalanx of digit I	Flexion of IP joint of digit I Plantar flexion of ankle and inversion of foot Assists in flexion of MTP joint of digit I	Tibial $L_5, S_{1,2}$

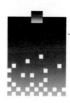

Table 6-8. Muscles extrinsic to the foot—cont

Muscles	Origins	Insertions	Actions	Nerves and root
Tibialis anterior	Anterior surface of tibia and interosseous membrane	Dorsal surface of medial cuneiform and base of first metatarsal	Dorsiflexion of ankle Assists in inversion of foot	Deep peroneal $L_{4,5}$
Extensor digitorum longus	Lateral condyle of tibia, antero-proximal surface of fibula	Via four tendons on dorsal surface, extensor expansions into middle and distal phalanges of digits II-V	Extension of MTP and IP joints of digits II-V Assists in dorsiflexion and eversion	Deep peroneal $L_{4,5}, S_1$
Extensor hallucis longus	Distal portion of anteromedial shaft of fibula	Dorsal surface of base of distal phalanx of digit I	Extension of IP joint Assists in extension of MTP joint of digit I Assists in dorsiflexion and inversion	Deep peroneal $L_{4,5}, S_1$
Peroneus tertius	Anterodistal surface of fibula	Base of fifth metatarsal	Ankle dorsiflexion and eversion of the foot	Deep peroneal $L_{4,5}, S_1$
Peroneus longus	Proximolateral shaft of fibula and lateral condyle of tibia	Tendon passes behind lateral malleolus to lateral aspect of first metatarsal base and medial cuneiform	Eversion of the foot Assists in plantar flexion	Superficial peroneal L_5, S_1
Peroneus brevis	Distolateral shaft of fibula	Behind lateral malleolus to tuberosity of base of fifth metatarsal	Eversion of the foot Assists in plantar flexion	Superficial peroneal L_5, S_1

MTP, Metatarsophalangeal; *IP*, interphalangeal.

Table 6-9. Muscles intrinsic to the foot

Muscles	Origins	Insertions	Actions	Nerves and root
Flexor digitorum brevis	Plantar surface of calcaneus	Via four tendons to middle phalanges of digits II-V; tendons are split at the MTP joint to allow the flexor digitorum longus tendons to attach	Flexion of proximal IP joints Assists in flexion of MTP joints of digits II-V	Medial plantar $L_{4,5}, S_1$
Flexor hallucis brevis	Plantar surfaces of cuboid and lateral cuneiform	Via two tendons into base of proximal phalanx of digit I	Flexion of MTP joints of digit I	Medial plantar $S_{1,2}$
Flexor digiti minimi brevis	Plantar aspect of base of fifth metatarsal and cuboid	Base of proximal phalanx of fifth digit	Flex MTP joint of digit V	Lateral plantar $S_{1,2}$
Extensor digitorum brevis	Dorsolateral surface of calcaneus (same as extensor hallucis brevis)	Via four tendons into lateral sides of extensor digitorum longus tendons of digits I-IV	Extension of MTP and IP joints of digits II-IV	Deep peroneal $L_{4,5}, S_1$
Extensor hallucis brevis	Dorsolateral surface of calcaneus (same as extensor digitorum brevis)	Proximal phalanx of digit I	Extension of MTP joint of digit I	Deep peroneal $L_{4,5}, S_1$
Lumbricals	Tendons of flexor digitorum longus	Medial side of digits II-V into the extensor hood on the dorsal surface of proximal phalanges	Flex MTP joints and extension of IP joints of digits II-V	Medial and lateral plantar $S_{1,2,3}$
Abductor hallucis	Inferomedial side of calcaneus	Medial base of proximal phalanx of digit I	Abduction and flexion of digit I	Medial plantar $S_{1,2}$
Adductor hallucis	*Oblique portion:* base of second and third metatarsals *Transverse portion:* third, fourth, and fifth MTP joint capsules	Lateral base of proximal phalanx of digit I	Adduction of digit I	Lateral Plantar $S_{1,2}$
Quadratus plantae	Plantar surface of calcaneus	Lateral aspect of flexor digitorum longus tendon	Assists in flexion of digits II-V	Tibial $S_{1,2}$

MTP, Metatarsophalangeal; *IP*, interphalangeal.

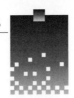

Exercise 6-6. Movement analysis: *muscles of the ankle and those extrinsic to the foot*

Indicate the movement(s) that can be performed by each muscle by marking an "X" under each correct action.

Muscles	Plantar flexion	Dorsiflexion	Inversion	Eversion
Gastrocnemius				
Plantaris				
Soleus				
Tibialis posterior				
Flexor digitorum longus				
Flexor hallucis longus				
Tibialis anterior				
Extensor digitorum longus				
Extensor hallucis longus				
Peroneus tertius				
Peroneus longus				
Peroneus brevis				

Exercise 6-7. Innervation analysis: *muscles of the ankle and those extrinsic to the foot*

Indicate the correct innervation for each muscle by marking an "X" under the correct columns.

Muscles	Tibial	Deep peroneal	Superficial peroneal
Gastrocnemius			
Plantaris			
Soleus			
Tibialis posterior			
Flexor digitorum longus			
Flexor hallucis longus			
Tibialis anterior			
Extensor digitorum longus			
Extensor hallucis longus			
Peroneus tertius			
Peroneus longus			
Peroneus brevis			

■■ ■ *Exercise 6-8. Movement analysis: intrinsic muscles of the foot*

Indicate the movement(s) that can be performed by each muscle by marking an "X" under each correct action.

Muscles	Flexion of MTP joints	Extension of MTP joints	Flexion of IP joints	Extension of IP joints	Abduction	Adduction
Flexor digitorum brevis						
Flexor hallucis brevis						
Extensor digitorum brevis						
Extensor hallucis brevis						
Lumbricals						
Abductor hallucis						
Adductor hallucis						
Flexor digiti minimi brevis						
Quadratus plantae						

MTP, Metatarsophalangeal; IP, interphalangeal.

■■ ■ *Exercise 6-9. Innervation analysis: intrinsic muscles of the foot*

Indicate the correct innervation for each muscle by marking an "X" under the correct columns.

Muscles	Deep peroneal	Medial plantar	Lateral plantar	Tibial
Flexor digitorum brevis				
Flexor hallucis brevis				
Extensor digitorum brevis				
Extensor hallucis brevis				
Lumbricals				
Abductor hallucis				
Adductor hallucis				
Flexor digiti minimi brevis				
Quadratus plantae				

Identify the muscles of the knee, lower leg, and foot on Figures 6-28, 6-29, 6-30, and 6-31.

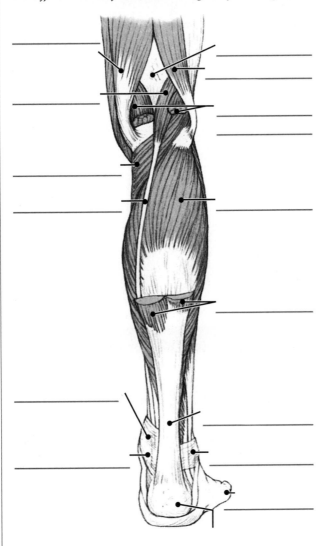

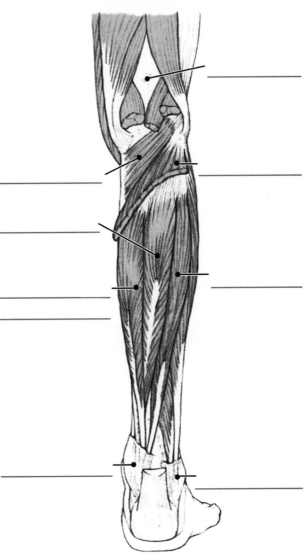

Figure 6-28. Muscles of the posterior lower leg, middle layer.
From Mathers et al: Clinical anatomy principles, St. Louis, 1996, Mosby.

Figure 6-29. Muscles of the posterior lower leg, deep layer.
From Mathers et al: Clinical anatomy principles, St. Louis, 1996, Mosby.

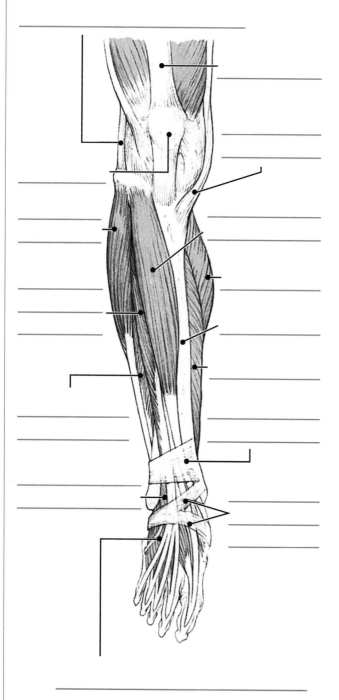

Figure 6-30. Muscles of the anterior lower leg.
From Mathers et al: Clinical anatomy principles, *St. Louis, 1996, Mosby.*

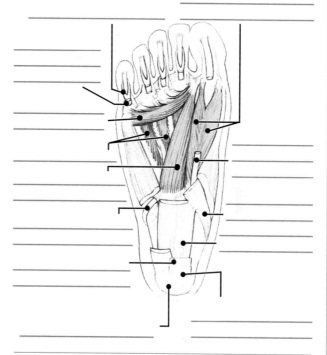

Figure 6-31. Muscles of the sole of the foot, layers three and four.
From Mathers et al: Clinical anatomy principles, *St. Louis, 1996, Mosby.*

■ **Exercise 6-11. Muscles of the hip and lower extremity**

Draw the muscle attachments with the correct origin and insertion on the illustrations provided on page 138; indicate the direction of the line of pull for the following items:

Posterior view	Anterior view
Gluteus maximus	Iliopsoas
Gluteus medius	Sartorius
Piriformis	Tensor fasciae latae
Gemellus inferior	Rectus femoris
Biceps femoris—long head	Pectineus
Biceps femoris—short head	Adductor magnus
Semitendinosus	Vastus medialis
Gastrocnemius	Vastus lateralis
Soleus	Tibialis anterior
Tibialis posterior	Extensor digitorum longus
Flexor digitorum longus	Extensor hallucis longus
Flexor hallucis longus	Peroneus longus
Flexor digitorum brevis	Peroneus brevis

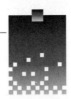

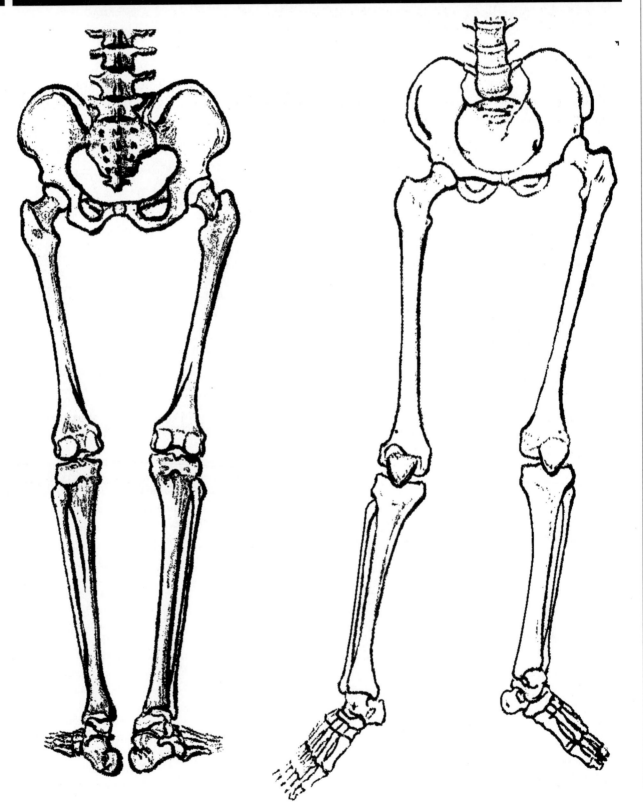

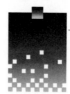

*With the list of 26 muscles in Exercise 6-11, attempt to palpate each muscle belly on your study
partner. With washable markers or adhesive labels, note the location of the muscle belly and its origin and insertion. Be sure to show the direction of the fibers of each muscle. Compare your accuracy with other classmates!*

Complete the following statements based on your familiarity with the muscles of this chapter.

1. What muscles perform trunk flexion on a fixed femur?

   _____

   _____

   _____

2. What muscles act directly to bring about hip abduction?

   _____

   _____

   _____

   _____

3. Name the hamstring muscles that insert on the lateral condyle of tibia.

   _____

   _____

4. Name the muscles that insert into the iliotibial band.

   _____

   _____

5. What is the action of piriformis?

   _____

6. What muscle of the adductor group is a two-joint muscle?

   _____

7. Knee extension is performed by what four muscles?

   _____

   _____

   _____

   _____

8. Which muscle group is innervated by the sciatic nerve?

   _____

   _____

   _____

9. Hip flexion and abduction and lateral rotation of the femur are all performed by which muscle?

   _____

10. What is the action of quadratus femoris?

   _____

11. In which plane does rectus femoris lie?

   _____

12. What is the innervation of the quadriceps femoris muscle group?

   _____

13. To which landmark does the patellar ligament attach?

   _____

14. Name the muscle with an origin on the anteromedial aspect of femur.

   _____

15. List the three muscles of the triceps surae muscle group.

   _____

   _____

16. Name the only single-joint flexor of the knee that rotates the tibia on the femur, as well as the femur on the tibia.

   _____

17. What is the innervation of tibialis posterior?

   _____

18. Which dorsiflexor muscle can be easily palpated over the anterior aspect of tibia?

   _____

19. Which extrinsic muscle inserts via four tendons into the plantar surfaces of the bases of distal phalanges?

   _____

Exercise 6-13. Muscles of the hip and lower extremity--cont

20. Name the muscle that is innervated by the deep peroneal nerve and has an insertion at the base of the fifth metatarsal.

_____

21. Name the muscle whose tendon hooks behind the lateral malleolus, crosses the plantar surface of the foot, and inserts on the first metatarsal?

_____

22. What intrinsic muscle of the foot flexes the fifth digit?

_____

23. Describe the action of the lumbricals of the foot.

_____

24. What other intrinsic muscle shares the same origin with extensor hallucis brevis?

_____

25. Name the muscle that inserts into the tendon of flexor digitorum longus and assists with its line of pull.

_____

Key Words

abductor hallucis
adductor brevis
adductor group
adductor hallucis
adductor longus
adductor magnus
ambulate
biceps femoris—long head
biceps femoris—short head
extensor digitorum brevis
extensor digitorum longus
extensor hallucis brevis
extensor hallucis longus
extensor retinaculum
extrinsic muscles of the foot
fixed
flexor digiti minimi brevis
flexor digitorum brevis
flexor digitorum longus
flexor hallucis brevis
flexor hallucis longus
flexor retinaculum
gastrocnemius

gemellus inferior
gemellus superior
gluteal group
gluteus maximus
gluteus medius
gluteus minimus
gracilis
hamstring group
iliacus
iliopsoas
iliotibial band
intrinsic muscles of the foot
lateral rotator muscles of the foot
lumbricals
movable
obturator internus
obturator externus
patellar ligament
pectineus
peroneal retinaculum
peroneus brevis
peroneus longus
peroneus tertius

piriformis
plantaris
popliteus
psoas major
psoas minor
quadratus femoris
quadratus plantae
quadriceps femoris
quadriceps tendon
rectus femoris
sartorius
semimembranosus
semitendinosus
soleus
tendocalcaneus
tensor fasciae latae
tibialis anterior
tibialis posterior
triceps surae muscles
vastus intermedius
vastus lateralis
vastus medialis

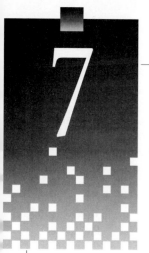

7

Muscles and Movement of the Abdomen, Vertebral Column, Face, and Temporomandibular Joint

❝This chapter will enable you to identify the individual muscles of the abdomen, vertebral column, face, and temporomandibular joint, their attachments to the skeleton, ensuing skeletal movements, and innervations that affect these movements, as well as to enable you to compare and contrast these elements through written exercises.❞

Chapter objectives

The student will be able to:

1. Identify each muscle of the abdomen, vertebral column, face, and temporomandibular joint.

2. Identify the specific skeletal attachment of each muscle.

3. Recognize the innervation of each muscle.

4. Identify the movement created by each muscle as it relates to its skeletal attachment.

5. Discuss the functional significance of each muscle as it relates to the surrounding muscles.

Muscles of the Abdomen

The muscles of the abdomen are responsible for trunk movements such as flexion, lateral flexion, and rotation around the vertebral column. Since these muscles wrap around the trunk like a corset, they stabilize the vertebral column and internal organs from abnormal movement and maintain their normal positions.

Aside from the muscles of the pectoral girdle, the anterior and lateral trunk is covered by four abdominal muscles: rectus abdominis, external oblique, internal oblique, and transverse abdominis. Each has right and left halves that are connected anteriorly by the **linea alba.** This tendinous sheath runs from the pubic symphysis to the xiphoid process and is the central attachment for all the abdominal muscles (Fig. 7-1).

Rectus abdominis, commonly the center of attention to exercise enthusiasts, is a segmented muscle that runs from the rib cage to the pelvis, parallel to midline. It is a multibellied muscle that lays end to end and is separated by segments of tendon. The most common action of this muscle is that of pulling the rib cage toward a somewhat fixed pelvis (Fig. 7-2).

Lateral to rectus abdominis, the other three abdominal muscles lie in layers with **external oblique** most superficial, followed by **internal oblique,** and finally **transverse abdominis** (see Figs. 7-1 and 7-2). When both the right and left halves of each muscle contract simultaneously, the action is trunk flexion. However, if only one side contracts, the action will be some degree of lateral trunk flexion and rotation.

The fibers of the external and internal oblique muscles lie in an angular fashion as their names imply with their

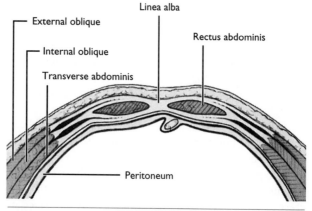

Figure 7-1. Layers of the abdominal wall.
From Mathers et al: Clinical anatomy principles, *St. Louis, 1996, Mosby.*

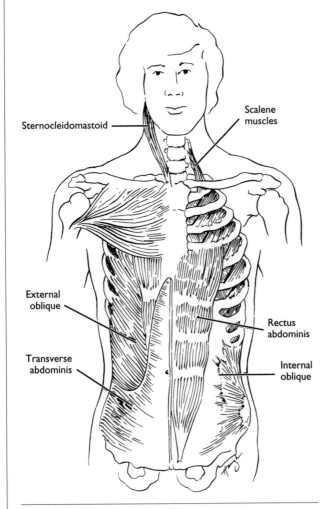

Sternocleidomastoid

Scalene
muscles

External
oblique

Rectus
abdominis

Transverse
abdominis

Internal
oblique

Figure 7-2. Anterior trunk muscles.
From Frownfelter, Dean: Principles and practice of cardiopulmonary physical
therapy, ed 3, St. Louis, 1996, Mosby.

lines of pull in opposition to one another. External oblique performs trunk rotation to the side opposite the contracting muscle; internal oblique performs trunk rotation to the same side of the contracting muscle. Therefore lateral flexion and rotation to the right require contraction of both the left external oblique and right internal oblique, assisted by the right rectus abdominis.

Reverse action of rectus abdominis and both oblique muscles is to pull the pelvis toward the ribs. The abdominal muscles are responsible for maintaining pelvic stabilization, or proper orientation of the pelvis, with regard to the alignment of the low back and femurs. Choosing the iliac crest as a reference landmark, the pelvis is described as moving into an anterior tilt if the coxal bones tip forward and the ischial tuberosities roll posteriorly. Tightening the

abdominal muscles can contribute to a posterior pelvic tilt with the iliac crest moving posteriorly and the ischial tuberosities moving in an anterior direction. Exaggerated abnormal posterior tilt is demonstrated by a sway-back posture.

The fibers of transverse abdominis lie in the horizontal plane and do not have a great impact on trunk movement. This muscle is important as a stabilizer to the abdominal visceral, the largest structure dedicated to holding the internal organs such as the stomach and intestines in place.

Since none of the abdominal muscles cross the hip joint, it is not possible for this muscle group to perform movement specifically at the hip joint. Unfortunately, hip flexion is commonly mistaken for pelvic movement when the abdominal muscles are the focus of an exercise. Improper movement of the femur may, in some cases, detract from the intended pelvic movement, thus the abdominal muscles are often neglected in their conditioning.

Functional significance

The abdominal muscles are used to bring the upper body forward over the lower extremities to achieve a sitting position. Turning to face a different direction with the upper body while seated is also a demonstration of this muscle group. During upright activities such as ambulation, the abdominal muscles participate in controlling the position of the upper trunk over the base of support through the lower extremities. If the head and shoulders lean too far to one side or backward, the abdominal muscles help bring the segments back in line.

Since this group is antagonistic to muscles performing extension of the vertebral column, the abdominal muscles contribute to correct posture in the area of the lower back. Adequate abdominal muscle strength aids in good pelvic alignment and protects against abnormal movement of the lumbar vertebrae, which could lead to injury.

Compression of the internal viscera is important during exhalation and in the evacuation of the intestinal tract. Paralysis of these muscles can lead to complications that involve inadequate breathing or intestinal dysfunction. A summary of the abdominal muscles is provided in Table 7-1.

Muscles of the Vertebral Column

Most of the muscles that control the vertebral column have relatively small muscle bellies when compared with those of the abdominal region, pectoral girdle, or lower extremity. Often, individual muscles are classified into groups according to similarity in bony attachment along the vertebral column. As with the abdominal muscles, those of the vertebral column are found in pairs. Simultaneous contraction of both the

Table 7-1. Muscles of the abdomen

Muscles	Origins	Insertions	Actions	Nerves and root
Rectus abdominis	Superior edge of pubic body and symphysis	Ribs 5-7 and their cartilage and xiphoid process of sternum	Trunk flexion	Thoracic spinal nerves T_{7-12}
External oblique	Last eight ribs and costal cartilages	Iliac crest and linea alba	*Bilaterally:* trunk flexion *Unilaterally:* lateral flexion and rotation to opposite side	Thoracic spinal nerves T_{8-12}
Internal oblique	From inguinal ligament over iliac crest and cartilage of last six ribs	Superior crest of pubis, linea alba, and inferior border of last three ribs	*Bilaterally:* trunk flexion *Unilaterally:* lateral flexion and rotation to same side	Thoracic spinal nerves T_{8-12}
Transversus abdominis	From inguinal ligament over iliac crest and cartilage of last six ribs	Linea alba via a broad aponeurosis to pubic crest	Compresses abdominal wall and viscera Upper portion helps decrease angle of ribs in expiration Stabilizes linea alba, permitting better action by other trunk muscles	Thoracic spinal nerves T_{7-12}

Exercise 7-1. Movement and innervation analysis: abdominal muscles

Indicate the correct movement and innervation for each muscle by marking an "X" under the correct columns.

Muscles	Trunk flexion	Lateral trunk flexion	Rotation same side	Rotation opposite side	Trunk stabilization	Nerves
Rectus abdominis						
External oblique						
Internal oblique						
Transverse abdominis						

right and left halves of a pair of muscles is referred to as **bilateral** contraction. **Unilateral** contraction generally results in lateral flexion or a rotation of the vertebral column.

Palpated anterolateral to the throat, the **sternocleidomastoid** muscle and the three **scalenus** muscles (anterior, medius, posterior) participate in flexion and rotation of the cervical region of the vertebral column (Fig. 7-3). Sternocleidomastoid is named for its three skeletal attachments. When working unilaterally, the sternocleidomastoid has a line of pull that results in rotation of the head and face away from the contracting side, whereas the scalenes muscles perform rotation toward the same side as the contracting muscle. Remember, insertion moves toward a fixed origin.

Previously discussed as a scapular stabilizer, **upper trapezius** (Fig. 7-4) can affect movement on the cervical vertebrae when its insertion on the scapula is fixed. Here also, rotation to the opposite side refers to the movement where the face turns away from the side that is contracting.

Similarly, **levator scapulae** (see Fig. 7-4) depend upon fixed scapulae to affect movements on the cervical vertebrae. Its rotational component is such that when it draws its movable end inferiorly, the face turns toward the same side as the contracting muscle. Bilateral contraction of any pair of muscles posterior to the vertebrae produces extension within the sagittal plane.

Splenius capitis, splenius cervicis, semispinalis capitis, semispinalis cervicis, and **semispinalis thoracis** *(not shown)* (Fig. 7-5) are all overlapping muscles that perform extension of the cervical vertebrae and rotation toward the same side. These muscles lie deep to upper trapezius and can only be palpated indirectly as part of the muscle mass that lies parallel to the vertebral spinous processes. Such muscles are often referred to as the *paraspinal* muscles.

An important muscle of the lower back is **quadratus lumborum** (not to be confused with quadratus femoris). It is a deep muscle that runs from the iliac crest to the lumbar vertebrae and ribs and is a strong lateral flexor of the lumbar

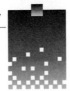

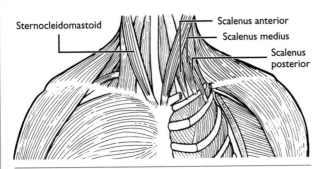

Sternocleidomastoid
Scalenus anterior
Scalenus medius
Scalenus posterior

Figure 7-3. Scalenes muscles.
Adapted from Scanlon, Spearman, Sheldon: Egan's fundamentals of respiratory
care, *ed 6, St. Louis, 1995, Mosby.*

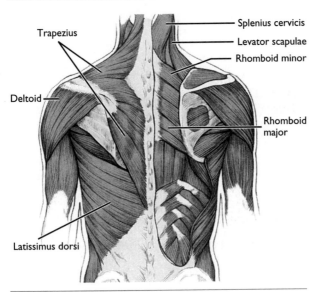

Trapezius
Splenius cervicis
Levator scapulae
Rhomboid minor
Deltoid
Rhomboid major
Latissimus dorsi

Figure 7-4. Back musculature.
From Mathers et al: Clinical anatomy principles, *St. Louis, 1996, Mosby.*

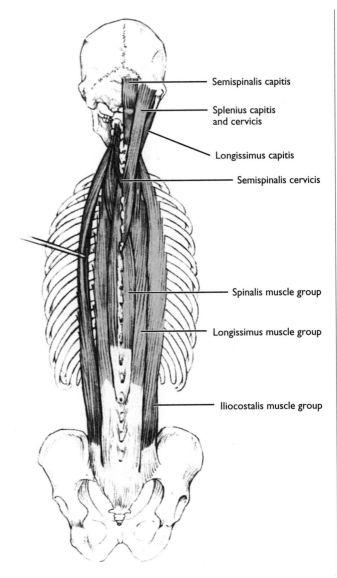

Semispinalis capitis
Splenius capitis and cervicis
Longissimus capitis
Semispinalis cervicis
Spinalis muscle group
Longissimus muscle group
Iliocostalis muscle group

Figure 7-5. Erector spinae muscles.
From Mathers et al: Clinical anatomy principles, *St. Louis, 1996, Mosby.*

region (Fig. 7-6). The unilateral reverse action of this muscle
is referred to as *hip hiking*, whereby one side of the pelvis is
lifted toward the rib cage.

The deepest muscles that surround the vertebral column are the **multifidus, rotatores, interspinales** *(not shown)*,
and **intertransversarii** (Figs. 7-7 and 7-8). Each of these
muscles crosses a limited number of vertebrae or from only
one vertebra to the next. Individually, their actions are not
strong enough to affect a significant change in the position of
the skeleton, but when contracted in concert with other larger
muscles they contribute significant movement and stability to
the vertebral column. Larger muscles that work with these
smaller muscles are latissimus dorsi and quadratus lumborum. Again, these muscles participate in vertebral extension,
lateral flexion, and rotation. A summary of the muscles of the
vertebral column is provided in Table 7-2.

The **erector spinae** muscle group is a collection of long,

thin muscles that runs somewhat parallel to the vertebral column but also has attachments on the ribs, pelvis, and sacrum.
By name, these muscles are referred to as the **iliocostalis,
longissimus,** and **spinalis** groups with more specific segments according to location. These muscles are much longer
than the previous group and may span across several ribs,
from the pelvis to the rib cage or from the ribs to the occipital
bone (see Fig. 7-5). The erector spinae muscles are more
superficial than the smaller muscles, such as multifidus and
rotatores, but they lie deep to the larger trapezius, rhomboids,
and latissimus dorsi. A summary of the erector spinae muscle
group is provided in Table 7-3.

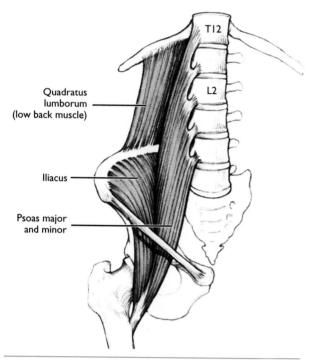

Figure 7-6. Quadratus lumborum.
From Mathers et al: Clinical anatomy principles, *St. Louis, 1996, Mosby.*

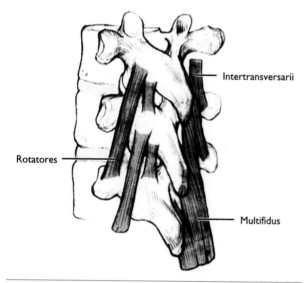

Figure 7-7. Rotatores and multifidus.
From Mathers et al: Clinical anatomy principles, *St. Louis, 1996, Mosby.*

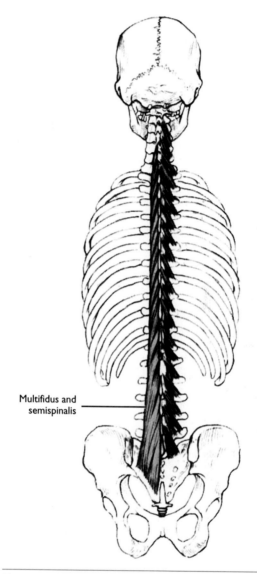

Figure 7-8. Deep muscles of the vertebral column.
From Mathers et al: Clinical anatomy principles, *St. Louis, 1996, Mosby.*

Functional significance

Though the sternocleidomastoid and scalenes group obviously helps control head position by performing cervical flexion, it also helps keep the eyes level with the environment by adjusting the head position in various degrees of lateral flexion and simultaneous rotation. A full field of vision is available through adequate length of these muscles. They also control head position when the trunk is no longer vertical, such as when leaning to lie down in bed. Proper head alignment is a rather complex coordination of events. The sternocleidomastoid and scalenes also perform as accessory muscles of respiration by helping lift the rib cage during inhalation. This action is necessary during strenuous activity or in individuals with long-term respiratory illness.

Upper trapezius, levator scapulae, and the splenius and semispinales groups all perform extension to the cervical and thoracic vertebrae. Their control of postural alignment is

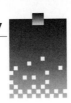

Table 7-2. Muscles of the vertebral column

Muscles	Origins	Insertions	Actions	Nerves and root
Sternocleidomastoid	*Sternal head:* superior part of manubrium *Clavicular head:* superomedial part of clavicle	Mastoid process	*Bilaterally:* flexion of cervical spine *Unilaterally:* lateral flexion and rotation to opposite side	Spinal accessory 11th cranial nerve

Scalenus
  anterior
  medial
  posterior
	Transverse processes of cervical vertebrae	*Anterior and medial:* 1st rib anteriorly
		Posterior: 2nd rib anteriorly
			Bilaterally: elevate first two ribs, assisting with inspiration
			Assist in cervical flexion
			Unilaterally: assist in lateral flexion to same side
				Spinal nerves C_{4-8}

Trapezius (upper)	External occipital protuberance Crest and superior curved line of occipital bone	Lateral clavicle and acromion process of scapula	*Insertion fixed and bilaterally:* cervical extension *Insertion fixed and unilaterally:* cervical extension, lateral flexion, and rotation to opposite side	Spinal accessory $C_{2,3,4}$
Levator scapulae	Transverse processes of C_{1-4}	Vertebral border of scapula between superior angle and root of spine	*Insertion fixed and bilaterally:* cervical extension *Insertion fixed and unilaterally:* lateral flexion and rotation to same side	Dorsal scapular $C_{4,5}$
Splenius capitis	Spinous process of C_7 to T_4 and posterior cervical ligament	Lateral portion of superior curved line of occipital bone and mastoid process of temporal bone	*Bilaterally:* cervical extension *Unilaterally:* lateral flexion and rotation to same side	Spinal nerves C_{3-5}
Splenius cervicis	Spinous processes of T_{3-6}	Transverse processes of C_{2-5}	*Bilaterally:* cervical extension *Unilaterally:* lateral flexion and rotation to same side	Spinal nerves C_{4-8}

Semispinalis
  capitis
  cervicis
  thoracis
	In overlapping layers
	Transverse processes of thoracic vertebrae and C_7
		Occipital bone and spinous processes of C_2 to T_4	*Bilaterally:* cervical extension
			Unilaterally: lateral flexion and rotation to same side
				Spinal nerves C_{3-8}

Quadratus lumborum	Posterior aspect of iliac crest	Last rib near vertebral attachment and transverse processes of lumbar vertebrae	Lateral flexion of trunk in lumbar region Assists with trunk extension *Reverse action:* elevation of pelvis	Lumbar plexus T_{12} to L_3
Multifidus	Transverse processes of C_4 to L_5 to iliac crest	Each crossing two to four vertebrae, attaching to spinous process of vertebrae above from L_5 to C_1	*Bilaterally:* trunk extension *Unilaterally:* rotation to opposite side	Adjacent spinal nerves
Rotatores	Transverse processes of all vertebrae	Lamina of vertebrae above	*Bilaterally:* trunk extension *Unilaterally:* Rotation to opposite side	Adjacent spinal nerves
Interspinales	In pairs, superior surface of all spinous processes	Inferior aspect of spinous process superior to vertebra of origin	Trunk extension	Adjacent spinal nerves
Intertransversarii	Transverse processes of all vertebrae	Transverse process of vertebrae superior to vertebra of origin	Lateral flexion of the vertebral column	Adjacent spinal nerves

important for the correct horizontal placement of the eyes but includes the proper positioning of the mouth and throat during swallowing and breathing.

Quadratus lumborum is recognized as a lateral flexor of the trunk, useful when reaching away from a stable base of support. Control by this muscle can, for short periods, assist in maintaining a position with the upper trunk outside a base of support. As a *hip hiker*, quadratus lumborum is active when one wishes to scoot one hip forward in a chair without completely leaning to the opposite direction. The hip must first be lifted before it can be pulled forward. During ambulation, the *hip hiker* helps lift the pelvis of the lower extremity that is swinging, especially when there is insufficient hip and knee flexion. Stair climbing is another event often dependent upon quadratus lumborum for hip elevation.

Multifidus, rotatores, interspinales, and intertransversarii, as well as the erector spinae muscle group, are all similar in their significance to activities of daily living. These muscles make upright trunk posture possible. Weakness in these groups results in poor posture and abnormal bony alignment as a result of the effects of gravity pulling the body downward. These postural muscles are contracting constantly in all activi-

ties, even during sleep to some extent. Since most functional activity takes place in either a sitting or standing upright position, there is almost no time when these muscles are not providing stability or facilitating trunk position upon which the extremities can move. Even activities performed while lying down require vertebral extension to lift the hips as often occurs when dressing the lower body or positioning the body in bed. After an illness or injury to any part of the body, it is the postural muscles that are first challenged and must be rehabilitated before other activities can be attempted!

Table 7-3. Muscles of the erector spinae

Muscles	Origins	Insertions	Actions	Nerves
Iliocostalis cervicis thoracis lumborum	In layers from posterior aspect of ribs and spinous processes of lower vertebrae to iliac crest and sacrum	To posterior aspect of ribs more proximal, transverse processes of cervical vertebrae	*Bilaterally:* extension of vertebral column *Unilaterally:* lateral flexion	Adjacent spinal nerves
Longissimus capitis cervicis thoracis	In layers from transverse processes of cervical, thoracic, and lumbar vertebrae	To transverse processes of vertebrae superior to vertebra of origin and mastoid process of temporal bone	*Bilaterally:* extension of vertebral column *Unilaterally:* lateral flexion and rotation to same side	Adjacent spinal nerves
Spinalis capitis cervicis thoracis	In layers from spinous processes of lumbar, thoracic, and cervical vertebrae Blends with semispinalis capitis	Spinous processes of thoracic and cervical vertebrae to occipital bone and mastoid process of temporal bone	*Bilaterally:* extension of vertebral column *Unilaterally:* lateral flexion and rotation to same side	Adjacent spinal nerves

Exercise 7-2. Movement and innervation analysis: vertebral column

Indicate the correct movement and innervation for each muscle by marking an "X" under the correct columns.

Muscles	Extension	Flexion	Rotation same side	Rotation opposite side	Lateral flexion	Assists with inspiration	Nerves
Sternocleidomastoid							
Scalenes (anterior, medial, posterior)							
Trapezius (upper)							
Levator scapulae							
Splenius (capitis, cervicis)							
Semispinalis (capitis, cervicis, thoracis)							
Quadratus lumborum							
Multifidus							
Rotatores							
Interspinales							
Intertransversarii							
Iliocostalis (cervicis, thoracic, lumborum)							
Longissimus (capitis, cervicis, thoracis)							
Spinalis (capitis, cervicis, thoracis)							

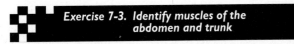

Exercise 7-3. Identify muscles of the abdomen and trunk

Identify the muscles of the abdomen and trunk on Figure 7-9.

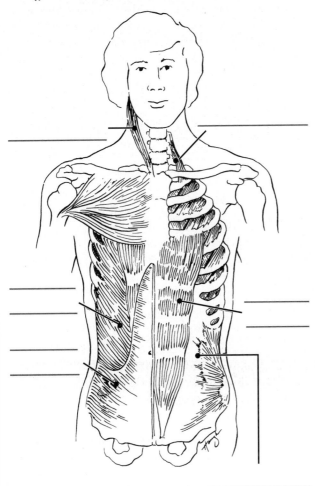

Figure 7-9. Anterior trunk muscles (note direction of fibers).
From Frownfelter, Dean: Principles and practice of cardiopulmonary physical therapy, *ed 3, St. Louis, 1996, Mosby.*

Muscles of Primary Respiration

The primary muscle of respiration is the **diaphragm,** innervated by the phrenic nerve. Contraction of this muscle is both a voluntary and involuntary event so that breathing may be constant. This roundish muscle forms a canopy of sorts between the thoracic and abdominal regions. Its only bony attachments are to the lumbar vertebrae posteriorly and to the lower ribs. The tendinous insertion allows it to contract in a circular fashion, drawing the highest center of the canopy downward (Fig. 7-10). The temporary vacuum created inside the thoracic cavity causes the air outside the body to be sucked into

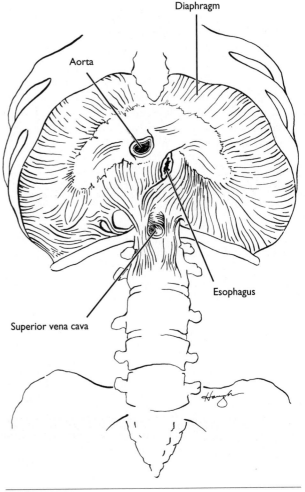

Figure 7-10. Diaphragm.
From Frownfelter, Dean: Principles and practice of cardiopulmonary physical therapy, *ed 3, St. Louis, 1996, Mosby.*

the lungs for gas exchange. This is referred to as **inspiration.** Once the diaphragm relaxes, it returns to its original position and air is forced out of the lungs. During normal breathing, **expiration** is a passive event (Figs. 7-11 and 7-12).

The process of inspiration is furthered by the **external intercostal** and **internal intercostal** muscles, which help lift the rib cage away from the downward contracting diaphragm (Fig. 7-13). This action increases the volume of space available in the thoracic cavity and increases the volume of air to be inhaled.

Since the ribs are the sole protection for the lungs against outside forces, the intercostal muscles serve to brace these bones together. Stability of the rib cage allows the ribs to move as a unit while guarding the fragile tissues beneath.

During strenuous activity the diaphragm and intercostal muscles are not able to rapidly exchange large volumes

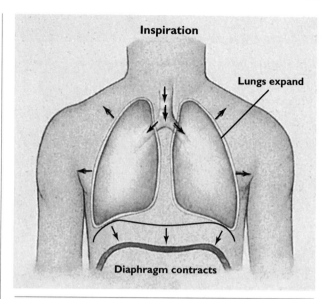

Inspiration

Lungs expand

Diaphragm contracts

Figure 7-11. Mechanics of breathing, inspiration.
From Thibodeau, Patton: Structure and function of the body, *ed 10, St. Louis, 1996, Mosby.*

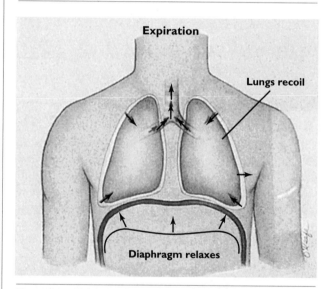

Expiration

Lungs recoil

Diaphragm relaxes

Figure 7-12. Mechanics of breathing, expiration.
From Thibodeau, Patton: Structure and function of the body, *ed 10, St. Louis, 1996, Mosby.*

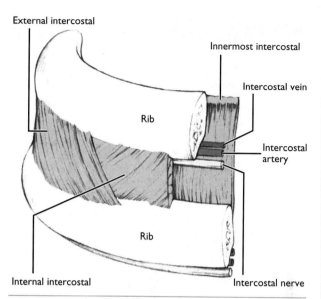

External intercostal

Innermost intercostal

Intercostal vein

Rib

Intercostal artery

Rib

Internal intercostal

Intercostal nerve

Figure 7-13. Intercostal muscles.
From Mathers: Clinical anatomy principles, *St. Louis, 1996, Mosby.*

upper extremities be fixed distally or repositioned for efficient performance, such as bracing against a chair or holding the arms overhead.

Some muscles further assist by changing the position of the vertebral column in either flexion or extension and changing the relative position of the thoracic and abdominal regions to one another. For instance, taking a very deep breath is accomplished by extending the trunk and cervical vertebrae and retracting the shoulders. Thus the trapezius and erector spinae muscles are able to impact the ability to inhale deeply.

Accessory muscle use is not exclusive to inspiration. For example, to inhale a new, large volume of fresh air, the depleted air must be quickly expelled from the lungs. Expiration is assisted by the abdominal muscles. Occasionally, the activity of forced respiration may be so pronounced that the individual will demonstrate obvious alternating trunk extension and flexion to promote air exchange. A summary of the primary muscles of respiration is provided in Table 7-4.

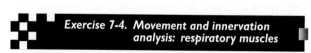

Exercise 7-4. Movement and innervation analysis: respiratory muscles

Indicate the correct movement and innervation for each muscle by marking an "X" under the correct columns.

Muscles	Inspiration	Expiration	Nerves
Diaphragm			
External intercostals			
Internal intercostals			

of air on their own. For assistance, other skeletal attachments help raise and lower the rib cage and are referred to as **accessory muscles of respiration..** To do so, these muscles are often working in reverse action—insertion fixed and origin mobile. Sternocleidomastoid, scalenes, serratus anterior, pectoralis major, and pectoralis minor all have attachments on the rib cage, sternum, or clavicle and assist in lifting the rib cage. In some instances this activity may require that the

Exercise 7-4 continued on page 152

Accessory muscles	Inspiration	Expiration	Nerve
Sternocleidomastoid			
Scalenes (anterior, medial, posterior)			
Serratus anterior			
Pectoralis major			
Pectoralis minor			

Accessory muscles	Inspiration	Expiration	Nerve
Trapezius (upper, middle, lower)			
Erector spinae			
Rectus abdominis			
External oblique			
Internal oblique			
Transversus abdominis			

Table 7-4. Primary muscles of respiration

Muscles	Origins	Insertions	Actions	Nerves and root
Diaphragm	Bodies of lumbar vertebrae one to three and medial surfaces of last four to six ribs on xiphoid process	A central tendon within the diaphragm; no bony insertion	Principle muscle of inspiration Upon contraction, draws inferiorly, creating a temporary vacuum within thoracic cavity, facilitating inspiration Relaxes and returns to original position	Phrenic nerve C_{2-5}
External and internal intercostals	Inferior border of ribs and costal cartilages Internal intercostals are deep to external intercostals	Superior border of rib below the rib of origin	Elevation of ribs during inspiration Stabilizes the rib cage	Intercostal nerves

Muscles of the Face and Temporomandibular Joint

Facial muscles and the muscles of the **temporomandibular joint** contribute to verbal and nonverbal communication, the expression of emotions, eye protection, and improved breathing and vision, as well as eating and manipulating food and liquids in the mouth. Although muscles of the axial and appendicular skeleton attach to two or more bones to cause movement, facial muscles are attached to one another, to deep connective tissues, or to superficial connective tissues such as skin. Most facial and jaw muscles are quite superficial with the most complex layers existing around the cheek and temporomandibular joint area (Fig. 7-14). Refer to Tables 7-5 and 7-6 for the movement of each muscle.

The act of chewing food is called **mastication.** Muscles of the temporomandibular joint are also known as the muscles of mastication, and they possess great strength and mechanical advantage in their line of pull across the temporomandibular joint. The actions at this joint include elevation of the mandible to close the mouth and depression of the mandible to open the mouth. Protraction, thrusting the mandible forward, is antagonistic to retraction, or

pulling the mandible posteriorly. Lateral movements are also necessary for proper chewing. Three of the strongest muscles of the temporomandibular joint are dedicated to the act of closing the mouth and clamping down to chew or crush food. **Temporalis, masseter,** and **medial pterygoid** participate in the elevation of the mandible. The **lateral pterygoid** is responsible for depressing the mandible but is somewhat assisted in this activity by the facial muscle, **platysma** (Figs. 7-15 and 7-16). Summaries of muscles of the face and temporomandibular joint are provided in Tables 7-5 and 7-6.

Summary

Chapter 7 concludes the discussion of the individual voluntary muscles that cause movements of the body. Remember, practice, practice, practice, not memorization, will make this information familiar and useful. Even veterans who rely regularly on their knowledge of human anatomy require an occasional review to maintain an accurate foundation of material such as this! Repeat performance of the exercises within this text will prove to be beneficial.

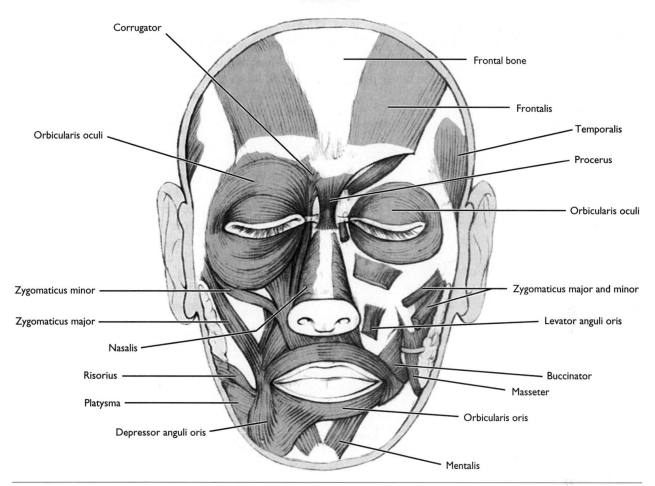

Corrugator

Frontal bone

Frontalis

Temporalis

Orbicularis oculi

Procerus

Orbicularis oculi

Zygomaticus minor

Zygomaticus major and minor

Zygomaticus major

Levator anguli oris

Nasalis

Risorius

Buccinator

Platysma

Masseter

Depressor anguli oris

Orbicularis oris

Mentalis

Figure 7-14. Facial muscles.
From Mathers: Clinical anatomy principles, *St. Louis, 1996, Mosby.*

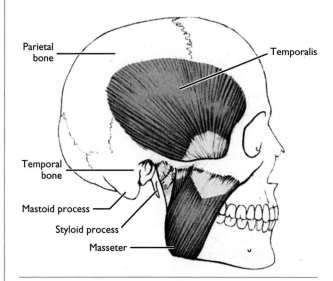

Parietal bone

Temporalis

Temporal bone

Mastoid process

Styloid process

Masseter

Figure 7-15. Temporalis and masseter.
From Mathers: Clinical anatomy principles, *St. Louis, 1996, Mosby.*

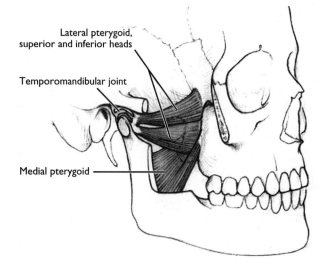

Lateral pterygoid, superior and inferior heads

Temporomandibular joint

Medial pterygoid

Figure 7-16. Medial and lateral pterygoid.
From Mathers: Clinical anatomy principles, *St. Louis, 1996, Mosby.*

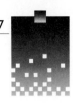

Table 7-5. Muscles of the face

Facial muscles surrounding mouth	Locations	Actions	Nerves
Buccinator	Deep muscle of cheek	Compresses cheeks	Facial
Depressor anguli oris	Inferior to edges of mouth	Pulls angle of mouth downward	Facial
Levator anguli oris	Above angle of mouth toward zygomatic arch	Pulls angle of mouth up	Facial
Mentalis	Covers chin	Protracts lower lip (pouting)	Facial
Orbicularis oris	Wraps around mouth	Closes lips (whistling muscle)	Facial
Platysma	Covers mandible and throat	Flattens bottom lip and tightens skin over throat	Facial
Risorius	From angle of mouth transverse across cheek	Pulls angle of mouth straight backward	Facial
Zygomaticus major	From angle of mouth to zygomatic arch	Raises angle of mouth (smiling)	Facial
Facial muscles surrounding eyes and nose			
Corrugator	Superior to and between orbits	Pulls eyebrows together	Facial
Frontalis	Covers forehead	Raises eyebrows and wrinkles forehead	Facial
Nasalis	From midline of nose to base of nostrils	Flares nostrils	Facial
Orbicularis oculi	Wraps around orbit	Closes eye (winking)	Facial
Procerus	Runs superior to inferior over bridge of nose	Wrinkles up nose	Facial

Table 7-6. Muscles of the temporomandibular joint

Muscles	Origins	Insertions	Actions	Nerves
Temporalis	Temporal region	Coronoid process and ramus of mandible	Elevation and retraction	Trigeminal
Masseter	Zygomatic arch	Angle of mandible	Elevation and assists with protraction	Trigeminal
Medial pterygoid	Palatine bone and maxilla	Medial aspect of angle of mandible	Elevation and assists with protraction	Trigeminal
Lateral pterygoid	Sphenoid bone	Runs transversely to anterior aspect of condyle of mandible	Depression after initial relaxation of temporalis, masseter, and medial pterygoid Lateral movement	Trigeminal

▦ ■ □ Exercise 7-5. Movement and innervation analysis: facial muscles

Indicate the correct movement and innervation for each muscle by marking an "X" under the correct columns.

Muscles	Movement	Nerves
Buccinator		
Depressor anguli oris		
Levator anguli oris		
Mentalis		
Orbicularis oris		

■ ■ ■ *Exercise 7-5. Movement and innervation analysis: facial muscles—cont*

Muscles	Movement	Nerves
Platysma		
Risorius		
Zygomaticus major		
Corrugator		
Frontalis		
Nasalis		
Orbicularis oculi		
Procerus		

■ ■ ■ *Exercise 7-6. Muscles of the face and temporomandibular joint*

Identify the muscles of the face and temporomandibular joint on Figures 7-17, 7-17, and 7-19.

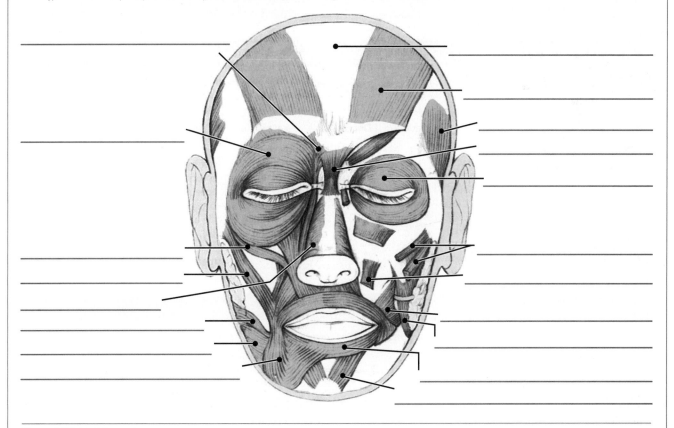

Figure 7-17. Facial muscles.
From Mathers: Clinical anatomy principles, St. Louis, 1996, Mosby.

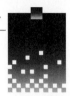

■■■ *Exercise 7-6. Muscles of the face and temporomandibular joint—cont*

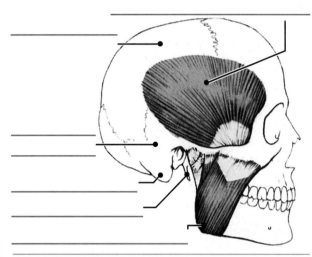

Figure 7-18. Muscles of mastication.
From Mathers: Clinical anatomy principles, *St. Louis, 1996, Mosby.*

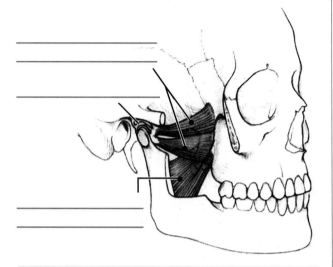

Figure 7-19. Muscles of mastication.
From Mathers: Clinical anatomy principles, *St. Louis, 1996, Mosby.*

■■■ *Exercise 7-7. Movement and innervation analysis: muscles of the temporomandibular joint*

Indicate the correct movement and innervation for each muscle by marking an "X" under the correct columns.

Muscles	Elevation	Depression	Retraction	Protraction	Lateral movement	Nerves
Temporalis						
Masseter						
Medial pterygoid						
Lateral pterygoid						

■■■ *Exercise 7-8. Illustrate the muscles of the abdomen and trunk*

On the illustrations provided, draw the muscle attachments with the correct origin and insertion; indicate the direction of the line of pull for each of the following muscles (Figs. 7-20 and 7-21).

Posterior view		**Anterior view**	
Upper trapezius	Splenius capitis and cervicis	Pectoralis minor	Scalene muscles
Lower trapezius	Longissimus muscle group	Rectus abdominus	Sternocleidomastoid
Semispinalis capitis	Quadratus lumborum	External oblique	External intercostal muscles

CHAPTER 7   *Muscles and movement of the abdomen, vertebral column, face, and temporomandibular joint*

■■ ■ **Exercise 7-8. Illustrate the muscles of the abdomen and trunk—cont**

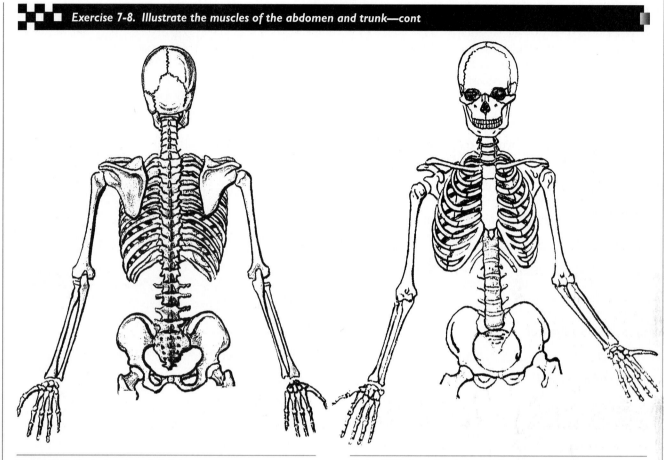

Figure 7-20. Posterior view of skeleton.
From Mathers: Clinical anatomy principles, *St. Louis, 1996, Mosby.*

Figure 7-21. Anterior view of skeleton.
From Mathers: Clinical anatomy principles, *St. Louis, 1996, Mosby.*

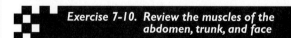
Exercise 7-9. Palpate the muscles of the abdomen, trunk, and face

With the list of 12 muscles in Exercise 7-8, try to palpate each muscle belly on your study partner. With washable markers or adhesive labels, note the location of the muscle belly and its origin and insertion. Show the direction of the fibers of each muscle. Compare your accuracy with other classmates!

Exercise 7-10. Review the muscles of the abdomen, trunk, and face

1. Name the multibellied muscle that performs trunk flexion.

2. Name the structure that joins the abdominal muscles and runs from the pubic symphysis to the xiphoid process.

Exercise 7-10. Review the muscles of the abdomen, trunk, and face—cont

3. Name the abdominal muscle that performs rotation to the opposite side.

4. Name the muscle that stabilizes the scapula and performs cervical extension bilaterally and rotation to the same side unilaterally.

5. List the three actions of quadratus lumborum

157

Exercise 7-10 continued on page 158

■ ■ *Exercise 7-10. Review the muscles of the abdomen, trunk, and face—cont*

6. Name the very short paraspinal muscle that runs from the spinous process of one vertebra to the spinous process of the next, causing trunk extension bilaterally and rotation to the opposite side unilaterally

_____

7. List the common actions of the erector spinae group.

_____

_____

8. What is the innervation of the diaphragm?

_____

9. When the diaphragm is in its lowest position, is it completely relaxed or completely contracted?

_____

10. What is the action of mentalis?

_____

11. Describe the location of the corrugator muscle.

_____

12. What is the action of platysma?

_____

13. Describe the location of zygomaticus major.

_____

14. What is the action of procerus?

_____

15. What is the action of orbicularis oculi?

_____

16. What is the innervation of the muscles of mastication?

_____

17. What muscle performs strong elevation and retraction of the mandible?

_____

18. What muscle depresses the mandible?

_____

19. What is the origin of medial pterygoid?

_____

20. What is the insertion of masseter?

_____

Key Words

bilateral
buccinator
corrugator
depressor anguli oris
diaphragm
erector spinae
expiration
external oblique
external intercostals
facial muscles
frontalis
hip hiker
iliocostalis (cervicis, thoracis, lumborum)
inspiration
internal oblique
internal intercostals
interspinales
intertransversarii

lateral pterygoid
levator anguli oris
levator scapulae
linea alba
longissimus (capitis, cervicis, thoracis)
mastication
masseter
medial pterygoid
mentalis
multifidus
muscles of mastication
nasalis
orbicularis oculi
orbicularis oris
pectoralis major
pectoralis minor
platysma
procerus

quadratus lumborum
rectus abdominis
risorius
rotatores
scalenus (anterior, medial, posterior) muscles
semispinalis (capitis, cervicis, thoracis)
serratus anterior
splenius: (capitis, cervicis)
splinalis (cervicis, thoracis)
sternocleidomastoid
temporalis
temporomandibular joint
transverse abdominis
trapezius (upper, middle, lower)
unilateral
zygomaticus major

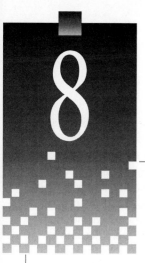

8 Nervous System

This chapter will enable you to identify the primary elements of the nervous system as they affect human movement.

Chapter objectives

The student will be able to:

1. Identify the elements that make nerve tissue unique in its function.

2. Understand the physiologic events that are necessary to nerve impulse transmission.

3. Identify the components of the central nervous system.

4. Identify the components of the peripheral nervous system.

5. Describe the reflex arc.

6. Identify the elements of the muscle spindle.

As previously examined, the musculoskeletal system is a conglomeration of contractile units, each capable of performing many individual tasks with limited value. Through careful coordination and integration of abilities, the mastery of complex movements can begin. The **nervous system** controls all functions in the body, both **voluntary** and **involuntary,** including the musculoskeletal system and all other organ systems.

Function and Structure of a Neuron

Nerve tissue possesses two distinct qualities—**irritability** and **conductivity.** Irritability refers to being sensitive and responsive to stimuli. A stimulus can trigger a reaction in nerve tissue that begins near the initial stimulus and then transfers throughout the tissue. Conductivity is the ability to transmit a response along itself toward the next receptor. Nerve tissue is a one-way delivery system by which the human organism communicates within itself.

The simplest component of the nervous system is the **neuron.** By function, there are three categories—the **efferent (motor) neuron, afferent (sensory) neuron,** and **association neuron** (Fig. 8-1). An efferent neuron carries an impulse from the brain to the limbs and organs, affecting a change

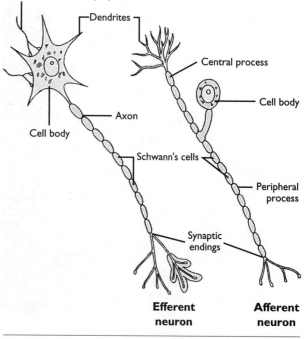

Incoming axons and synapses

Dendrites

Central process

Cell body

Axon

Cell body

Schwann's cells

Peripheral process

Synaptic endings

Efferent neuron

Afferent neuron

Figure 8-1. Efferent and afferent neurons.
From Mathers et al: Clinical anatomy principles, *St. Louis, 1996, Mosby.*

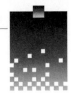

such as movement. An afferent neuron receives information and sends it toward the brain to be processed. An association neuron carries an impulse from one neuron to another.

A typical neuron consists of many **dendrites** that extend from the cell body and act like antennae, receiving stimuli and then transferring them on to a **cell body.** From here, each stimulus becomes an impulse that moves down the **axon** and on to a **terminal branch** or end of the neuron. Most large diameter axons are coated by a **myelin sheath,** an insulation-like lipid material that speeds the transmission of **nerve impulses** (Figs. 8-2, *A* and 8-2, *B*).

At this stage, this single neuron may communicate its impulse to one or many neurons across a **synapse** (Fig. 8-3).

There exists a small space between neurons called the **synaptic cleft.** There are areas in the terminal branches, referred to as **synaptic vesicles,** which store special chemical substances called **neurotransmitters.** Many different chemicals serve as neurotransmitters in the human body; most are specialized as to their location and intended function. When the impulse or action potential reaches a terminal branch, a synaptic vesicle is stimulated and releases its neurotransmitter into the synaptic cleft to be picked up by a **receptor.** The receptor is a specialized area on adjacent tissue; this area may be another neuron, a muscle fiber, or an organ.

The most frequently discussed neurotransmitter is **acetylcholine,** which stimulates skeletal muscle fibers. Acetylcholine is released by the synaptic vesicles of efferent (motor) neurons into the synaptic cleft near the **motor end plate** on a motor or skeletal muscle fiber. In this case the intersection between the neuron and muscle fiber is called a **neuromuscular junction.** The neuromuscular components required to cause a skeletal muscle fiber contraction include the efferent neuron, synaptic vesicles, neurotransmitter, synapse, synaptic cleft, motor end plate, and motor fiber. These components are collectively referred to as the **motor unit** (Fig. 8-4).

Neurons can also be classified by structure, that is, the arrangement of the dendrites, cell body, and axon. The three different arrangements of neurons are **multipolar, unipolar,** and **bipolar,** depending on the location of the cell body to the axon. A multipolar neuron has its dendrites attached directly

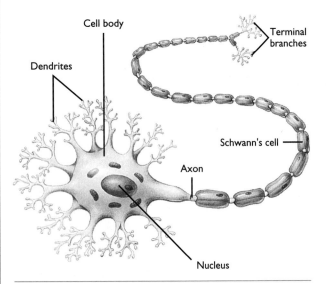

Figure 8-2, A. Typical efferent neuron.
From Thibodeau, Patton: Structure and function of the body, ed 10, St. Louis, 1996, Mosby.

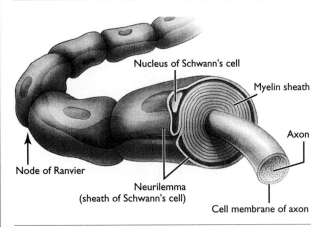

Figure 8-2, B. Myelinated neuron segment.
From Thibodeau, Patton: Structure and function of the body, ed 10, St. Louis, 1996, Mosby.

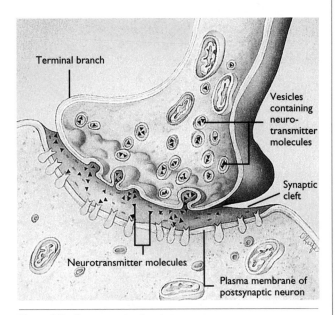

Figure 8-3. Components of a synapse.
From Thibodeau, Patton: The human body in health & disease, ed 2, St. Louis, 1992, Mosby.

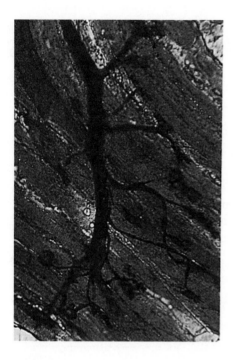

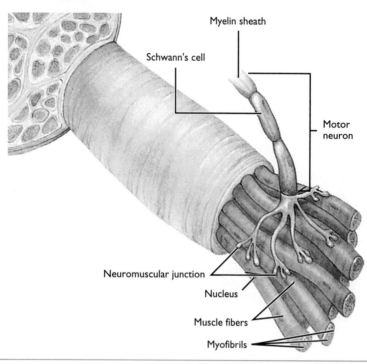

Myelin sheath

Schwann's cell

Motor
neuron

Neuromuscular junction

Nucleus

Muscle fibers

Myofibrils

Figure 8-4. Components of a motor unit.
From Thibodeau, Patton: The human body in health & disease, *ed 2, St. Louis, 1992, Mosby.*

to the cell body and to the long axon; its impulses are carried out to the terminal branches. This is the configuration of most motor neurons. Unipolar neurons receive stimuli through dendrites, which then carry an impulse along a short axon that slightly branches off before attaching to the cell body. The impulse is then carried by the same branch to the last portion of the axon to the terminal branches. Thus unipolar refers to one entrance and exit point from the cell body.

Many sensory neurons are unipolar in structure. Bipolar neurons receive stimuli similar to unipolar neurons; however, the axon enters the cell body at one side and exits the cell body on the opposite side. Also sensory in nature, bipolar neurons are often associated with the senses of sight, smell, and taste.

Impulse Transmission

In its resting state a neuron has a chemical balance, whereby the exterior of the axon holds a high concentration of **sodium ions** that set up a positive charge. Inside the cell membrane there is a high concentration of **potassium ions** that create a negative charge. Without stimulation there is a natural balance between the positive and negative charges, and the neuron is referred to as **polarized** or having a **resting potential.**

A polarized, resting neuron must receive a certain level of stimuli to become active to change this resting state. These stimuli may come from a single source or accumulate

through the contributions of many incoming neurons to the dendrites. The minimum level of stimuli required to change the resting potential is called the **threshold stimulus.**

The impulse is initiated by the stimulus that is causing a change in the **polarity** of the neuron. The positive sodium ions are then able to cross the cell membrane, driving the negative ions outside. This reverses the locations of the high concentrations of both ions, **depolarizing** the neuron (Fig. 8-5, *A*) Depolarization is a chemical-electric change that occurs sequentially along the wall of the axon until it reaches the terminal branches. This sequential depolarization is called the **action potential** of the neuron.

Once a threshold stimulus for a neuron is reached, the resulting impulse travels on the axon, an *all-or-none* response similar to the response of a single muscle fiber contraction. The impulse either travels the length of the axon to the terminal branches or it does not. There is no weak or partial conduction of an impulse.

After depolarization, the sodium and potassium return to their original positions via the **sodium-potassium pump,** or **active transport system.** When this *reset* phase is accomplished, the neuron is considered to be **repolarized.** Without a correction of the ions, the neuron cannot respond to another stimulus until after the repolarization is complete. This creates a brief moment called the **refractory period,** a time when a neuron is unable to respond to stimuli.

161

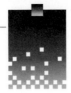

Saltatory Conduction

In the case of large axons covered by a myelin sheath, impulses travel by **saltatory conduction,** a process whereby the change in polarity of the wall of an axon takes place only at the gaps in the myelin sheath called the **nodes of Ranvier** (Fig. 8-5, *B*). The myelin sheath consists of repeating **Schwann's cells** that are wrapped around the axon with its outer membrane, referred to as the **neurilemma.** In a sense, the Schwann's cells and nodes of Ranvier intercept an impulse and greatly increase the speed of transmission to the end of the axon, allowing the impulse to *skip* over myelinated segments of the axon. Saltatory conduction cannot occur on unmyelinated axons. When the myelin sheath is damaged, the nerve impulses can be severely slowed.

Exercise 8-1. Elements of nerve tissue and impulse transmission

Complete the statements based on your familiarity of the nerve tissue and impulse transmission.

1. Two distinctive qualities of nerve tissue are
   _____ and _____.

2. Stimuli are received by a neuron through the
   _____.

3. Neurons that carry impulses from the brain toward the muscles and organs are _____.

4. Neurons that carry impulses from the body toward the brain are _____.

5. The insulation coating on an axon that speeds impulse transmission is the _____.

6. Impulses move along an axon to the
   _____ and then to the
   _____.

7. The point at which a neuron links up with other neurons or effector/affector tissues is the _____.

8. The chemical substances released by synaptic vesicles in the terminal branches are _____.

9. The most common neurotransmitter that affects skeletal muscle contraction is _____.

10. The receptor on a skeletal muscle fiber is the
    _____.

11. The efferent neuron, synapse, acetylcholine, motor end plate, and motor fiber collectively make up the
    _____.

Exercise 8-1. Elements of nerve tissue and impulse transmission—cont

12. The structure of most efferent neurons is
    _____.

13. The structure of most sensory neurons is
    _____.

14. A neuron at rest is referred to as _____.

15. The minimum level of stimuli sufficient to trigger an impulse within a neuron is the _____
    _____.

16. When there is a reverse in the chemical ion concentrations along the wall of an axon, the neuron is
    _____.

17. Carrying an impulse along an axon by sequential depolarization is called the _____
    _____ of the neuron.

18. When the *reset* phase is accomplished and the ions have returned to their original positions, the neuron is considered to be _____.

19. Sodium and potassium return to their original positions via the _____
    or _____.

20. The repeating portions of the myelin sheath, which the impulse *skips* over, are referred to as _____
    _____.

21. The gaps between the Schwann's cells where the impulse travels along the axon are called the _____
    _____.

22. After carrying an impulse, the _____
    _____ is the brief period when the neuron is incapable of firing again.

23. The outer membrane of the myelin sheath is the
    _____.

24. The speedy process of nerve impulse transmission that involves myelinated axons is called
    _____.

25. The portion of the body that controls both involuntary and voluntary functions is the _____
    _____.

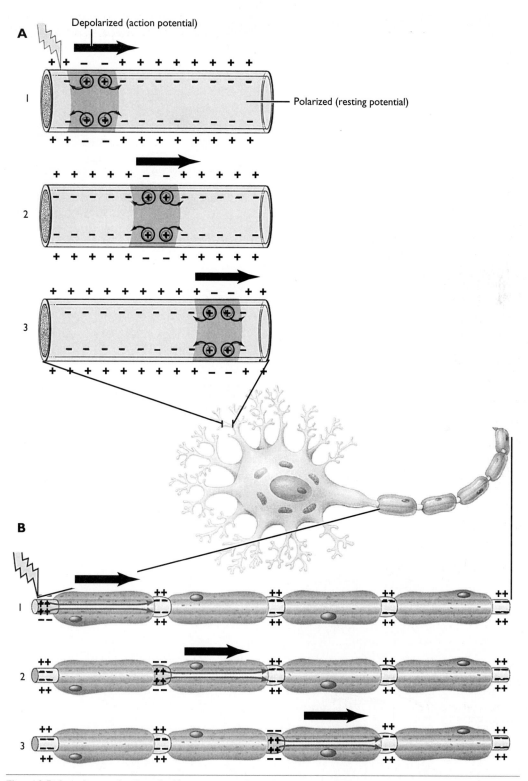

A

Depolarized (action potential)

Polarized (resting potential)

B

Figure 8-5. Impulse conduction. *A,* Along an unmyelinated neuron. *B,* Along a myelinated neuron—saltatory conduction.

From Thibodeau, Patton: Structure and function of the body, ed 10, St. Louis, 1996, Mosby.

163

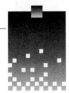

■ *Exercise 8-2. Structure of a neuron*

Identify the structure of a neuron on Figs. 8-6, A, 8-6, B, and 8-7.

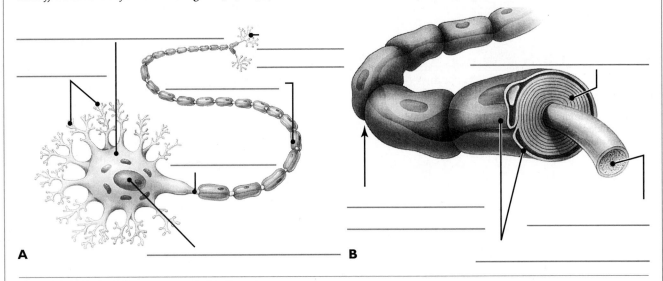

A   **B**

Figure 8-6, A. Typical efferent neuron. B. Myelinated neuron segment.
From Thibodeau, Patton: Structure and function of the body, ed 10, St. Louis, 1996, Mosby.

■ *Exercise 8-3. Nerve impulse transmission*

*In the space provided, illustrate the process of nerve impulse transmission on a **nonmyelinated** neuron, complete with positive and negative ionic changes. Illustrate the process of nerve impulse transmission on a **myelinated** neuron, complete with the elements required and positive and negative ionic changes.*

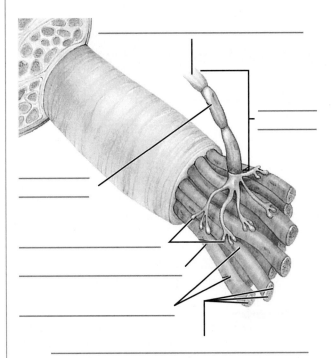

Figure 8-7. Components of a motor unit.
From Thibodeau, Patton: The human body in health & disease, ed 2, St. Louis, 1992, Mosby.

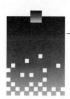

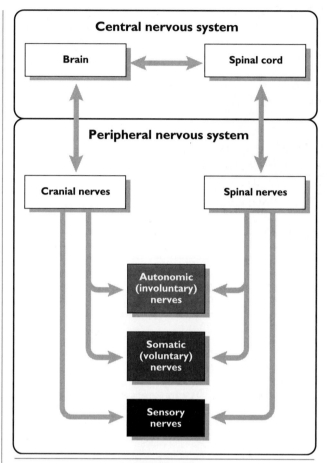

Figure 8-8. Divisions of the nervous system.

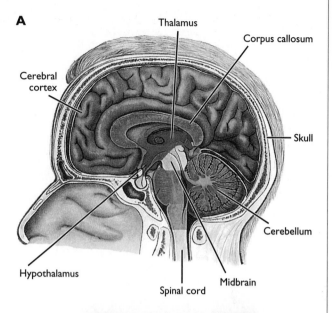

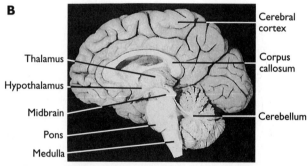

Figure 8-9. *A,* Major regions of the central nervous system. *B,* Section of a preserved brain.
From Thibodeau, Patton: Structure and function of the body, *ed 10, St. Louis, 1996, Mosby.*

Central Nervous System

Nerve tissue is divided into two primary categories: **central nervous system (CNS)** and **peripheral nervous system (PNS)** (Fig. 8-8). The CNS consists of the **brain** and **spinal cord.** The PNS consists of nerves (efferent and afferent), which extend outside the brain and spinal cord.

Brain

The brain is, of course, the supercomputer that controls all body functions, integrates the senses, responds to stimuli, and reasons and creates emotions. The areas of the brain most critical to voluntary movement are in the **cerebrum** and the **cerebellum.**

The cerebrum is the largest portion of the brain and is divided into two **hemispheres** and several **lobes.** The **longitudinal fissure** divides the right and left hemispheres of the brain. Deep inside the brain the two hemispheres are connected via a bridge called the **corpus callosum** (Fig. 8-9).

Primarily, the cerebrum is made of two types of nerve tissue, **gray matter** and **white matter.** A thin layer of gray

matter covers the outer surface of the cerebrum and is called the **cerebral cortex.** Deep to the gray matter is white matter, which makes up the largest portion of the cerebrum. Gray matter is composed primarily of neuron cell bodies, whereas white matter is mostly myelinated axons.

The lobes of the cerebrum divide the brain into areas that describe its function. These names correspond to the bones of the cranium. The **frontal lobes** contain areas that control the contraction of voluntary muscles, critical thought processes (reasoning), and motor control of speech (Fig. 8-10). The **parietal lobes** are the areas where sensory information is received and where language is comprehended. In the **temporal lobes,** sensory information is interpreted and memory is stored. Controlling vision and processing visual information takes place in the **occipital lobe.**

Deep within the brain are the **basal ganglia, thalamus,** and **hypothalamus.** The basal ganglia controls voluntary

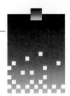

A

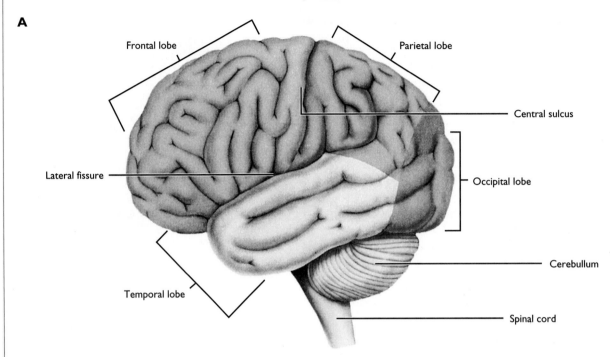

Frontal lobe

Parietal lobe

Central sulcus

Lateral fissure

Occipital lobe

Cerebellum

Temporal lobe

Spinal cord

B

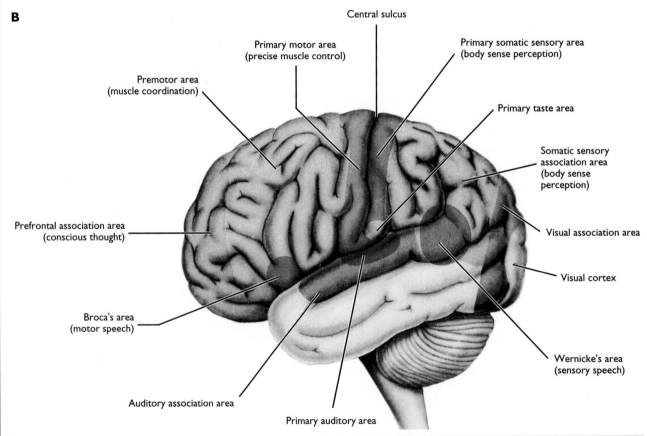

Central sulcus

Primary motor area
(precise muscle control)

Primary somatic sensory area
(body sense perception)

Premotor area
(muscle coordination)

Primary taste area

Somatic sensory
association area
(body sense
perception)

Prefrontal association area
(conscious thought)

Visual association area

Visual cortex

Broca's area
(motor speech)

Wernicke's area
(sensory speech)

Auditory association area

Primary auditory area

Figure 8-10. *A,* Lobes of the brain. *B,* Functional regions of the brain.
From Thibodeau, Patton: Structure and function of the body, *ed 10, St. Louis, 1996, Mosby.*

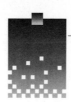
motor function, whereas the thalamus directs sensory information within the brain. The hypothalamus has several internal components that involve a variety of functions, such as regulating body temperature, appetite, and gastrointestinal activity, releasing of hormones from the pituitary gland, and controlling strong emotions, such as fear.

Within the cerebrum, there are several open areas known as **ventricles,** which produce and contain **cerebrospinal fluid. Choroid plexus,** which are specialized cells in the cerebrum, produce the fluid. The clear cerebrospinal fluid provides nutrients to the CNS and circulates from the ventricles down through the **central canal** of the spinal cord.

The cerebellum is a separate region posterior and somewhat inferior to the cerebrum. The cerebellum interacts with various areas of the cerebrum, processing sensory and motor information that controls posture, repetitive motion, and accuracy of skeletal movement.

Spinal cord

The spinal cord consists of long segments of neural tissue that reach from the brainstem through the **foramen magnum** of the occipital bone, down through the consecutive **vertebral canal,** approximately to the level of the second lumbar vertebrae (L_2). The distal end of the spinal cord is called the **conus medullaris.** From here, there are many branches of spinal nerves known as the **cauda equina,** or *horse's tail,* that continue through the vertebral canal.

A cross-section of the spinal cord shows the butterfly-shaped gray matter surrounded by white matter (Fig. 8-11). This arrangement is opposite that found in the cerebrum. The gray matter of the spinal cord is divided into **anterior** and **posterior horns** with an intermediate area connecting the two. These areas correspond to a variety of different specialized tracts of neural tissue, which correspond with the brain. The anterior horn is actually the location of cell bodies

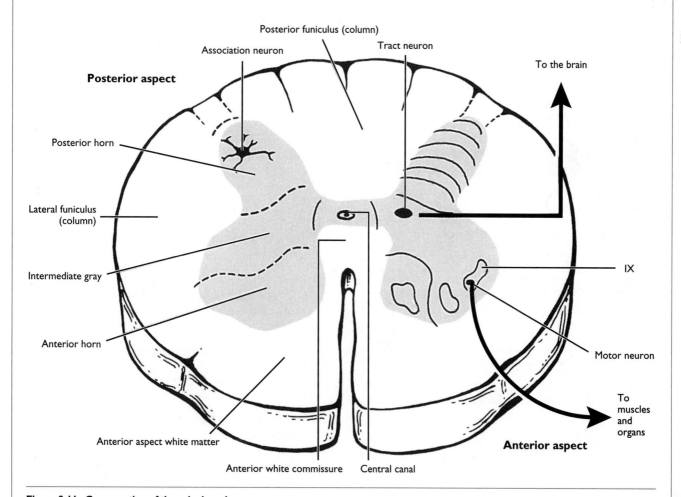

Figure 8-11. Cross-section of the spinal cord.
From Cramer, Darby: Basic and clinical anatomy of the spine, spinal cord, and ANS, *St. Louis, 1995, Mosby.*

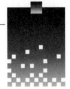

of efferent neurons, which innervate skeletal muscle. The posterior horns are dedicated to receiving incoming sensory information. The anterior and posterior horns connect to the anterior and posterior nerve roots, respectively, which exit from the spinal cord.

Inside the white matter of the spinal cord, there are nerve tracts that run to and from the brain and peripheral body parts. Some tracts are myelinated and some are unmyelinated. The afferent **ascending tracts** carry sensory impulses toward the brain, whereas efferent **descending tracts** carry impulses to muscles and body organs. Each tract has a specific name and serves a particular section of the body's normal functions. For example, the **spinocervicothalamic tract** is an afferent tract that is associated with touch and vibration. The **corticospinal tract** carries impulses to voluntary skeletal muscles.

Meninges

The CNS is wrapped by three layers of connective tissue called **meninges.** Named from most superficial to deep, the layers are the **dura mater, arachnoid mater,** and the **pia mater.** The dura mater is the toughest of the three layers and attaches to the inside of the cranial bones. The arachnoid mater is a thin membrane that holds the cerebrospinal fluid around the brain. The pia mater has blood vessels that provide nutrients to nearby tissues of the brain and spinal cord.

■ ■ ■ Exercise 8-4. Central nervous system

Complete the following statements based on your familiarity with the central nervous system.

1. The two divisions of the nervous system are the
   _____ and
   _____.

2. The _____ and
   _____ make up the CNS.

3. The _____ and
   _____ are two areas of
   the brain critical to voluntary movement.

4. The _____ is the largest
   portion of the brain and is divided into two hemispheres.

5. The _____ is the
   portion of the brain that deals with accuracy of movement.

6. The _____
   separates the two hemispheres of the cerebrum.

7. The two hemispheres of the cerebrum are attached via
   the _____.

8. The cerebral cortex is primarily made up of
   _____.

9. The _____ lobe of the
   cerebrum controls reasoning and voluntary motor control.

10. Interpretation of sensory information and memory storage occurs in the _____ lobe.

11. The _____ is
    an area deep inside the brain that also controls voluntary motor activity.

12. The _____ is
    an area deep inside the brain that controls body temperature and appetite.

13. Cerebrospinal fluid is produced by the
    _____ in the
    _____.

14. The _____
    interacts with various areas of the cerebrum and process sensory and motor information to control posture, repetitive motion, and accuracy of skeletal movement.

15. The spinal cord ends at the _____ vertebral level.

16. The distal end of the spinal cord is known as the
    _____.

17. The collection of spinal nerves at the end of the cord are called the _____.

18. There are _____ pairs of spinal nerves,
    whereas there are _____ vertebrae.

19. The butterfly shape in the cross-section of the spinal cord is made up of _____.

20. The _____
    of the spinal cord are the locations where cell bodies of efferent neurons innervate skeletal muscle.

21. The _____ of the spinal cord
    are dedicated to receiving incoming sensory information.

22. Pathways that carry impulses toward the brain are called the _____.

23. Pathways that carry impulses from the brain to the muscles and organs are the _____.

24. The _____ is the
    most superficial covering over the brain and spinal cord.

25. The _____
    is the deepest covering over the brain and spinal cord.

Exercise 8-5. *Structures of the brain and spinal cord*

Identify the structures of the brain and spinal cord in Figures 8-12, 8-13, and 8-14.

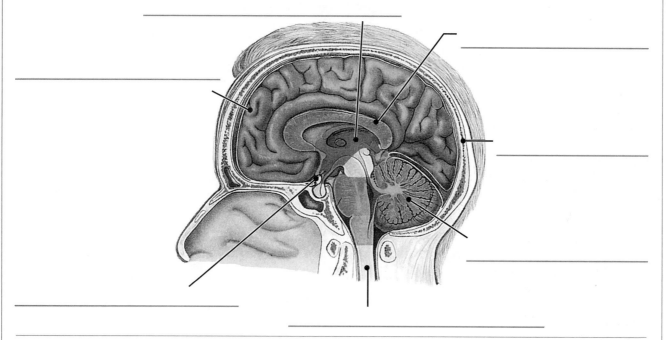

Figure 8-12. Major regions of the central nervous system.
From Thibodeau, Patton: Structure and function of the body, *ed 10, St. Louis, 1996, Mosby.*

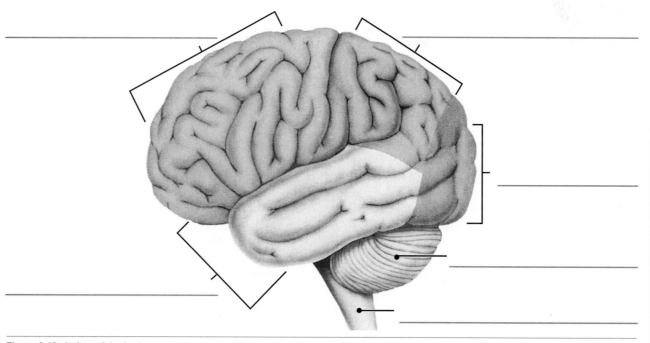

Figure 8-13. Lobes of the brain.
From Thibodeau, Patton: Structure and function of the body, *ed 10, St. Louis, 1996, Mosby.*

Exercise 8-5 continued on page 170

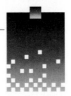

Posterior aspect

To _____

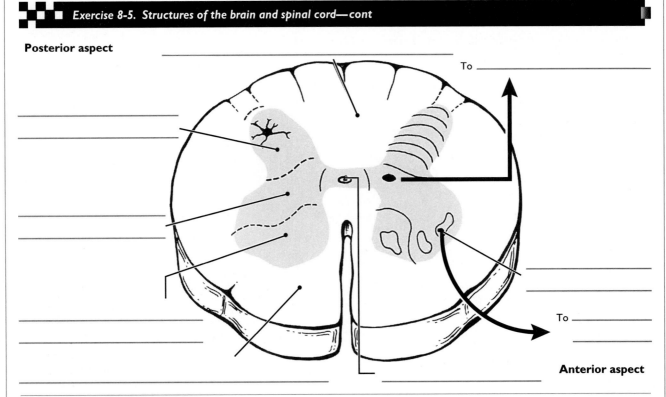

To _____

Anterior aspect

Figure 8-14. Cross-section of the spinal cord.
From Cramer, Darby: Basic and clinical anatomy of the spine, spinal cord, and ANS, St. Louis, 1995, Mosby.

Peripheral Nervous System

Twelve pairs of **cranial nerves** and 31 pairs of **spinal nerves** branch off the brain and spinal cord. These structures lie outside the physical enclosures of the cranium and vertebral column. Both systems use the efferent (motor) and afferent (sensory) neurons to control the body and receive feedback from it.

Cranial nerves

The cranial nerves primarily innervate the special senses, such as sight, smell, taste, and hearing, as well as equilibrium, tongue movements, sensations in the throat, facial expressions, and the muscles of respiration (Table 8-1) (Fig. 8-15).

Table 8-1 Cranial nerves

Nerve	Function
I Olfactory	Sense of smell (sensory)
II Optic	Vision (sensory)
III Oculomotor	Muscles inside orbit that control eye movement and focus (motor)
IV Trochlear	Eye movement (motor)

Table 8-1 Cranial nerves—cont

Nerve	Function
V Trigeminal	Eyes, face, forehead, scalp, mouth, cheeks, lips, jaw (sensory)
	Muscles of the temporomandibular joint (motor)
VI Abducens	Eye movement (motor)
VII Facial	Muscles of the face (motor)
	Taste (sensory)
VIII Vestibulocochlear (acoustic)	Equilibrium and hearing (sensory)
IX Glossopharyngeal	Muscles of pharynx (motor)
	Taste (sensory)
X Vagus	Muscles of throat and respiration (motor)
	Thoracic and abdominal regions (sensory)
XI Spinal accessory	Muscles of cervical and thoracic spine (motor)
XII Hypoglossal	Muscles of tongue (motor)

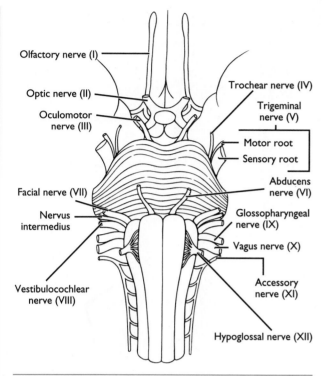

Figure 8-15. Cranial nerves.
From Greenstein: Clinical assessment of neuromusculoskeletal disorders, *St. Louis, 1997, Mosby.*

Labels for Figure 8-15:
- Olfactory nerve (I)
- Optic nerve (II)
- Oculomotor nerve (III)
- Trochear nerve (IV)
- Trigeminal nerve (V)
- Motor root
- Sensory root
- Abducens nerve (VI)
- Facial nerve (VII)
- Nervus intermedius
- Glossopharyngeal nerve (IX)
- Vagus nerve (X)
- Accessory nerve (XI)
- Vestibulocochlear nerve (VIII)
- Hypoglossal nerve (XII)

Study Note

To remember the cranial nerves by name, devise your own acrostic.

I	O	_____
II	O	_____
III	O	_____
IV	T	_____
V	T	_____
VI	A	_____
VII	F	_____
VIII	V(A)	_____
IX	G	_____
X	V	_____
XI	S(A)	_____
XII	H	_____

Spinal nerves

Spinal nerves are mixed in nature, carrying impulses to and from the CNS along paired motor and sensory neurons. Innervation of skeletal muscle by each nerve root level is labeled according to its **myotome,** whereas sensory innervation is labeled according to its **dermatome** (Fig. 8-16). Though the two patterns of innervation are similar, they are not identical. For motor nerve root innervation, refer to the discussion of each individual muscle.

As the name suggests, the spinal nerves directly branch off the spinal cord. Between the cranium and L_2, there are a total of *31 pairs of spinal nerves* that branch out from the spinal cord, exiting through the **intervertebral foramen** between each adjacent vertebra to become the roots of the PNS. All organ systems and skeletal muscles in the body can be controlled from these spinal nerves.

Spinal nerve roots are described by a number that corresponds to the vertebra where the nerve root exits the vertebral canal. Cervical nerve roots are labeled for the specific vertebra above which the nerve root passes, with the exception of C_8, which lies below the C_7 vertebra. All other spinal nerves are labeled for the specific vertebra below which the nerve passes. Therefore a spinal nerve level will actually be inferior to the actual vertebral level of the same number (Fig. 8-17).

In several specialized areas, spinal nerves branch off and then reattach to one another forming one of three intricate neural networks, each called a **plexus.** These three areas correspond to the upper and lower extremities and are known as the **cervical plexus, lumbosacral plexus,** and **brachial plexus** (Table 8-2) (Figs. 8-18 and 8-19). The spinal nerves in the thoracic region exit the intervertebral foramen and connect directly with their components.

The PNS is further divided into two more systems, delineating involuntary and voluntary control. These are the **autonomic nervous system** (ANS) and the **somatic nervous system** (SNS).

Table 8-2. Nerves of the upper and lower extremities

Brachial plexus	Lumbosacral plexus
Musculocutaneous	Superior and inferior gluteal
Median	Femoral
Ulnar	Obturator
Axillary	Sciatic
Radial	Tibial
	Common peroneal
	Pudendal

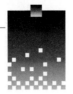

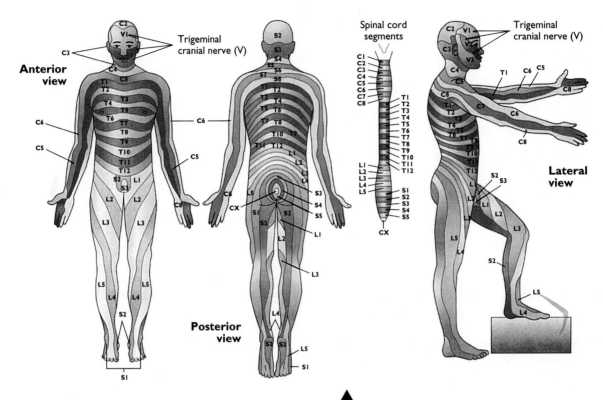

Anterior view

Posterior view

Lateral view

Trigeminal cranial nerve (V)

Spinal cord segments

▲

Figure 8-16. Dermatome chart
From Thibodeau, Patton: The human body in health & disease, ed 2, St. Louis, 1992, Mosby.

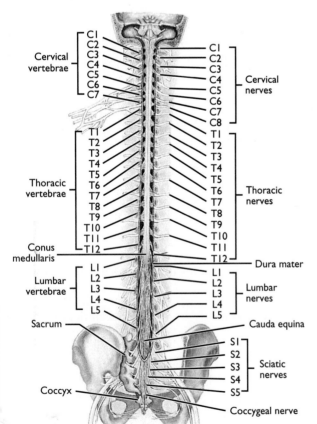

Cervical vertebrae

Cervical nerves

Thoracic vertebrae

Thoracic nerves

Conus medullaris

Dura mater

Lumbar vertebrae

Lumbar nerves

Sacrum

Cauda equina

Sciatic nerves

Coccyx

Coccygeal nerve

Figure 8-17. Spinal cord and spinal nerves.
From Thibodeau, Patton: The human body in health & disease, ed 2, St. Louis, 1992, Mosby.

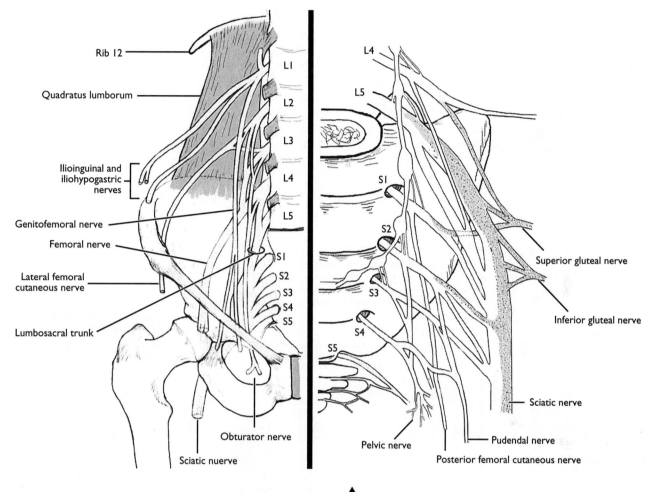

Rib 12

Quadratus lumborum

Ilioinguinal and
iliohypogastric
nerves

Genitofemoral nerve

Femoral nerve

Lateral femoral
cutaneous nerve

Lumbosacral trunk

L1
L2
L3
L4
L5
S1
S2
S3
S4
S5

Obturator nerve

Sciatic nuerve

L4
L5
S1
S2
S3
S4
S5

Superior gluteal nerve

Inferior gluteal nerve

Sciatic nerve

Pelvic nerve

Pudendal nerve

Posterior femoral cutaneous nerve

▲

Figure 8-18. Lumbosacral plexus.
From Mathers et al: Clinical anatomy principles, *St. Louis, 1996, Mosby.*

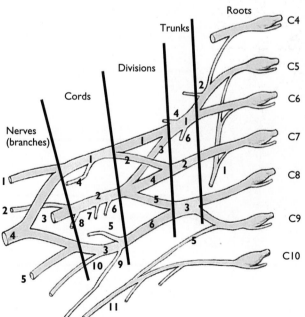

Roots
Trunks
Divisions
Cords
Nerves
(branches)

C4
C5
C6
C7
C8
C9
C10

◄ **Figure 8-19. Brachial plexus.**
From Mathers et al: Clinical anatomy principles, *St. Louis, 1996, Mosby.*

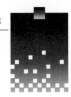

Autonomic Nervous System

The ANS controls the involuntary activities in the body, such as the **visceral** (organ) activities and responses via peripheral nerves. The ANS can cause changes in normal body functions, which are unconscious in nature. For example, it can speed up or slow down the rate of the heart beat and respirations, dilate or constrict the iris of the eye, and increase or decrease digestion. The ANS is an efferent system in that it causes a change in the activity of muscles or organs (Fig. 8-20).

The ANS can be further subdivided into the **sympathetic nervous system** and the **parasympathetic nervous system.** These two subsystems work in opposition with one another, each countering the other. The unconscious regulation of the body's systems relies on feedback received from the sensory organs throughout the body.

The sympathetic division prepares the body to defend itself in times of perceived stress by stimulating vital organs. The response to the stimulation is an increased heart rate, increased respiration and blood pressures, dilated pupils, and

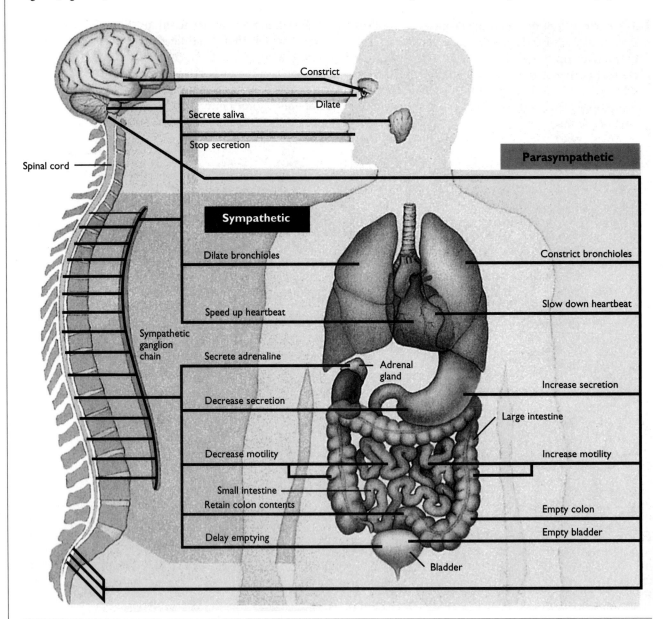

Figure 8-20. Autonomic nervous system.
From Thibodeau, Patton: Structure and function of the body, ed 10, St. Louis, 1996, Mosby.

a diversion of oxygenated blood to skeletal muscle and away from organs such as the stomach and intestines. This is the body's way of responding to threat and maximizing available oxygen in a mission of "fight or flight."

The parasympathetic division resets the body back to *normal*, or homeostasis. It is the responsibility of the parasympathetic division to return the body to its natural balance by normalizing blood pressure, calming respiration, and encouraging normal digestion and internal organ function. This division does not respond to emergency need but to the more regular, consistent activities performed by the body.

Somatic Nervous System

The SNS innervates voluntary skeletal muscles through large myelinated axons. With direction from the cerebrum and cerebellum, these activities can be fine tuned and carried out with precision and can improve with practice.

Neuromuscular Regulation of Movement

Not only does the nervous system alert the individual to pain and to changes in temperature and touch, as well as provide the capability to contract skeletal muscle, it has the intricate function of making the individual aware of the degree of movement and location of his or her body parts in space. This is accomplished by both sensory and motor neurons in specialized structures called muscle spindles, golgi tendon organs, and proprioceptors.

Muscle spindles

Within skeletal muscle, there is a sophisticated component known as the **muscle spindle,** which constantly relates information to the CNS about current muscle length, the speed of muscle contraction, and the stretch to which a muscle tissue may be subjected.

Long muscle fibers responsible for skeletal movement are called **extrafusal fibers.** Smaller fibers within the muscle belly and surrounded by connective tissue are called **intrafusal fibers.** These intrafusal fibers are innervated by two sets of sensory neurons, called Ia- and II-type neurons, which wrap around the intrafusal fibers. These neurons are stimulated by changes in the diameter and length of the fibers during the activity of the muscle belly. As a muscle changes length, the sensory fibers are stimulated, sending information to the CNS.

A gamma motor neuron is attached to the ends of the intrafusal fiber group, causing a stretch to the intrafusal fiber group, even when the overall muscle length becomes shorter. This attachment allows the sensory fibers to constantly monitor the changes in muscle length during all types of activity.

A muscle spindle gets its name from its tapered or spindlelike shape. Postural muscles, whose lengths do not change significantly over a period of time, have few muscle spindles. However, muscles involved in fine, precise movements, such as those in the fingers or eyes, have many muscle spindles.

Golgi tendon organs

Also reporting to the CNS, specialized receptors exist in skeletal muscle tendons near where they attach to the muscle fibers. In some areas, terminal branches of sensory axons are wrapped around groups of collagen fibers. When the tendon is stretched, the terminal branches become compressed, triggering an impulse along the axon and returning afferent information on the degree of strain on the tendon back to the CNS. The afferent neurons and collagen fiber groups are called **golgi tendon organs.** Not all collagen tissue has afferent innervation.

Proprioception

Knowing where a body part is located in space without visually checking is the result of the sense of **proprioception,** or joint posture sense. This sense is the result of the integration of sensory information provided by muscle spindles, golgi tendon organs, and **joint receptors.** Joint receptors are afferent components located within the synovial joint capsules and ligaments. Collecting information from various stimulation allows a person to monitor the position of the head, trunk, and extremities while stationary, as well as to coordinate movements throughout the body.

Reflex arc

Occasionally, the body reacts to stimuli without conscious thought or higher brain function. This reaction is called a **reflex.** It is accomplished by a stimulus to an afferent (sensory) neuron at the periphery of the body that is carried to the spinal cord through the posterior horn. Via an association neuron, the stimulus then moves on to an effector (motor) neuron in the anterior horn and back to the effector, which is usually a skeletal muscle. Stimulus, such as pain or extreme temperature, can result in an immediate response to protect the body. Quickly withdrawing one's hand from a hot stove is an example of a reflex; a conscious decision is not needed to hasten the action in a healthy individual.

The chain of sensory neuron, association neuron, and effector neuron to the effector is called the **reflex arc** (Fig. 8-21). The reflex arc receives information and responds to stimuli before sending or receiving information along the ascending or descending tracts of the spinal cord. Examples of the reflex arc in action begin with stimulus such as extreme pain, sudden temperature change, or a muscle stretch, often resulting in skeletal muscle action.

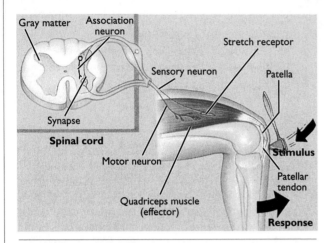

Figure 8-21. Patellar reflex.
From Thibodeau, Patton: Structure and function of the body, ed 10, St. Louis, 1996, Mosby.

Exercise 8-6. Peripheral nervous system

Complete the following statements based on your familiarity with the peripheral nervous system.

1. Peripheral nerves dedicated to the special senses such as hearing, sight, taste, and respiration are the

   _____.

2. Peripheral nerves that innervate the skeletal muscles and organs are _____.

3. The cranial nerve that is responsible for equilibrium and hearing is the _____

   _____.

4. The cranial nerve that is responsible for respiration and innervating the diaphragm is the

   _____.

5. A network of spinal nerves that innervate the upper extremity originates from the

   _____.

6. The "fight-or-flight" response comes from the

   _____

   division of the ANS.

7. Homeostasis is achieved by the

   _____

   division of the ANS.

Exercise 8-6. Peripheral nervous system—cont

8. To perform hip flexion and knee extension, contraction of the quadriceps femoris muscles occurs via the

   _____ nervous system.

9. An afferent impulse that immediately results in an efferent response is an example of the

   _____.

10. The structures that report tension on tendons are the

    _____.

11. The complex component that is made up of two afferent neurons and one motor neuron and reports muscle length is the _____.

12. Joint position sense is known as

    _____.

13. Elements involved in proprioception are

    _____,

    _____,

    and _____.

Exercise 8-7. *Identify components of the reflex arc*

Identify the components of the reflex arc on Figures 8-22 and 8-23.

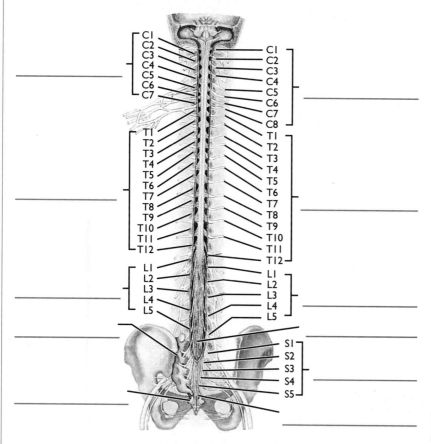

Figure 8-22. Spinal cord and spinal nerves.
From Thibodeau, Patton: The human body in health &
disease, *ed 2, St. Louis, 1992, Mosby.*

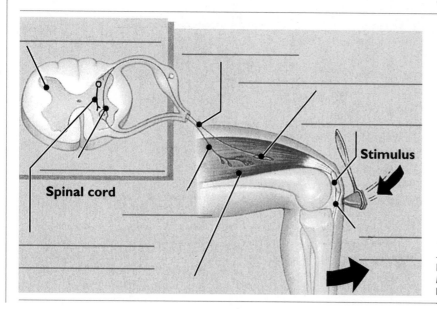

Stimulus

Spinal cord

Figure 8-23. Patellar reflex.
From Thibodeau, Patton: Structure and function of the
body, *ed 10, St. Louis, 1996, Mosby.*

Key Words

abducens nerve
acetylcholine
action potential
active transport system
afferent neuron
"all-or-none" response
anterior horn
arachnoid mater
ascending tracts
association neuron
autonomic nervous system
axillary nerve
axon
basal ganglia
bipolar neuron
brachial plexus
brain
cauda equina
cell body
central canal
central nervous system
central sulcus
cerebellum
cerebral cortex
cerebrospinal fluid
cerebrum
cervical plexus
choroid plexus
common peroneal nerve
conductivity
conus medullaris
corpus callosum
corticospinal tract
cranial nerves
dendrites
depolarized neuron
dermatome
descending tracts
dura mater
efferent neuron
extrafusal fibers
facial nerve
foramen magnum

frontal lobes
glossopharyngeal nerve
gluteal nerve, superior and inferior
golgi tendon organs
gray matter
hemispheres
hypoglossal nerve
hypothalamus
intervertebral foramen
intrafusal fibers
involuntary
irritability
joint receptors
lobes
longitudinal fissure
lumbosacral plexus
median nerve
meninges
motor end plate
motor neuron
motor unit
multipolar neuron
muscle spindle
musculocutaneous nerve
myelin sheath
myotome
nerve impulses
nervous system
neurilemma
neuromuscular junction
neuron
neurotransmitters
nodes of Ranvier
obturator nerve
occipital lobe
oculomotor nerve
olfactory nerve
optic nerve
parasympathetic nervous system
parietal lobes
peripheral nerves
peripheral nervous system
pia mater
plexus

polarity
polarized neuron
posterior horn
potassium ions
proprioception
pudendal nerve
radial nerve
receptor
reflex
reflex arc
refractory period
repolarized neuron
resting potential
saltatory conduction
Schwann's cells
sciatic nerve
sensory neuron
sodium ions
sodium-potassium pump
somatic nervous system
spinal accessory nerve
spinal cord
spinal nerves
spinocervicothalamic tract
sympathetic nervous system
synapse
synaptic cleft
synaptic vesicles
temporal lobes
terminal branches
thalamus
threshold stimulus
tibial nerve
trigeminal nerve
trochear nerve
ulnar nerve
unipolar neuron
vagus nerve
ventricles
vertebral canal
vestibulocochlear nerve
visceral
voluntary
white matter

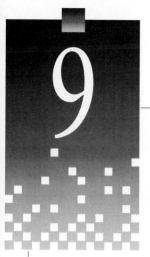

Cardiovascular System, Blood, and Lymphatic System

66 *This chapter will enable you to identify the primary elements of the cardiovascular and lymphatic systems as they affect human movement.* **99**

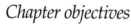

Chapter objectives

The student will be able to:

1. Identify the primary structures of the heart.

2. Identify the pathways of blood through the heart.

3. Identify the significant elements of cardiac muscle tissue.

4. Describe the electrical impulse mechanism as it controls cardiac muscle contraction.

5. Identify primary vascular structures.

6. Describe the physical characteristics of blood.

7. Identify the significant structures and their functions within the lymphatic system.

Internal Anatomy of the Heart

The supply line that carries oxygen and nutrients to the body depends on pressure for propulsion through the vascular system. This pressure is maintained by the pumping action of the heart and rhythmic cardiac muscle contractions. The heart is located in the thoracic cavity between the **lungs** in an area called the **mediastinum,** which is between the sternum and vertebrae. The **base** of the heart is the wider, superior portion; its **apex** is the narrow inferior tip, which is slightly left of the sternum. The entire heart lies between the second and sixth ribs (Fig. 9-1).

The heart is an enclosed structure with four **chambers.**

It receives blood into its right side and expels it from its left. The thick walls are primarily cardiac muscle that encircles the chambers and, upon contraction, compresses the blood inside each chamber, forcing it into the next open chamber or into a blood vessel. There is a one-way path for the blood, with backwash prevented by **valves** that are between the chambers and in some blood vessels.

The heart itself is contained inside a flexible double membranous sac called the **pericardium.** The innermost membrane is called the **visceral pericardium,** or **epicardium,** and it is also the most external layer of the heart itself. The outside membrane of the sac is more fibrous and is known as the **parietal pericardium.** The two membranes are separated by a thin layer of clear fluid that allows them to move independently over one another as the heart expands and contracts.

Heart chambers

The four chambers of the heart begin with the right and left **atria** (atrium, *singular*), located most superiorly. The inferior pair of chambers are the right and left ventricles, which are much larger than the atria and located where the myocardium is thickest. This is especially true of the left ventricle where the pressure on the blood from cardiac muscle contraction is greatest. The two atria are separated by the **interatrial septum,** whereas the right and left ventricles are separated by the **interventricular septum** (see Fig. 9-1).

The wall of each chamber has several layers, which can be examined from superficial to deep. Deep to the epicardium is the **myocardium**, or **cardiac muscle.** The internal lining of the heart is the **endocardium,** which has a smooth surface continuous with the inner lining of the arteries and veins and with the valves between each chamber (see Fig. 9-1).

Since the heart is essentially a bag with walls made of constantly contracting muscle fibers, it makes sense that the

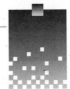

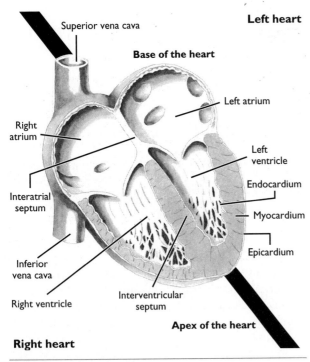

Left heart

Base of the heart

Superior vena cava

Left atrium

Right atrium

Left ventricle

Interatrial septum

Endocardium

Myocardium

Epicardium

Inferior vena cava

Right ventricle

Interventricular septum

Apex of the heart

Right heart

Figure 9-1. Internal anatomy of the heart.
From Huszar: Basic dysrhythmias: interpretation and management, *St. Louis, 1988, Mosby.*

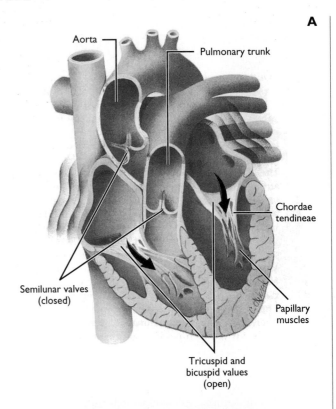

A

Aorta

Pulmonary trunk

Chordae tendineae

Semilunar valves (closed)

Papillary muscles

Tricuspid and bicuspid valves (open)

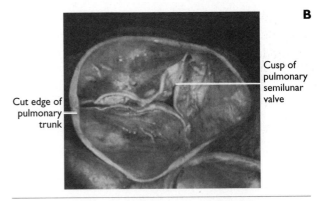

B

Cut edge of pulmonary trunk

Cusp of pulmonary semilunar valve

Figure 9-2. A, Heart valves; B, pulmonary semilunar valve.
From Thibodeau, Patton: Structure & function of the body, ed 9, *St. Louis, 1992, Mosby.*

muscle tissue must have a fixed source of attachment or origin; otherwise, it might be inclined to collapse and then be unable to receive any quantity of blood. To remain open between contractions, there is a semirigid fibrous framework near the large openings within the heart, which continues transversely through the walls of each chamber. This framework is called the **skeleton of the heart.**

Heart valves

The valves within the heart prevent the reversal of the blood flow along its intended path. There are two types of valves: **atrioventricular** (AV) and **semilunar.** The two AV valves are actually large multiple folds of endothelium located at the entrance to each ventricle. The valve between the right atrium and right ventricle is called the **tricuspid valve,** named for its three flaps; the valve between the left atrium and left ventricle is called the **mitral,** or **bicuspid valve,** named for its two flaps. These valves are prevented from collapsing by the **chordae tendineae,** or stringlike attachments, that connect them to the ventricular walls via **papillary muscles** (Fig. 9-2).

A heart valve opens as blood flows from the atrium into the ventricle. The valve then closes when the pressure on the blood inside the ventricle increases as the myocardium in the ventricle wall begins its contraction and the area available

inside the ventricle becomes smaller. This muscle contraction squeezes the blood, forcing it out the only exit, which is the blood vessel that is connected to either the lungs or the body's vascular network. The closed valves prevent the high pressure blood from flowing back into the atria.

Semilunar valves, also made of endothelium, are small pouches with interlocking flaps. These valves differ from AV valves in that they have no chordae tendineae or papillary muscles. They prevent blood from returning to the ventricles from the pulmonary arteries and aorta. The **pulmonary** semilunar valves are inside the **pulmonary trunk** before it branches into the **pulmonary arteries.** The **aortic semilunar valve** is found at the opening of the **aorta.**

Pathway of Blood through the Heart

From the large blood vessels called the **inferior and superior venae cavae,** deoxygenated blood enters the heart at the right atrium; it passes over the right AV valve (tricuspid) and moves to the right ventricle. The powerful compressive forces push the blood out toward the lungs through the pulmonary trunk, past the first semilunar valve, and through the pulmonary arteries to the lungs. The carbon dioxide is exchanged for oxygen, and the blood reenters the heart through the **pulmonary veins** into the left atrium. The now oxygenated blood is pushed on to the left ventricle by passing the left AV valve (bicuspid). A strong left ventricular contraction forces the blood out of the heart through the aorta, past the second semilunar valve. This entire process occurs very quickly as a

result of the simultaneous contraction of the mycardium within both atria, followed by simultaneous contraction of the mycardium within both ventricles (Fig. 9-3).

Monitoring the Activity of the Heart

Since the constant availability of oxygen is critical to the life of all body tissues, it is important to assess the current activity and efficiency of the heart. Simple techniques make it possible to gather information on this activity so that valuable data can be documented and sudden changes or abnormalities can be reported.

Heart rate

The number of cardiac muscle contractions per minute is called the **heart rate** (HR), and it is recorded as beats per minute (bpm). It is possible to feel the HR by placing the hand over the anterior thoracic region, inferior to the clavicle, and left of the sternum. The normal HR for the average adult

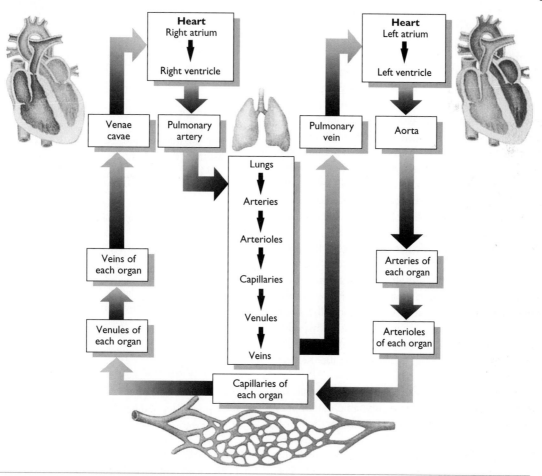

Figure 9-3. Blood flow in the circulatory system.
From Thibodeau, Patton: Structure & function of the body, ed 9, St. Louis, 1992, Mosby.

at rest is 70 bpm. If the resting HR of an adult is greater than 100 bpm, it is referred to as **tachycardia,** or rapid HR. When the resting HR of an adult is less than 60 bpm, it is referred to as **bradycardia,** or slow HR.

With the contraction of the ventricles, there is an intermittent rhythmic surge in the pressure against the walls of the arteries. This surge is known as the **pulse,** and it can be felt in arteries that lie close to the surface of the body. Aside from listening with a stethoscope, it is possible to monitor the HR by palpating the pulse. The most common locations where the pulse can be monitored are the **common carotid artery** and the **radial artery** (see Fig. 9-10).

The volume of blood that is pumped out of the heart through the aorta with each contraction is called the **stroke volume** (SV), and it is recorded in milliliters per beat (mpb). Sophisticated equipment is required to monitor the SV. The overall efficiency of the heart is called the **cardiac output** (CO), and it is calculated by multiplying the HR by the SV:

$$CO = HR \times SV$$

Blood pressure

As previously discussed, the transport of oxygen and nutrients through the vascular system depends on the pressure that propels the blood forward. The blood pressure is the force that is exerted on the walls of the blood vessels; it is dependent upon the quantity of blood present, the strength of the contractions of the heart, and the peripheral resistance in the vascular system. **Peripheral resistance** is the opposition to the blood flow through a vessel and may differ with the blood viscosity (free-flowing quality) and the length and diameter of the vessels. Damage to the vessel walls or blockage can seriously decrease the diameter of the vessels.

During a series of ventricular contractions, the pressures within the aorta will rhythmically increase and decrease. When the ventricle contracts and blood rushes through the aorta, the pressure is at its peak. This value is known as the **systolic pressure.** As the contraction subsides and the aortic semilunar valve closes, the arterial pressure drops. This value is known as the **diastolic pressure.** While the ventricle is relaxed, it is refilling with blood in preparation for the next contraction.

Blood pressure is measured by using a device called a **sphygmomanometer,** which has an inflatable cuff that is wrapped around the upper extremity; it monitors the blood flow in the brachial artery. With a **stethoscope,** one can listen to the change in sound after the pressure from inflating the cuff is sharply increased and then slowly decreased. The numbers giving value to the systolic and diastolic pressures are recorded one over the other as if it were a fraction and

labeled in millimeters of mercury (Hg). The average blood pressure in a healthy adult is 120/80 mmHg. Abnormally high blood pressure is referred to as **hypertension,** whereas abnormally low blood pressure is **hypotension.**

Heart sounds

The heart beat that can be heard as a *lub-dub* through a stethoscope is actually the sound of the heart valves closing. The first sound, and usually the loudest of the two, is made by the mitral and tricuspid valves closing almost simultaneously. This is followed by the closing of the aortic pulmonary semilunar valves, the second heart sound. The actual blood flow and the contractions of the chambers are silent events.

Exercise 9-1. Structures of the heart

Complete the following statements based on your familiarity with the structures of the heart as discussed in this chapter.

1. The two structures that supply deoxygenated blood to the heart are the _____ and _____.

2. The space in which the heart is located is called the _____.

3. There are _____ chambers in the human heart.

4. The two inferior chambers of the heart, where the strongest cardiac muscle contractions occur, are the _____.

5. _____ divides the right and left ventricles.

6. The primary muscle layer of the heart is the _____.

7. The smooth inner layer of the heart, arteries, and veins, which also forms the heart valves, is the _____.

8. The rigid rings that prevent the chambers and valves from collapsing is the _____.

9. The valve located between the left atrium and left ventricle is the _____.

10. Blood vessels that carry deoxygenated blood away from the heart are called the _____ and _____.

■ *Exercise 9-1. Structures of the heart—cont*

11. The structure that prevents blood from flowing back into the right ventricle from the pulmonary trunk is the

    _____.

12. The first chamber to receive oxygenated blood is the

    _____.

13. The chamber with the thickest layer of myocardium and the strongest contraction is the

    _____.

14. The stringlike attachments that prevent the valves from collapsing when ventricular pressures increase are the

    _____.

15. The single structure through which oxygenated blood leaves the heart on its way to the body is the

    _____.

16. The structures that control the chordae tendineae as they attach to the ventricular wall are the

    _____.

17. A device used to listen to the heart and lung sounds is a

    _____.

18. The number of times the heart beats in a minute is called the _____.

19. Blood pressure is dependent upon three basic elements; they are _____,

    _____,

    and _____.

20. When the HR is greater than 100 bpm, it is referred to as

    _____.

21. Blood pressure is measured by using a

    _____.

22. The pressure value during ventricular contraction is known as the

    _____.

23. HR multiplied by the SV equals

    _____.

24. The pressure value during ventricular relaxation is known as _____.

25. Abnormally high blood pressure is referred to as

    _____.

■ *Exercise 9-2. Internal anatomy of the heart*

Identify the internal anatomy of the heart on Figures 9-4 and 9-5.

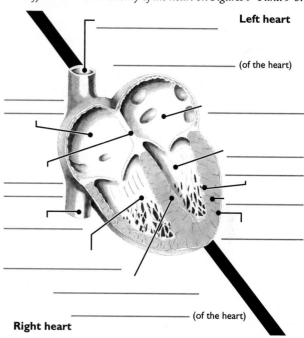

Left heart

_____ (of the heart)

Right heart

Figure 9-4. Internal anatomy of the heart.
From Huszar: Basic dysrhythmias: interpretation and management, *St. Louis, 1988, Mosby.*

_____ (of the heart)

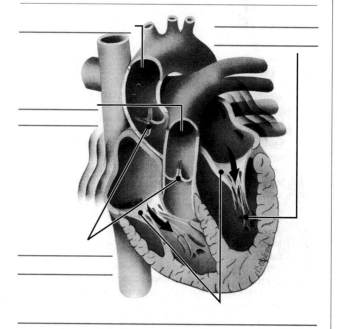

Figure 9-5. Heart valves.
From Thibodeau, Patton: Structure & function of the body, *ed 9, St. Louis, 1992, Mosby.*

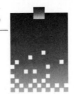

Exercise 9-3. Path of a blood through the heart

Beginning with deoxygenated blood approaching the heart, list the 14 areas through which a drop of blood must pass to complete the cardiac cycle, becoming oxygenated and ready for use by the body systems. Spaces have been designated where the names of certain valves should be included.

1. _____

2. _____

3. _____ *(valve)*

4. _____

5. _____

6. _____ *(valve)*

7. _____

8. _____

9. _____

10. _____

11. _____ *(valve)*

12. _____

13. _____ *(valve)*

14. _____

Cardiac Muscle Fibers

Cardiac muscle tissue is similar to skeletal muscle tissue in that both have striations and operate via sliding myofilaments. However, skeletal muscle fibers are separate structures, whereas cardiac muscle fibers are connected via **intercalated disks.** These disks allow direct transmission of depolarizing impulses to be communicated throughout the cardiac muscle fibers. Thus the entire myocardium layer can contract as a single functional unit. In skeletal muscle contraction the impulses are isolated to individual fibers. In cardiac muscle the impulses are shared, and an *all-or-none* response occurs throughout the entire organ, not just in the muscle fiber.

Electrical Stimulation of Cardiac Muscles

The impulse that stimulates the contraction of the cardiac muscle originates within the heart itself in a highly specialized area in the right atrium known as the **sinoatrial** (SA) **node,** also known as the **pacemaker of the heart.** The SA node is located on the superior wall of the right atrium. In this small area the depolarization of the cardiac muscle tissue repeatedly occurs at a rate of 70 to 80 times per minute. A wave of depolarization then travels throughout both atria and then to the **atrioventricular** (AV) **node** (Fig. 9-6).

The AV node is located on the interatrial septum on the inferior portion of the right atrium. Here, the impulse pauses while the atria contract simultaneously. The AV node is the only connection that carries an impulse between the atria and ventricles. The impulse continues down a pathway within the interventricular septum, which is called the **atrioventricular** (AV) **bundle** (bundle of His), to the apex of the heart. The AV bundle has two branches, one for each ventricle. From here the impulse spreads over the **Purkinje's fibers,** which penetrate deep into the myocardium of the ventricles from the apex of the heart. In this way the muscle tissue of the ventricles becomes innervated from the apex back toward the atria in a way that forces the blood up and out of the pulmonary arteries from the right ventricle and out of the aorta from the left ventricle. Like the atria, both ventricles are stimulated and contract simultaneously.

The changes in electrical activity in the heart can be monitored on an **electrocardiogram** (ECG). This activity is represented as a series of waves and spikes in an otherwise consistent level of electrical current, which is evidence of the depolarization and repolarization of chamber walls (Fig. 9-7).

Various landmarks on the normal wave pattern have been given labels by which they can be referenced. The first landmark is called the **P wave;** it represents the depolarization of the atria. This landmark is followed by the depolarization of the ventricles, known as the **QRS complex.** This event is quite significant, and the change in polarity is much more drastic than that of the P wave.

The repolarization of the atria occurs during the same time as the strong depolarization of the ventricles and, therefore, cannot be represented on an ECG. The repolarization of the ventricles follows the QRS complex and is represented as the **T wave.** This normal pattern is known as a **sinus rhythm.**

As the initiation of the electrical impulse occurs within the heart, which causes cardiac muscle contraction, the **autonomic nervous system** (ANS) controls the impulses that increase or decrease the rate of contraction. During exercise, the **sympathetic division** of the ANS arouses the body and dramatically increases the HR, increasing the delivery of oxygen to skeletal muscles. To correct, the **parasympathetic division** sends impulses to calm the heart and decrease its rate of contractions, thus maintaining **homeostasis.**

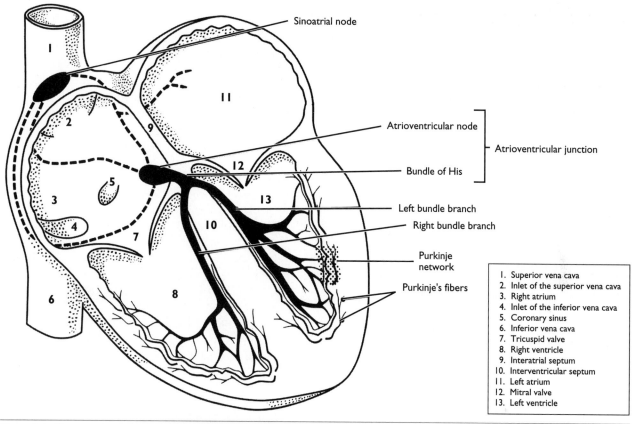

Figure 9-6. Electrical conduction system of the heart.
From Huszar: Basic dysrhythmias: interpretation and management, *St. Louis, 1988, Mosby.*

Exercise 9-4. *Cardiac impulse transmission*

Complete the following statements based on your familiarity with the structures of the heart as discussed in this chapter.

1. The structures present in cardiac muscle tissue that aids in the transmission of depolarizing impulses is called the

   _____.

2. What landmark appears on an ECG just before the contraction of both ventricles?

   _____

3. A specialized area on the floor of the right atrium that receives an impulse from the SA node is known as the

   _____

4. The _____ is a device that monitors the electrical activity of the heart.

5. The pacemaker of the heart is the

   _____.

6. The Purkinje's fibers carry the impulse into the myocardium of the ventricles from the

   _____.

7. Repolarization of both ventricles causes the
   _____ on an ECG.

8. Depolarization of the atria is recognized on an ECG by the _____.

9. Normal electrical activity of the heart is known as

   _____.

10. The _____ cannot be measured on the ECG because another simultaneous and stronger electrical event.

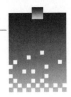

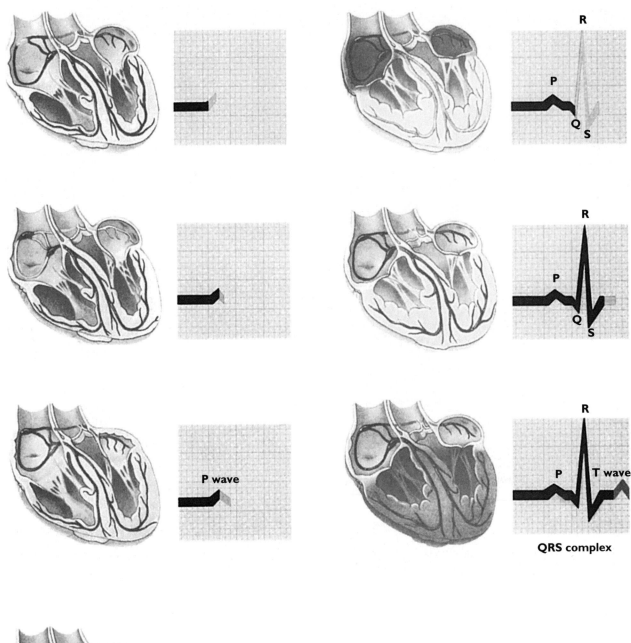

Figure 9-7. Events represented by the electrocardiogram (ECG).
From Thibodeau, Patton: Structure & function of the body, ed 9, St. Louis, 1992, Mosby.

Exercise 9-5. Identification of cardiac impulse activity

Identify cardiac impulse activity on Figure 9-8.

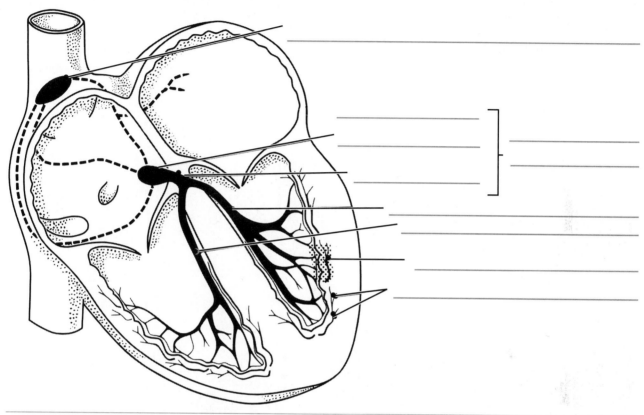

Figure 9-8. Electrical conduction system of the heart.
From Huszar: Basic dysrhythmias: interpretation and management, St. Louis, 1988, Mosby.

Exercise 9-6. Electrocardiographic wave pattern

Identify the following electrocardiographic wave pattern on Figure 9-9.

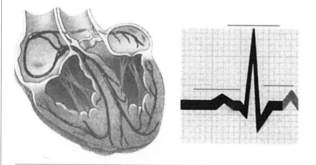

Figure 9-9. Electrical conduction system of the heart.
From Huszar: Basic dysrhythmias: interpretation and management, St. Louis, 1988, Mosby.

Exercise 9-7. Cardiac electrical activity

Complete the list of electrical events associated with cardiac function in the order in which they occur.

1. Impulse initiated in the

   _____.

2. _____depolarize and contract.

3. _____ is
   stimulated.

4. Impulse travels down the

   _____.

5. Impulse spreads throughout the

   _____.

6. _____ depolarize
   and contract.

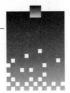

Blood Vessels

The blood vessels form a closed system
of circulation to and from the heart, as
well as to and from all organ systems
and tissues of the body (Figs. 9-10 and
9-11). These vessels include the **arteries, arterioles, capillaries, venules,** and
veins, by order of blood flowing
through them (see Fig. 9-3).

The walls of the blood vessels
have three layers, similar to the walls
of the heart, with the exception of the
capillaries (Fig. 9-12). The outermost
layer of a vessel is the **tunica adventitia,** which is made up of strong collagen fibers. In the arteries these collagen fibers prevent ruptures in the vessel wall. The middle layer is the **tunica media,** which contains smooth
muscle fibers and elastic connective
tissue. Contraction of this smooth
muscle causes **vasoconstriction,** or a
narrowing of the vessel. Relaxation of
the smooth muscle causes **vasodilation,** or an enlargement of the vessel.
The inner layer of the vessel is the
tunica intima; it is continuous with
the endocardium, which is quite
smooth, reducing friction as the blood
cells move through it. The hollow
opening created by the walls of the
blood vessel is called the **lumen,** and it
may vary in size according to the specific vessel or its state of vasodilation
or vasoconstriction.

Beginning at the aorta, arteries
are the vessels that carry oxygenated
blood to the organs and tissues, and
they are also the vessels of the circulatory system where the pressure of the
blood is greatest against its walls.
Arteries have the greatest quantity of
smooth muscle within their walls,
compared with any other blood vessel. Arterioles are the smaller branches of the arteries, about 0.5 mm in
diameter.

The vessels of the vascular system wherein the oxygen, nutrients, and
waste products of the tissues are
exchanged in the blood is at the level of

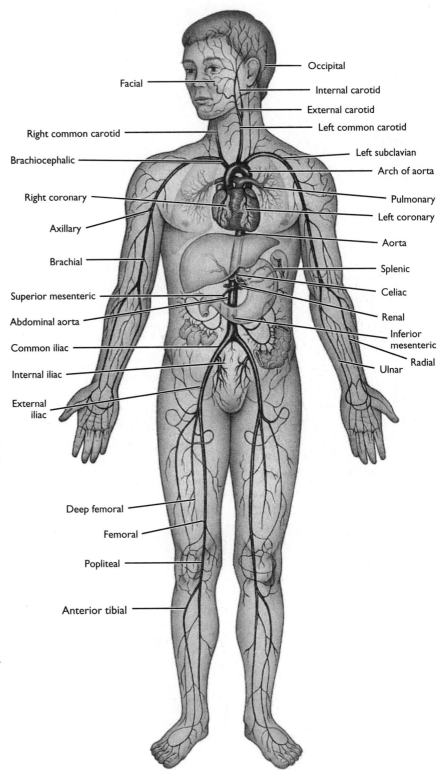

Figure 9-10. Principle arteries of the body.
From Thibodeau, Patton: The human body in health and disease, *ed 2, St. Louis, 1997, Mosby.*

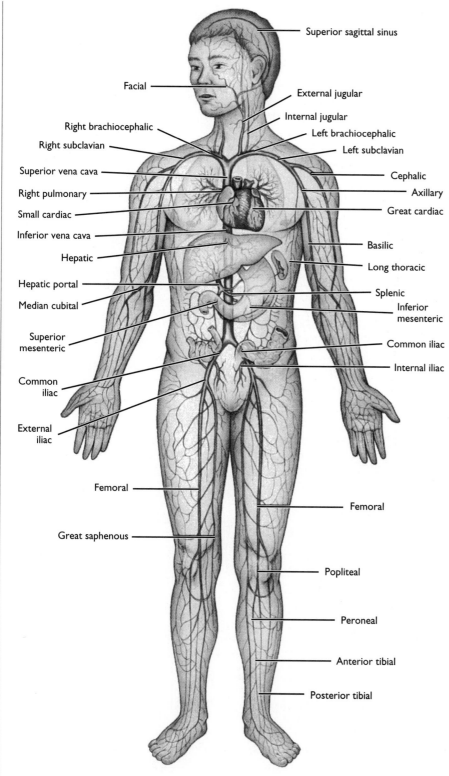

Figure 9-11. Principle veins of the body.
From Thibodeau, Patton: The human body in health and disease, *ed 2, St. Louis, 1997, Mosby.*

Labels (left side, top to bottom): Facial, Right brachiocephalic, Right subclavian, Superior vena cava, Right pulmonary, Small cardiac, Inferior vena cava, Hepatic, Hepatic portal, Median cubital, Superior mesenteric, Common iliac, External iliac, Femoral, Great saphenous

Labels (right side, top to bottom): Superior sagittal sinus, External jugular, Internal jugular, Left brachiocephalic, Left subclavian, Cephalic, Axillary, Great cardiac, Basilic, Long thoracic, Splenic, Inferior mesenteric, Common iliac, Internal iliac, Femoral, Popliteal, Peroneal, Anterior tibial, Posterior tibial

the capillaries. Each capillary consists of a single layer of tunica intima and measures only about 1 mm in length, and its lumen measures 0.01 mm in diameter. This allows room for only one red blood cell to slip through at a time. Capillaries form intricate microscopic networks called **capillary beds,** which infiltrate most of the tissues of the body.

Venules are enlargements in the vascular system that collect blood from the deoxygenated sides of the capillary beds. As a venule becomes larger, it forms veins that also have layers of tunica adventitia, tunica media, and tunica intima. The first significant difference in these layers from those found in arteries, however, is the thinner layer of smooth muscle (see Fig. 9-12). Vasoconstriction is not a strong quality of the blood vessels that return deoxygenated blood to the heart. Second, the tunica intima forms valves that prevent the backwash of blood in the low pressure venous system. These valves are similar to the semilunar valves of the heart. Within the vascular system, the pressure of the blood against the vessel walls is lowest in the veins; therefore the valves are necessary to return the blood to the right side of the heart and to prevent the pooling of blood as it returns.

Most of the venous structures of the body must carry blood against gravity in the upright individual. Venous blood flow is assisted by skeletal muscle contraction, which squeezes the tissues that lie between the muscles, thus helping the blood along its low-pressure path. The veins terminate at the **inferior** and **superior venae cavae** leading into the right atrium.

The forceful contraction of the heart muscle propels the blood through the body, and the pressure required to accomplish this can be measured at the arterial level. This pressure varies according to the dis-

189

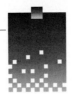

tance from the opening of the heart where blood is expelled (Fig. 9-13). Aortic pressure is the greatest, since it is so near the strong left ventricle. In the capillaries the pressure is approximately 25 to 35 mmHg and continues to drop in the venous system. By the time the blood reaches the inferior and superior venae cavae, there is almost no pressure exerted on the blood.

Blood supply to the cardiac muscle

Once oxygenated blood leaves the left ventricle through the aorta, two **coronary arteries** immediately branch off, carrying blood to the cardiac muscle itself. These two arteries are the beginning of a complex system that makes the heart one of the most vascular organs of the body (Figs. 9-14 and 9-15). After pumping blood through its own network of smaller arteries and capillaries, the blood is picked up by the **coronary veins** and returned to the right atrium via the **coronary sinus.**

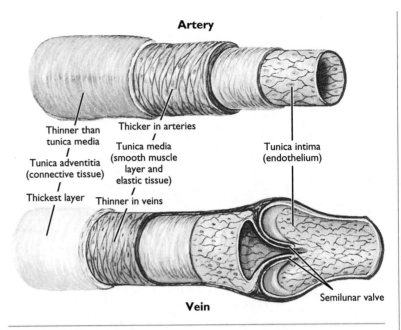

Figure 9-12. Artery and vein.
From Thibodeau, Patton: Structure & function of the body, ed 10, St. Louis, 1997, Mosby.

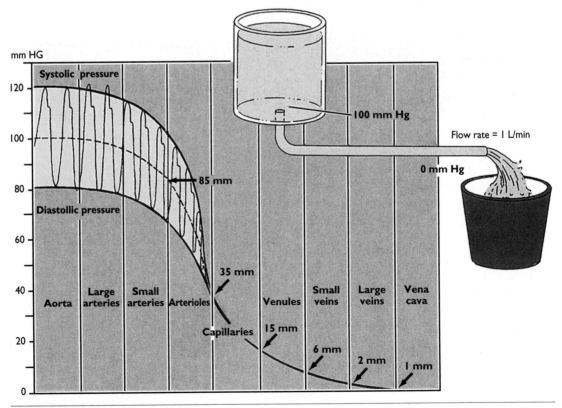

Figure 9-13. Pressure gradients in blood flow.
From Thibodeau, Patton: Structure & function of the body, ed 10, St. Louis, 1997, Mosby.

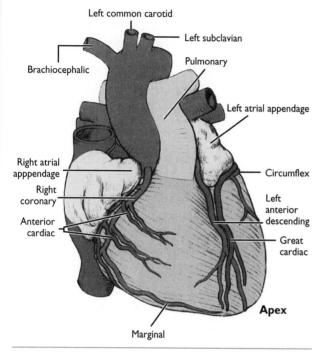

Figure 9-14. Coronary vessels (anterior view).
From Mathers et al: Clinical anatomy principles, *St. Louis, 1996, Mosby.*

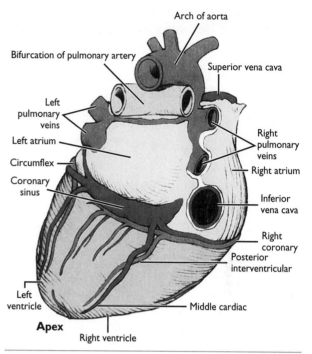

Figure 9-15. Coronary vessels (posterior view).
From Mathers et al: Clinical anatomy principles, *St. Louis, 1996, Mosby.*

■ Exercise 9-8. *Blood vessels*

Complete the following statements based on your familiarity with the blood vessels of the body as discussed in this chapter.

1. The blood vessels that carry oxygenated blood from the arteries to the capillaries are the

   _____.

2. Smooth muscle in the walls of the blood vessels are found in a layer called the

   _____.

3. The blood vessels that are made up of only tunica intima and are only large enough for one blood cell are the

   _____.

4. The significant difference in the tunica intima in the venous system, when compared with the arterial system, is the presence of

   _____.

5. The pulse in the carotid or radial arteries is actually the

   _____.

6. The network of blood vessels directly responsible for delivering oxygen and nutrients to the tissues is the

   _____.

7. The open area in a blood vessel is called the

   _____.

8. A decrease in the size of the open area within a blood vessel is called _____.

9. The _____
   carry oxygenated blood from the aorta to the cardiac muscle.

10. Deoxygenated blood returns to the right atria via the

    _____ and

    _____.

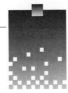

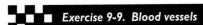
Exercise 9-9. Blood vessels

Identify the blood vessels on Figure 9-16.

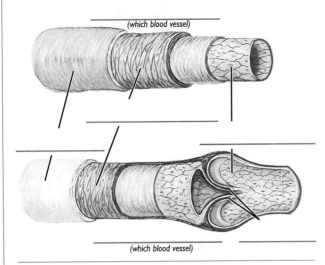

(which blood vessel)

(which blood vessel)

Figure 9-16. Artery and vein.
From Thibodeau, Patton: Structure & function of the body, ed 10, St. Louis, 1997, Mosby.

Blood

Blood transports oxygen, water, nutrients, hormones, antibodies, carbon dioxide, and other necessary substances to and from body tissues. Blood under pressure causes the valves of the heart to close (heart beat); blood is also necessary for the heart to perform its mechanical activity. The volume of blood within the heart is needed to fill and provide a slight stretch to the ventricle walls just before their contraction, which assists with efficient cardiac output.

Blood is one of the connective tissues. Though it is very mobile within the cardiovascular system, it consists of a variety of solid elements suspended in fluid (Fig. 9-17). These specialized elements include red and white blood cells and fragments called platelets, which together make up about 45% of the total blood volume. The other 55% is made up of the straw-colored **plasma** that is mostly water. The average adult contains approximately 5 L, or just less than 5 quarts of blood.

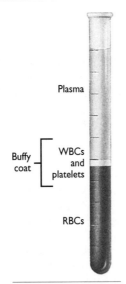

Plasma

Buffy coat | WBCs and platelets

RBCs

**Figure 9-17.
Components of blood.**
From Thibodeau, Patton: Structure & function of the body, ed 10, St. Louis, 1997, Mosby.

Red blood cells

Red blood cells carry oxygen throughout the body. A single red blood cell, also known as an **erythrocyte,** has a unique round flat disk shape and is **biconcave,** or dimpled, on both sides (Fig. 9-18). This shape allows the cell to fold or twist through narrow capillaries. Red blood cells have no nuclei. Approximately one third of a red blood cell's content is **hemoglobin,** a pigment that carries oxygen and carbon dioxide. When a red blood cell is rich in oxygen, its color is bright red, as opposed to low oxygen concentrations that result in a much darker color.

As discussed in Chapter 4, red blood cells are formed in the red bone marrow in areas such as the epiphyses of the femur and humerus and in the flat bones of the sternum and cranium—a process known as **hematopoiesis.** Typical red blood cell count can range from 4,200,000 to 6,200,000 cells per cubic millimeter (cc).

White blood cells

White blood cells differ from red blood cells in that they possess nuclei but do not specialize in carrying respiratory gases. White blood cells, also known as **leukocytes,** perform a variety of tasks. One such task is **phagocytosis,** a process that destroys microorganisms and particles harmful or foreign to the body. Another task is tissue repair. Vital to the maintenance of the body's immune system, white blood cells carry antibodies that resist infection.

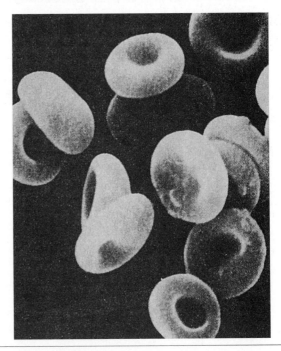

Figure 9-18. Red blood cells.
From Bevelander, Ramaley: Essentials of histology, ed 8, St. Louis, 1979, Mosby.

There are five types of leukocytes: **neutrophils, eosinophils, basophils, monocytes,** and **lymphocytes.** When diagnosing a patient, a physician will frequently check the number of white blood cells. A normal count might range from 5,000 to 10,000 cells per cubic millimeter of blood. Increases in the white blood cell count often indicate the presence of an infection or disease.

Platelets

Platelets are actually pieces of cells, which, like red blood cells, are round and lack a nucleus. A platelet is about one half the size of a red blood cell. Its function is to initiate the clotting process where a wound occurs to the circulatory system. Platelets release a substance called **serotonin,** which causes vasoconstriction of small blood vessels near the wound, decreasing blood loss. Platelets tend to stick to the edges of the damaged tissue and thus are able to block bleeding by forming a clot. In normal adults the count of platelets in the blood is approximately 130,000 to 360,000 per cubic millimeter of blood.

Blood plasma

When the red and white blood cells and platelets are removed from a quantity of blood, the remaining liquid is found to be approximately 92% water. This is known as **plasma,** and it is light gold or straw colored. The other 8% of the liquid is made up of proteins, nutrients (glucose, amino acids, lipids), nitrogenous wastes, and electrolytes including sodium, chloride, potassium, calcium, and magnesium—to name a few. Plasma is the medium that carries the solid particles through the vascular system.

▒▒ ■ ■ Exercise 9-10. Blood

Complete the following statements based on your familiarity with blood as discussed in this chapter.

1. The shape of a red blood cell is

   _____.

2. Another name for a red blood cell is

   _____.

3. Within a red blood cell, the hemoglobin serves to

   _____.

4. The process by which a red blood cell is formed is called

   _____.

5. A white blood cell is also known as

   _____.

▒▒ ■ ■ Exercise 9-10. Blood—cont

6. The destruction of harmful or foreign substances within the body by white blood cells is called

   _____.

7. The five types of leukocytes are:

   _____,

   _____,

   _____,

   _____,

   _____.

8. The function of a platelet is to

   _____.

9. The substance that causes vasoconstriction of small blood vessels is

   _____.

10. The primary ingredient of plasma is

   _____.

Lymphatic System

The **lymphatic system** is similar to the cardiovascular system in that it carries excess fluid, or **lymph,** through its vessels away from tissues, participating in the body's immune system. This network begins with its own capillaries, vessels, nodes, and large ducts, all collecting the lymph and directing it to the venous portion of the vascular system. This network has no arterial portion since its only function is to collect lymph and carry it away from the tissues (Fig. 9-19).

Lymph begins as excess **intercellular fluid** or **interstitial fluid**—mostly water that is not collected by the capillaries that carry blood. Lymph also contains excess material dissolved in the water and waste products from the tissues. The lymphatic capillaries begin in almost all the tissues of the body, networking alongside capillaries that carry blood. Absorbing fluid through its membrane-thin walls, the capillaries merge and become larger vessels, which often have valves that prevent backwash, as do the veins that carry blood.

Lymph nodes, or lymph glands, are specialized organs that contain lymphocytes and **macrophages,** which are cells that destroy bacteria and foreign substances that are harmful to the body. The nodes are like tiny filters that clean the lymph and fight disease. Large numbers of nodes are found in the groin and axillary regions.

After leaving the nodes, lymph vessels merge with one another to form larger **lymphatic trunks,** located primarily in

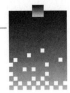

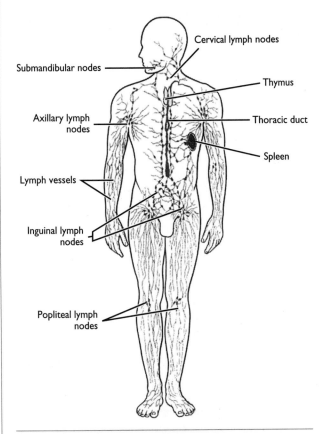

Cervical lymph nodes

Submandibular nodes

Thymus

Axillary lymph nodes

Thoracic duct

Spleen

Lymph vessels

Inguinal lymph nodes

Popliteal lymph nodes

Figure 9-19. Principle organs of the lymphatic system.
From Thibodeau, Patton: Structure & function of the body, ed 10, St. Louis, 1997, Mosby.

the torso. The trunks, in turn, deposit their contents into one of two collecting ducts known as the **thoracic duct** and **right lymphatic duct.** These ducts empty their contents into the left and right **subclavian veins** of the vascular system.

Within the lymphatic system, the fluid is under very little pressure and does not easily flow along its intended path, especially against gravity. When the interstitial fluid accumulates in the tissues, it is unable to adequately enter the lymphatic capillaries and vessels. This accumulation is known as **edema.** Excess fluid in the tissues can decrease the efficiency of the cardiovascular system by compressing surrounding tissues and structures. Prolonged edema can cause tissue death, known as **necrosis.**

An activity that can assist the movement of lymph is skeletal muscle contraction, which inadvertently applies pressure to surrounding tissues and effectively *milks out* any excess fluid. Active respiratory muscles also help push the fluid through the thoracic cavity with its repetitive contract-relax motion. Gravity, which often opposes lymph flow, can assist the flow when the extremities are placed in an antigravity

position (elevating them for a period of time). This position allows the fluid to drain toward the torso.

The **thymus gland** and **spleen** are also lymphatic organs. The thymus gland secretes hormones called **T-lymphocytes,** whereas the spleen produces phagocytic cells; both defend against infectious elements that are present in the body.

◼◻◼◻ Exercise 9-11. Lymphatic system

Complete the following statements based on your familiarity with the lymphatic system discussed in this chapter.

1. Lymph is made up of _____ and _____.

2. Components of the lymphatic system that carry lymph are:

   _____,
   _____,
   _____,
   _____.

3. Lymph is collected and returned to the vascular system at the _____.

4. Excess fluid not absorbed by the capillaries of the vascular or lymphatic systems is called _____.

5. Two organs of the lymphatic system are the

   _____,
   and _____.

Key Words

aorta
aortic semilunar valve
apex
arterioles
arteries
atrioventricular bundle
atrioventricular node
atrioventricular valve
atrium (*pl.* atria)
base
basophils
biconcave
bicuspid valve
bradycardia
bundle of His
capillaries
capillary beds
cardiac muscle
cardiac output
chambers
chordae tendineae
common carotid artery
coronary arteries
coronary sinus
coronary veins
diastolic pressure
edema
electrocardiogram
endocardium
eosinophils
epicardium
erythrocyte
heart rate
hematopoiesis
hemoglobin
hypertension

hypotension
inferior vena cava
interatrial septum
intercalated disks
intercellular fluid
interstitial fluid
interventricular septum
leukocytes
lumen
lungs
lymph
lymph glands
lymph nodes
lymphatic system
lymphatic trunks
lymphocytes
macrophages
mediastinum
mitral valve
monocytes
myocardium
necrosis
neutrophils
P wave
pacemaker of the heart
papillary muscles
parietal pericardium
pericardium
phagocytosis
plasma
platelets
pulmonary artery
pulmonary semilunar valves
pulmonary trunk
pulmonary veins
pulse

Purkinje's fibers
QRS complex
radial artery
red blood cells
right lymphatic duct
semilunar valve
serotonin
sinoatrial node
sinus rhythm
skeleton of the heart
sphygmomanometer
spleen
stethoscope
stroke volume
subclavian veins
superior vena cava
systolic pressure
T-lymphocyte
T wave
tachycardia
thoracic duct
thymus gland
tricuspid valve
tunica adventitia
tunica intima
tunica media
valves
vasoconstriction
vasodilation
veins
ventricles
venules
visceral pericardium
white blood cells

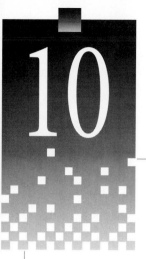

10

Respiratory System

This chapter will enable you to identify the primary elements of the respiratory system as it affects human movement.

Chapter objectives

The student will be able to:

1. Identify the primary structures of the respiratory system.

2. Describe the physical characteristics of lung tissue.

3. Identify the skeletal muscles involved in respiration.

4. Describe the principles involved in air exchange within the lungs.

5. Explain the basic physiologic aspects of gas exchange between the cardiac, vascular, and pulmonary systems.

All human activity is dependent upon the collection of oxygen, the efficient transport of oxygen to the cellular level by exchanging it for carbon dioxide, and finally the removal of the carbon dioxide from the body. This process is called **respiration,** and it occurs not only via the act of breathing but also within tissues of the body. The cardiovascular system can efficiently transport oxygen only if there is oxygen available. An examination of the structures of the respiratory system includes its passageways, the lung tissue, and the principles of air and gas exchange.

Anatomy of the Respiratory System

The event of air entering and exiting the body is called **ventilation.** The passageways to the lungs are called the **upper respiratory tract** and consist of the nose, nasal cavity, pharynx, larynx, and trachea (Fig. 10-1). The branches to the lungs, including the lungs themselves, are referred to as the **lower respiratory tract** and include the bronchial tree, bronchioles, alveolar ducts, and alveoli.

The initial portal into the body is the **nose.** Projecting slightly from the face, the nose is made up of two soft passageways supported by a piece of thin cartilage. On its way into the **nasal cavity,** air must pass over a fragile membrane that excretes a thin layer of moisture, or **mucus.** This membrane is carpeted by **cilia,** or tiny hairlike projections, as well as mucus. Together, they help filter out large particles of unwanted matter in the respiratory system. The mucus also helps add water to the dry air before it is inhaled further. This membrane contains an extensive **capillary network** that brings warm blood close to the tissue surface to warm the inhaled air. The nasal cavity is supported by a maze of tiny bones called the **nasal conchae,** which provide an extensive surface area for the capillary bed and ciliated mucous membrane.

From the nasal cavity, the air moves to a three-part chamber called the **pharynx** (see Fig. 10-1). The subdivisions are the **nasopharynx** behind the nasal cavity, the **oropharynx** just behind the mouth, and the **laryngopharynx,** which is the most inferior portion leading to the larynx. From the nose and nasal cavity, air must pass over the continuous ciliated mucous membrane through each of the three subdivisions of the pharynx and on to the **larynx, trachea,** and **lungs.** In comparison, food entering from the mouth passes through the oropharynx and laryngopharynx and on to the **esophagus** and stomach.

The opening to the larynx is protected by the flaplike structure called the **epiglottis.** Within the larynx are the **vocal cords,** which are actually folds in the mucous membrane, and the opening between the cords is a called the **glottis.** Air passes through the glottis and over the vocal cords, which are controlled by small muscles whose contractions change their length and tension, thereby changing the tone and quality of the voice. Other laryngeal muscles control swallowing.

The larynx precedes the trachea. Also known as the *windpipe*, the trachea is a long tube held open by many rings of cartilage. Approximately 12 cc in length, this flexible passageway lies anterior to the esophagus and is palpable on the anterior side of the throat. In the thoracic cavity, the trachea divides into the two-part **bronchial tree,** which consists of the left and right **bronchi** that branch off toward the lungs. Each bronchus (singular) quickly divides into smaller **bronchioles,** each of which are dedicated to a specific portion of its respective lung.

In the lungs, the passageways from the bronchioles become **alveolar ducts** that lead to clusters of **alveoli** (see Fig. 10-1). The wall of each alveolus is made of an extremely thin membrane across which gasses must be easily transported. Each alveolar cluster is covered by an **alveolar sac** that contains the capillaries from the pulmonary arteries and veins. Adult lungs contain thousands of alveoli; if their surface area were spread out flat, they would cover an area of about 75 square meters. This vast surface area is necessary to make available the exchange of oxygen and carbon dioxide in quantities large enough to meet the needs of the entire body.

The lungs have distinct separations in the tissue called **lobes;** the left lung has two lobes and the right lung has three (Fig. 10-2). Each lobe is further divided into **lobules,** each receiving air through its own bronchiole. The lungs are covered by a double enclosed membrane called the **pleura** (Fig. 10-3). The **visceral pleura** lies closest to the lungs, whereas the **parietal pleura** lies next to the rib cage; between both

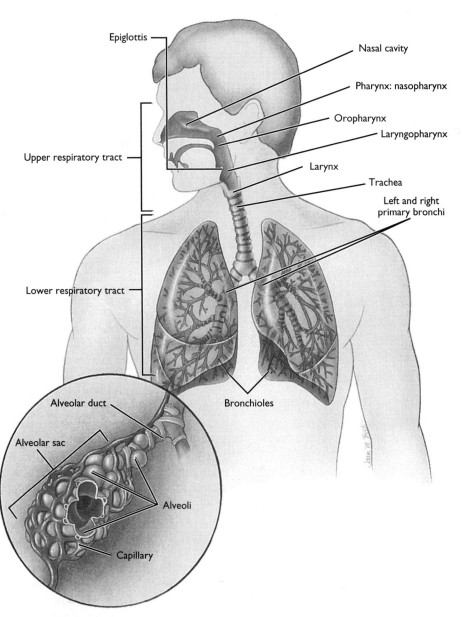

Figure 10-1. Anatomy of the respiratory system.
From Thibodeau, Patton: Structure & function of the body, ed 10, St. Louis, 1997, Mosby.

pleurae is the **pleural cavity.**

Lung tissue, in its normal state, is moist, extremely soft, and cannot withstand the pulling and pushing forces of the thoracic cavity without collapsing and tearing. Thus the visceral and parietal pleurae respond and help maintain the shape and integrity of fragile lung tissue. Since the two pleural layers are not directly attached to one another, their efficiency depends on the **surface tension** created by a thin layer of serous or watery fluid that lies between the two. The moist pleural membranes move together like two layers of wet cello-

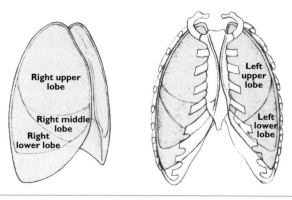

Figure 10-2. Lobes of the right and left lungs.
From Mathers et al: Clinical anatomy principles (C.L.A.S.S. Series, Stanford Project), *St. Louis, 1996, Mosby.*

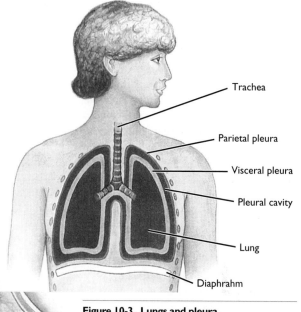

- Trachea
- Parietal pleura
- Visceral pleura
- Pleural cavity
- Lung
- Diaphrahm

Figure 10-3. Lungs and pleura.
From Thibodeau, Patton: Structure & function of the body, *ed 9, St. Louis, 1992, Mosby.*

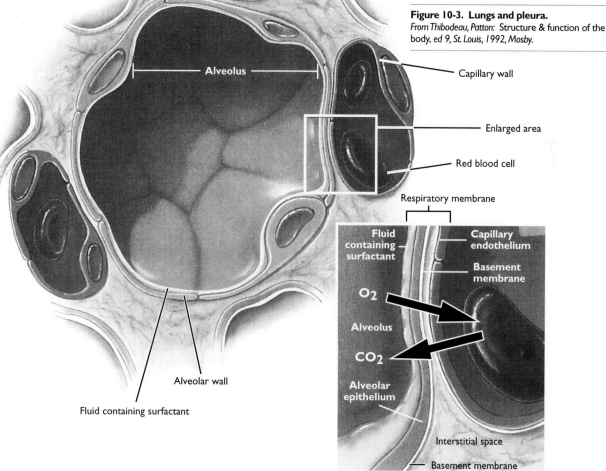

Capillary wall

Enlarged area

Red blood cell

Respiratory membrane

Fluid containing surfactant

Capillary endothelium

Basement membrane

O_2

Alveolus

CO_2

Alveolar epithelium

Interstitial space

Basement membrane

Alveolus

Alveolar wall

Fluid containing surfactant

Figure 10-4. Lungs and pleura.
From Thibodeau, Patton: Structure & function of the body, *ed 9, St. Louis, 1992, Mosby.*

phane plastic wrap. The ease with which the lungs are able to inflate and remain open is called **compliance.** Diseased lung tissue or damaged respiratory passageways can contribute to poor compliance.

Though this clingy attachment is necessary outside the lungs, such surface tension can collapse the thin walls of the alveoli where gas exchange occurs. Here, the surface tension is corrected by a fluid called **surfactant,** which is secreted within the alveoli; it prevents the walls of the alveoli from sticking together (Fig. 10-4).

The capillary network that surrounds the alveoli is quite extensive. Each individual alveolus is wrapped by a tiny vascular structure that brings deoxygenated blood to the membrane of the alveolus where oxygen and carbon dioxide are exchanged. The oxygen is absorbed by the blood plasma and carried in the red blood cells by the **hemoglobin.** The carbon dioxide is released into the alveoli to be expelled from the body.

Inferior to the lungs and pleurae lies the primary muscle of respiration, the **diaphragm,** innervated by the **phrenic nerve** (see Fig. 10-3). As discussed in Chapter 7, this broad thin muscle is attached like a canopy between the thoracic and abdominal regions. Its contraction is responsible for the ability to draw air into the lungs.

Exercise 10-1. Anatomy of the respiratory system

Complete the following statements based on your familiarity with the respiratory system.

1. The process of exchanging oxygen and carbon dioxide within the tissues of the body is called

   _____.

2. The process of air entering and exiting the body is called

   _____.

3. The nasal cavity is lined by a membrane covered with _____ and _____ to help rid the body of unwanted particles.

4. The purpose of the capillary network within the nasal cavity is to _____.

5. The three divisions of the pharynx are:

   _____

   _____

   _____

6. The _____ protects the opening of the larynx.

Exercise 10-1. Anatomy of the respiratory system—cont

7. The vocal cords are located within the

   _____.

8. The air passage behind the nasal cavity is the

   _____.

9. Areas where both air and food must pass are:

   _____

   _____

10. The *windpipe* that lies anterior to the esophagus is the

    _____.

11. The trachea divides into two parts called the

    _____.

12. The right lung has _____ lobes, whereas the left lung has _____ lobes.

13. The _____ is the membrane that covers the lungs.

14. The pleural cavity is the

    _____.

15. Bronchioles further divide into

    _____,

    leading to the _____.

16. In the lungs, gas exchange takes place across the thin walls of the _____.

17. The ease with which the lungs are able to inflate and remain open is

    _____.

18. The fluid produced inside the alveoli that reduces internal surface tension is called

    _____.

19. The primary muscle of respiration is the

    _____,

    innervated by the

    _____.

20. The blood from the pulmonary circulatory system is brought closest to the alveoli at the

    _____.

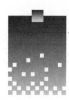

■ ■ ■ **Exercise 10-1.** *Anatomy of the respiratory system—cont*

21. The upper respiratory tract consists of:

_____

_____

_____

_____

_____

22. The lower respiratory tract consists of:

_____

_____

_____

_____

■ ■ ■ **Exercise 10-2.** *Identification of the anatomy of the respiratory system*

Identify the anatomy of the respiratory system on Figures 10-5 and 10-6.

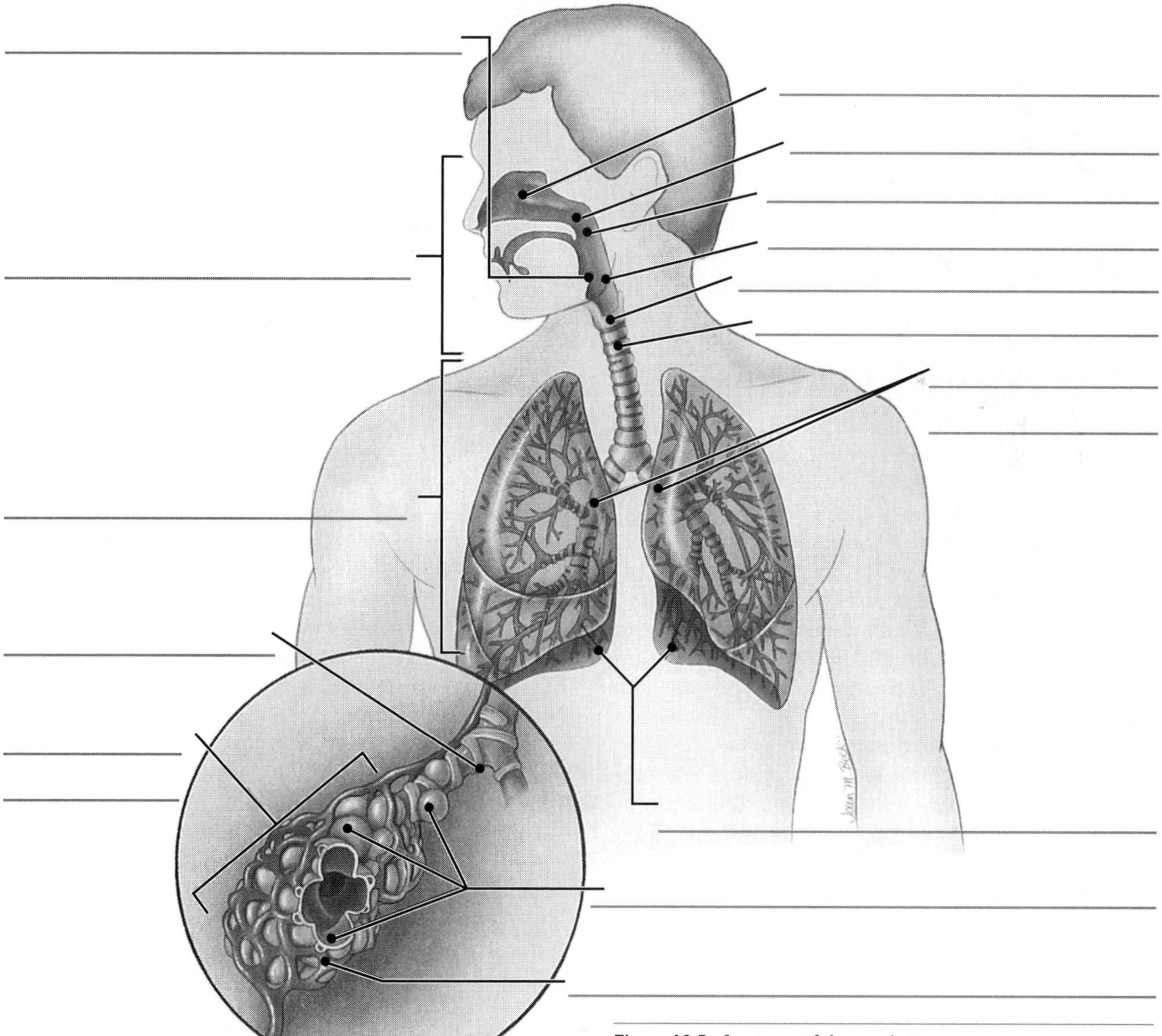

Figure 10-5. Anatomy of the respiratory system.
From Thibodeau, Patton: Structure & function of the body, ed 10, St. Louis, 1997, Mosby.

Exercise 10-2 continued on page 202

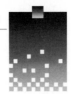

■■ ■ Exercise 10-2. Identification of the anatomy of the respiratory system—cont

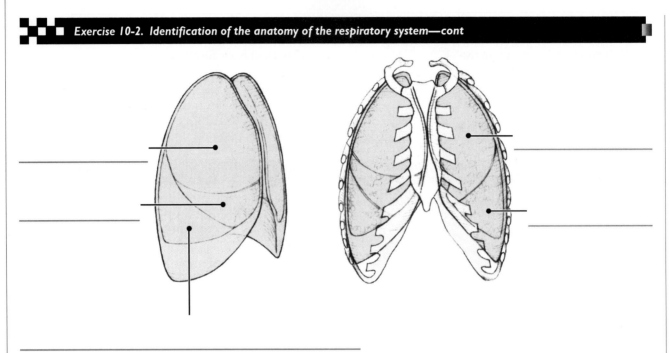

Figure 10-6. Lobes of the right and left lungs.
From Mathers et al: Clinical anatomy principles (C.L.A.S.S. Series, Stanford Project), *St. Louis, 1996, Mosby.*

Mechanical Principles of Air Exchange

The ability to draw air inside the lungs is called **inspiration,** or inhalation, whereas expelling air from the lungs is **expiration,** or exhalation. As defined earlier, ventilation is the alternating inspiration and expiration in a rhythmic pattern, an activity that occurs as a result of significant pressure changes within the thoracic cavity as compared with the atmospheric pressure that externally surrounds the body. Rhythmic ventilation is measured by counting the number of breaths per minute (bpm); one inspiration and expiration equals one breath. As with the cardiovascular system, pressures are measured in terms of millimeters of mercury (mm Hg).

Without actively breathing, the atmospheric and internal thoracic cavity pressures would be approximately the same and would not naturally exchange air. Thoracic cavity pressure is adjusted by changes in the position of the diaphragm and rib cage. When the pressure in the sealed thoracic cavity decreases in a temporary vacuum, the air outside the body rushes in, in an attempt to even out the difference. This event is inspiration. When the pressure in the thoracic cavity is increased by compressing the air inside the respiratory tracts, the air rushes out to the area of lower pressure. This is expiration.

Inspiration is facilitated by the contraction of the diaphragm, pulling it downward and away from the lungs

(Fig. 10-7). At the same time the external **intercostal muscles** pull the ribs upward, lifting the rib cage away from the diaphragm. This separation increases the volume of the thoracic cavity, creating a temporary vacuum since more air is now required to fill the larger empty space. When the passageways of the upper respiratory tract are open, air is allowed to flow into the lungs, normalizing the pressure.

Expiration is typically a passive event whereby the relaxation of the diaphragm causes it to return to its original canopy-like position, and relaxation of the intercostal muscles allow the rib cage to fall back to its lower position. This decrease in space between the diaphragm and rib cage causes the air inside the thoracic cavity to be compressed, thus the pressure increases and the high pressure air is forced out through the upper respiratory tract into the atmosphere. Expiration is assisted by the elastic quality of the tissues involved. When stretched during inspiration, a quality of **elastic recoil** in the lungs and connective tissues promotes the expelling of air from the area.

Skeletal Muscles of Respiration

Normal ventilation during rest or quiet activity occurs simply by the contraction of the diaphragm and external intercostal muscles. Restful expiration requires no active muscle activity.

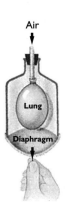

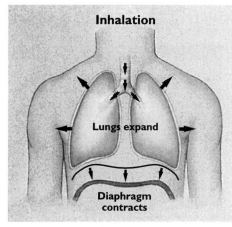

Inhalation

Air

Lung

Diaphragm

Lungs expand

Diaphragm contracts

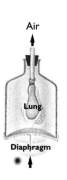

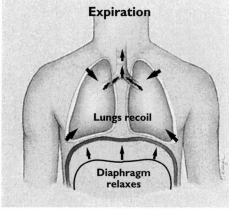

Expiration

Air

Lung

Diaphragm

Lungs recoil

Diaphragm relaxes

Figure 10-7. Mechanical principles of air exchange.
From Thibodeau, Patton: Structure & function of the body, ed 9, St. Louis, 1996, Mosby.

During activities where the oxygen demand is greater, the rate of ventilation must rapidly increase. Simple inspiration and passive expiration cannot meet the body's needs; additional assistance from surrounding skeletal muscles is required. The muscles that participate in this additional workload are called **accessory muscles** of respiration (Box 10-1).

Inspiration is assisted by muscles that have a line of pull that results in more powerful lifting of the rib cage and increasing the area of the anterior thoracic region. This assistance involves the muscles of the cervical and pectoral regions, as well as those that perform extension of the trunk.

Expiration is assisted by forcibly pulling the rib cage downward, quickly increasing the interthoracic pressure, and forcing the air out of the body. Often, the activity of an accessory respiratory muscle is accomplished by stabilizing what would otherwise be the insertion of a muscle to move the thorax or rib cage. Stabilization of the vertebral column, scapula, and upper extremities assists in this activity.

Box 10-1. Accessory muscles of respiration

Inspiration

Pectoralis major
Pectoralis minor
Sternocleidomastoid
Scalenes
Trapezius
Rhomboids
Levator scapula
Erector spinae
Serratus anterior
Quadratus lumborum

Expiration

Rectus abdominus
Internal and external obliques
Transverse abdominus
Latissimus dorsi

Cycle of Respiratory Air Volumes

To exchange oxygen and carbon dioxide in the capillaries, the volume of air in the lungs must be frequently changed. The measurement of these volumes is called **spirometry,** and the volumes are measured in cubic centimeters (cc) (Fig. 10-8). The *Pulmonary Function Test* is the complete evaluation of an individual's respiratory status.

The air that is exchanged during normal breathing, such as when sitting quietly, is known as the **tidal volume.** Beyond the tidal volume, it is possible to actively and forcibly inhale a larger quantity of air, a value known as the **inspiratory reserve volume.** Beginning again from the tidal volume range, it is possible to exhale forcibly an additional quantity of air, a value known as the **expiratory reserve volume.** These two additional volumes of air are commonly called upon during stressful exercise. At all times, there is a quantity of air that remains unchanged in the lungs; it is called the **residual volume,** and it maintains the inflation of the lungs.

Measurements of these four lung volumes make it possible to calculate the four elements of **respiratory capacity.** These elements are used to evaluate the quality of respiratory effort. The sum of the tidal volume and the inspiratory reserve volume is the **inspiratory capacity.** The vital capacity is the sum of the tidal volume and both the inspiratory and expiratory reserve volumes (see Fig. 10-8). The **functional reserve capacity** can be calculated by adding the expiratory reserve volume to the residual volume. An individual's **total lung capacity** is the sum of the vital capacity and the residual volume, or the total of all four categories of lung volume. Changes in these values may reflect the effects of disease and or medical treatment on the respiratory system.

Control of Respiration

The regulation of respiration occurs in the **midbrain,** more specifically, the pons, medulla, and hypothalamus (Fig, 10-9). In the **pons** and **medulla,** efferent neurons maintain the rhythmic pattern of ventilation. This primitive portion of the central nervous system (CNS) also responds to sensory impulses such as sensitive chemical sensors in the blood vessels of the neck, which indicate high levels of carbon dioxide and hydrogen in the blood. Reaction to such stimuli results in an increase in the depth of each breath, thus ventilating more air and expelling the carbon dioxide. One side effect of deeper breathing is increased oxygen absorption, but it is actually the carbon dioxide and hydrogen levels that are monitored by the brain. The pattern of deeper breathing and increased rate of breathing is called **hyperventilation.**

Other areas of the brain influence respiration in response to strong emotion, temperature change, or pain. This influence occurs in the **hypothalamus.** Since the muscles that participate in respiration are skeletal and can be voluntarily controlled, it is possible to intentionally manipulate breathing patterns. This ability allows an individual to change ventilation patterns while talking, eating, or singing. Voluntary muscle control comes from the higher areas in the **cerebral cortex,** similar to the motor patterns of other skeletal muscles. However, when the respiratory center in the midbrain receives impulses that alert it to significant compromise of appropriate carbon dioxide levels, it will override the cortex and attempt to resume normal ventilation.

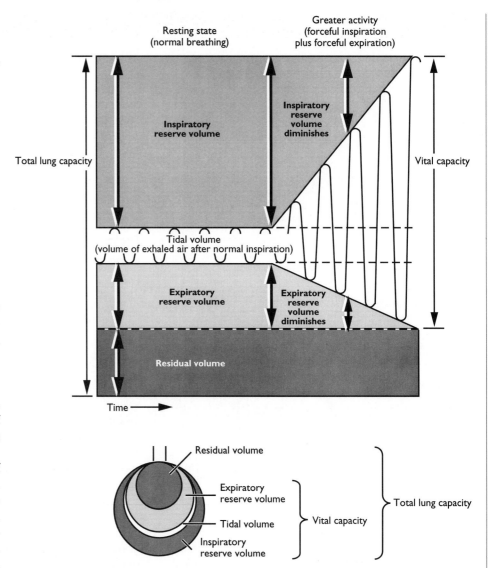

Figure 10-8. Pulmonary ventilation volumes.
From Thibodeau, Patton: Structure & function of the body, ed 10, St. Louis, 1997, Mosby.

Exercise 10-3. Respiration

Complete the following statements based on your familiarity with respiration.

1. A decrease in the pressure in the thoracic cavity and lungs precedes _____.

2. An increase in the pressure in the thoracic cavity and lungs precedes _____.

3. During inspiration, the diaphragm is pulled _____, whereas the rib cage is pulled _____.

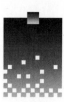

4. Calm expiration is a

_____

event in terms of skeletal muscle activity.

5. Expiration is assisted by the

_____

of tissues stretched during inspiration.

6. The muscles of quiet inspiration include:

_____

_____

7. Accessory muscles of inspiration that assist in lifting the rib cage are:

_____

_____

_____

_____

8. Accessory muscles of inspiration that increase the space in the thoracic region by extending the vertebral column and scapular retraction are:

_____

_____

_____

_____

9. Accessory muscles of expiration are:

_____

_____

_____

_____

10. Spirometry is a method of measuring

_____.

11. The four volumes of normal respiration are:

_____

_____

_____

_____

12. The four measurements of respiratory capacity are:

_____

_____

_____

_____

13. The volume of air exchanged during normal inhalation and expiration is the _____.

14. Forcible inhalation requires

_____.

15. The volume of air that is always present in the lungs is the

_____.

16. The functional reserve capacity is calculated by adding:

_____

_____

17. The vital capacity is the sum of:

_____

_____

_____

18. Efferent neurons from the _____ and _____ maintain the rhythmic pattern of ventilation.

19. The _____ responds to strong emotion, temperature change, or pain by adjusting the respiratory system.

20. Increase in depth and rate of respirations is referred to as

_____.

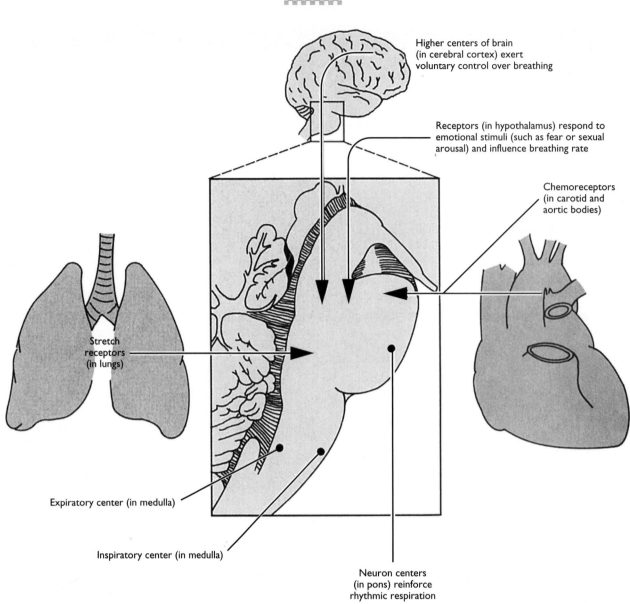

Higher centers of brain (in cerebral cortex) exert voluntary control over breathing

Receptors (in hypothalamus) respond to emotional stimuli (such as fear or sexual arousal) and influence breathing rate

Chemoreceptors (in carotid and aortic bodies)

Stretch receptors (in lungs)

Expiratory center (in medulla)

Inspiratory center (in medulla)

Neuron centers (in pons) reinforce rhythmic respiration

Figure 10-9. Regulation of respiration.
From Thibodeau, Patton: Structure & function of the body, ed 9, St. Louis, 1992, Mosby.

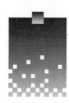

■ *Exercise 10-4. Respiratory system*

Identify the pulmonary ventilation volumes on Figure 10-10.

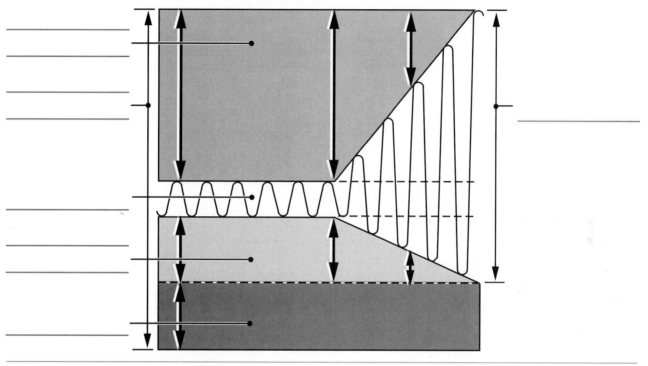

Figure 10-10. Pulmonary ventilation volumes.
From Thibodeau, Patton: Structure & function of the body, *ed 10, St. Louis, 1997 Mosby.*

Key Words

accessory muscles	glottis	mucus	rhomboids
alveolar ducts	hemoglobin	nasal cavity	scalenes
alveolar sac	hyperventilation	nasal conchae	serratus anterior
alveoli	hypothalamus	nasopharynx	spirometry
bronchi	inspiration	nose	sternocleidomastoid
bronchial tree	inspiratory capacity	oropharynx	surface tension
bronchioles	inspiratory reserve volume	parietal pleura	surfactant
capillary network	intercostal muscles	pectoralis minor	tidal volume
cerebral cortex	internal and external obliques	pectoralis major	total lung capacity
cilia	laryngopharynx	pharynx	trachea
compliance	larynx	phrenic nerve	transverse abdominus
diaphragm	latissimus dorsi	pleura	trapezius
elastic recoil	levator scapula	pleural cavity	upper respiratory tract
epiglottis	lobes	pons	ventilation
erector spinae	lobules	quadratus lumborum	visceral pleura
esophagus	lower respiratory tract	rectus abdominus	vital capacity
expiration	lungs	residual volume	vocal cords
expiratory reserve volume	medulla	respiration	
functional reserve capacity	midbrain	respiratory capacity	

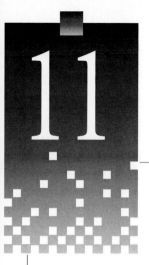

Functional Movement

> **"** *This chapter will enable you to demonstrate an understanding of musculoskeletal anatomy and normal movement by describing significant elements involved in the performance of functional tasks.* **"**

Chapter objectives

The student will be able to:

1. Recognize terminology that relates to functional movement.

2. Describe the joint movements that are necessary to perform a functional activity.

3. Identify each individual muscle and its innervation by functional muscle group.

4. Identify, through practice, the various components of functional activity.

Movement and Function

Now that the principle systems involved in making movement possible have been examined, they can be observed in action. During the performance of everyday tasks, the details of movement and their impact on the task can, with practice, be identified. The study of human movement is referred to as **kinesiology,** and it incorporates **biomechanics,** which involve elements such as gravity, mass, weight, force, levers, and direction of movement. The term **kinetic** refers to motion, whereas the suffix *-logy* means the study or science of the subject.

Functional movement refers to activity that results in the performance of a purposeful task, that is, any voluntary movement that requires planning and coordination with specific intent by the individual. Such activity requires joint range of motion, muscle strength, intact central and peripheral nervous systems, and adequate cardiopulmonary performance.

An individual's **functional ability** refers to the performance of **activities of daily living,** such as transferring from one position to another and feeding, bathing, toileting, and dressing one's self. Functional movements can be as simple as turning the face in the direction of a speaking voice or as complex as climbing a ladder.

Movement Identification

Since recalling that normal musculoskeletal movement can only occur where two or more bones articulate, the focus of this chapter is on the diarthrotic joints of the trunk and extremities. Accurate identification of the events that occur during functional movement requires strict attention to the smallest details. Not only must the moving body part be noted, but attention must also be given to events proximal and distal to the area where movement may contribute to or counteract the motion.

An individual may perform activities of daily living with relative simplicity without realizing that even small tasks, such as lifting a spoon to the mouth, combing hair, or taking a step, requires many different changes in the skeletal alignment. The focus is to break down these tasks into individual components and describe them using movement terminology. It may be necessary to review the movements available at the principle joints during these exercises. For example, when describing a person that is reaching to pick up a cup to drink, it is important to isolate the events as they occur in the trunk, shoulder, elbow, wrist, and hand, as well as in the jaw and cervical regions. If the lower extremities assist the performance, such as providing a base of support, the activity at the hips, knees, ankles, and feet should also be considered.

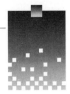

Further description of reaching for and drinking from a cup includes the starting position of sitting upright with the forearms resting on the lower extemities (Fig. 11-1). The hips and knees are flexed and relaxed, ankles are in a neutral or the anatomic position, and both forearms are pronated. (The lower extremities will not be included at this time.)

Concentrating only on joint movements, the subject begins by flexing the elbow, bringing the hand to the same height as the cup. The next motion is in the direction of supination but only to neutral, that is to the anatomic position at the radioulnar joint. Shoulder flexion, combined with elbow extension, places the hand near the cup. Abduction of the thumb and extension of digits II through IV preceeds gripping the cup, which requires opposition of the thumb and flexion of digits II through IV (Fig. 11-2). Bringing the cup toward the mouth requires shoulder and elbow flexion, as well as pronation (Fig. 11-3). Head position is adjusted by slight cervical extension, whereas the lower jaw is depressed. For this relatively simple task, twelve joint movements are listed.

Returning to the original position consists of elevation of the jaw and cervical flexion while supination to neutral rights the cup. Shoulder and elbow extension takes the cup back toward the table. The cup is released by reposition of the thumb and extension of the digits. Adduction along with flexion of the thumb and digits back to their original position occurs passively. The upper extremity returns to its resting position with elbow flexion and continued shoulder extension with pronation of the forearm.

This brief description greatly simplifies this activity, yet the movement and stabilization of the scapula have not been taken into account. However, for the purposes of this text, the gross movements required in this performance are successfully observed, and the muscle and nerve involvement can now be described. It may not always be necessary to perform the movements in the exact order discussed here. For instance, supination may occur earlier or perhaps just before grasping the cup. For the sake of uniform practice, the exercises in this chapter are discussed as if the participant is fully functional, with *normal* muscle strength and *normal* range of motion at each joint.

In most therapeutic environments, it is necessary to provide documentation to support observations. Although the method of documenting can take on a variety of formats, the data must always be accurate. Therefore it is important to be specific in all movement discussion, leaving few assumptions to the reader as to how the actual events occurred.

In time, only practice can lead to skill, improving accuracy and attention to detail. Rehearse this and similar simple movements while identifying the specific joint activities. It may be helpful to use a mirror and watch the performance of the activity in a slow and deliberate manner. Remember, practice makes permanent!

Exercise 11-1. Joint movement identification

Describe the following list of isolated events in terms of the joint involved and its specific movement. In this exercise, each movement is performed while seated, and the trunk is supported by a chair. List only the initial movements that are required to perform the task. For items 1 through 3, the joint designation has been provided. In items 4 and 5, decide from which joints the movements originate.

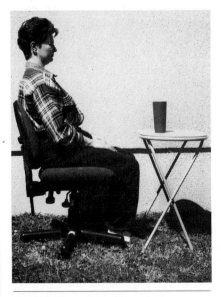

Figure 11-1

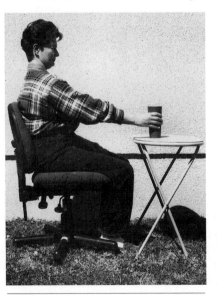

Figure 11-2

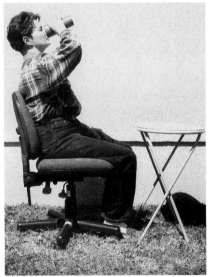

Figure 11-3

■ ■ *Exercise 11-1. Joint movement identification—cont*

1. Kick out with one foot (Fig. 11-4).

   a. Hip—_____

   b. Knee—_____

   c. Ankle—_____

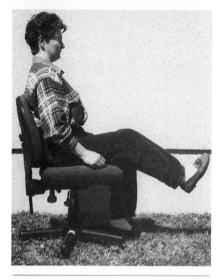

Figure 11-4

2. Fold both arms across the chest. All movements are bilateral (Fig. 11-5).

   a. Elbow—_____

   b. Shoulder—_____

   c. Shoulder—_____

   d. Shoulder—_____

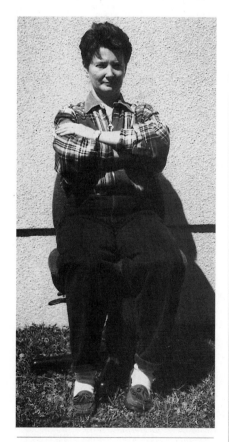

Remember, the starting position is the same as Figure 11-1.

Figure 11-5

211

Exercise 11-1 continued on page 212

■ ■   *Exercise 11-1. Joint movement identification—cont*

3. Cross one leg over the other at the knee (Fig. 11-6).

     a. Knee—_____

     b. Hip—_____

     c. Hip—_____

     d. Hip—_____

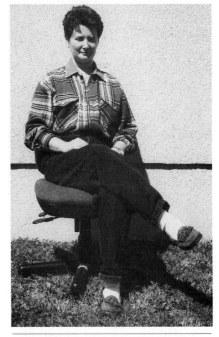

Figure 11-6

4. Reach up and touch the nose with outstretched fingers (Fig. 11- 7). Now indicate the correct joint and its movement.

     a. _____—_____

     b. _____—_____

     c. _____—_____

     d. _____—_____

     e. _____—_____

     f. _____—_____

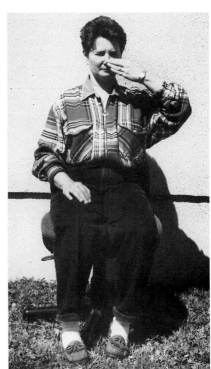

Figure 11-7

■■ ■ *Exercise 11-1. Joint movement identification—cont*

5. Lean forward and reach into hip pocket (Fig. 11-8).

a. _____ — _____

b. _____ — _____

c. _____ — _____

d. _____ — _____

e. _____ — _____

f. _____ — _____

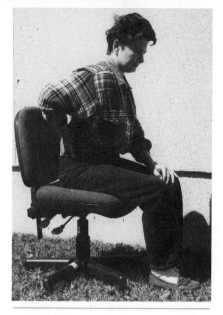

Figure 11-8

Functional Muscle Activity

Since functional activities rarely result from individual muscles acting alone, those muscles that act in concert with one another are listed as the **functional muscle groups.** A description of a specific movement provides the name of the functional muscle group. For example, psoas major, iliacus, and rectus femoris are members of the hip flexor group since all perform hip flexion. It is common to discuss muscles collectively by the description of their common action rather than by listing each individual muscle. Gross motor movements make use of broad synergistic patterns and are rarely the result of a singular muscle contraction. Once the joint and its movements are identified, the task of recognizing the participating muscle groups becomes easier.

It is important to remember the different types of muscle contractions. **Isometric** and **isotonic contractions** have already been defined and should be considered when observing and analyzing movement. The **fixators,** or stabilizing effects, of isometric contractions serve to hold the trunk or extremity in place while other movement occurs. The two varieties of isotonic muscle contraction, **concentric** and **eccentric,** perform most of the duties of skeletal movement.

It is also important to consider the different roles that active muscles, such as prime mover, synergist, fixator, or antagonist, will play. Abnormal movement often occurs as a result of inadequate muscle strength or length of connective tissue, resulting in a muscle incapable of fulfilling its appropriate role.

Familiarity with the origin, insertion, action, and innervation of all skeletal muscles is critical when discussing movement. It is important to recall the locations of the muscle bellies and how they overlap one another. Note the superficial muscles labeled in Figures 11-9 and 11-10.

Finally, it is necessary to be aware of the specific innervation of a muscle when, in the event of an injury, one must consider how the diminished quality or absence of impulses directly affect the resulting movement. The ability to isolate the spinal cord level, the peripheral nerve root, and the specific peripheral nerve responsible for a particular muscle can provide valuable information.

Remember, when discussing movement it is important to initially visualize the body in the anatomic position. It is important to examine the **normal movement** of a body that is free of injury and disease to identify *abnormal* movement in the individual with an injury requiring therapeutic intervention.

Again, accuracy and skill will develop only with practice. The following exercises will provide the beginning of an enjoyable exploration into the dynamic abilities of the human body!

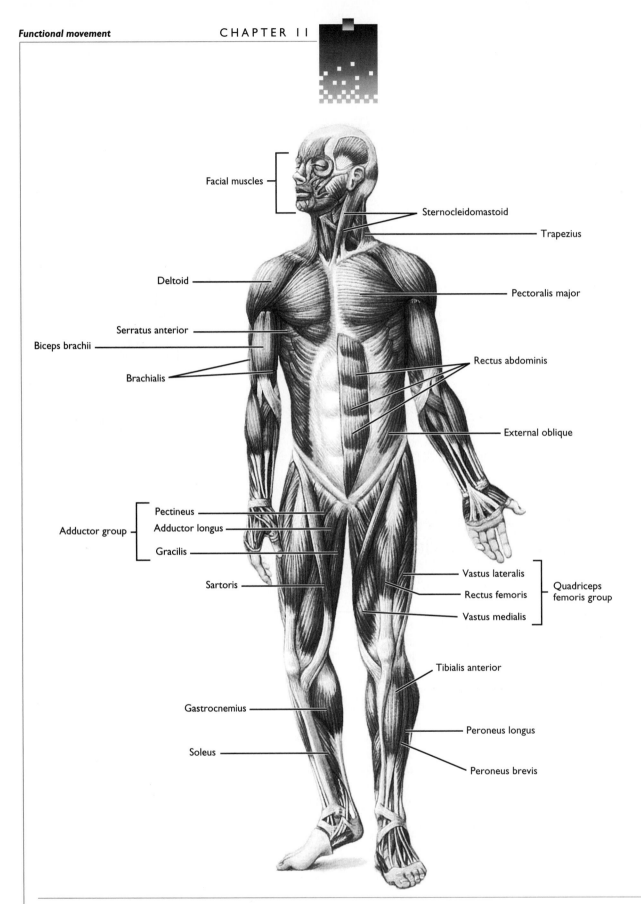

Figure 11-9. Major superficial muscles of the body (anterior view).
From Thibodeau, Patton: Structure & function of the body, ed 10, 1997, Mosby.

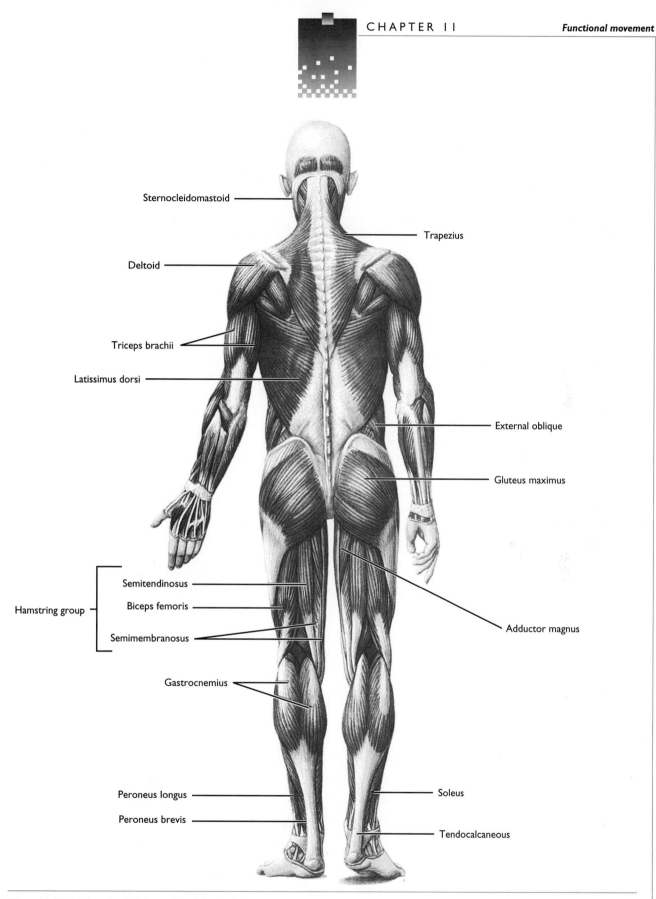

Figure 11-10. Major superficial muscles of the body (posterior view).
From Thibodeau, Patton: Structure & function of the body, *ed 10, 1997, Mosby.*

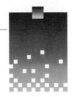

Components of Functional Activity: More Exercises

Since the movements for several simple activities have been identified in a previous exercise, provide the specific muscles as they correspond to the functional muscle groups and the nerves necessary to accomplish the task. Focus only on the active concentric movements. The starting position for Exercises 11-2, 11-3, and 11-4 is the same as in Figure 11-1.

■ Exercise 11-2. Muscle and nerve analysis

Cross one leg over the other, proximal to the knee (Fig. 11-11).

Joints	Movement	Specific muscles	Nerves
Knee	Extension	1. _____	1. _____
		2. _____	2. _____
		3. _____	3. _____
		4. _____	
		5. _____	
		6. _____	
Hip	Flexion	1. _____	1. _____
		2. _____	2. _____
		3. _____	3. _____
		4. _____	4. _____
		5. _____	
		6. _____	
		7. _____	
		8. _____	
		9. _____	
		10. _____	
		11. _____	
Hip	Lateral rotation	1. _____	1. _____
		2. _____	2. _____
		3. _____	3. _____
		4. _____	4. _____
		5. _____	5. _____
		6. _____	6. _____
		7. _____	
		8. _____	
		9. _____	
		10. _____	
Hip	Adduction	1. _____	1. _____
		2. _____	2. _____
		3. _____	3. _____
		4. _____	4. _____
		5. _____	
		6. _____	
		7. _____	
		8. _____	

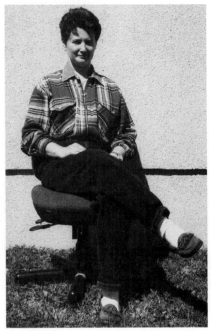

Figure 11-11

■ ■   *Exercise 11-3. Muscle and nerve analysis*

Reach up and touch nose with outstretched fingers (Fig. 11-12).

Joints	Movement	Specific muscles	Nerves
Elbow	Flexion	1. _____	1. _____
		2. _____	2. _____
		3. _____	3. _____
		4. _____	4. _____
		5. _____	
		6. _____	
		7. _____	
		8. _____	
Radio-ulnar	Supination to neutral	1. _____	1. _____
		2. _____	2. _____
		3. _____	
Shoulder	Flexion	1. _____	1. _____
		2. _____	2. _____
		3. _____	3. _____
		4. _____	4. _____
Shoulder	Medial rotation	1. _____	1. _____
		2. _____	2. _____
		3. _____	3. _____
		4. _____	4. _____
		5. _____	5. _____
			6. _____
Wrist	Extension	1. _____	1. _____
		2. _____	
		3. _____	
		4. _____	
		5. _____	
MCP joints (I-V)	Extension	1. _____	1. _____
		2. _____	
		3. _____	
		4. _____	
		5. _____	
IP joints (I-V)	Extension	1. _____	1. _____
		2. _____	2. _____
		3. _____	3. _____
		4. _____	
		5. _____	
		6. _____	
		7. _____	
		8. _____	

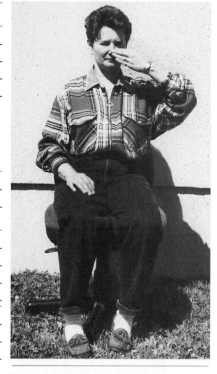

Figure 11-12

MCP, Metacarpophalangeal; *IP,* interphalangeal.

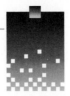

■ *Exercise 11-4. Muscle and nerve analysis*

Lean forward and reach into hip pocket (Fig. 11-13).

Joints	Movement	Specific muscles	Nerves
Trunk, Vertebral column	Maintain extension	1. _____ 2. _____ 3. _____ 4. _____ 5. _____ 6. _____ 7. _____ 8. _____ 9. _____	1. _____ 2. _____
Hip	Pelvis moves on fixed femurs	1. _____ 2. _____ 3. _____ 4. _____ 5. _____ 6. _____ 7. _____ 8. _____ 9. _____ 10. _____ 11. _____	1. _____ 2. _____ 3. _____ 4. _____
Shoulder	Abduction	1. _____ 2. _____	1. _____ 2. _____
Shoulder	Medial rotation	1. _____ 2. _____ 3. _____ 4. _____ 5. _____	1. _____ 2. _____ 3. _____ 4. _____ 5. _____ 6. _____
Elbow	Flexion	1. _____ 2. _____ 3. _____ 4. _____ 5. _____ 6. _____ 7. _____ 8. _____	1. _____ 2. _____ 3. _____ 4. _____
Wrist	Extension	1. _____ 2. _____ 3. _____ 4. _____ 5. _____	1. _____

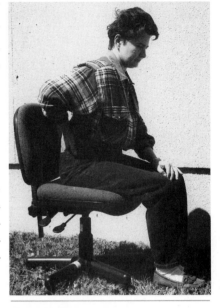

Figure 11-13

■■■ ■ *Exercise 11-4. Muscle and nerve analysis—cont*

Joints	Movement	Specific muscles	Nerves
MCP joints (I-V)	Extension	1. _____ 2. _____ 3. _____ 4. _____ 5. _____	1. _____
IP joints (I-V)	Extension	1. _____ 2. _____ 3. _____ 4. _____ 5. _____ 6. _____ 7. _____ 8. _____	1. _____ 2. _____ 3. _____
Radio-ulnar	Supination	1. _____ 2. _____ 3. _____	1. _____ 2. _____

MCP, Metacarpophalangeal; *IP,* interphalangeal.

■■■ ■ *Exercise 11-5. Movement and component analysis*

Consider the movements as sequentially presented in Figures 11-14 through 11-16. Provide the movements, muscles, and nerves required for each. Assume the upper extremities are passive in this exercise.

Joints	Movement	Specific muscles	Nerves	
Trunk, Vertebral column	1. _____	1. _____ 2. _____ 3. _____ 4. _____ 5. _____ 6. _____ 7. _____ 8. _____ 9. _____	1. _____ 2. _____	
Hip	1. _____ _____ _____	1. _____ 2. _____ 3. _____ 4. _____ 5. _____ 6. _____ 7. _____ 8. _____ 9. _____ 10. _____ 11. _____	1. _____ 2. _____ 3. _____ 4. _____	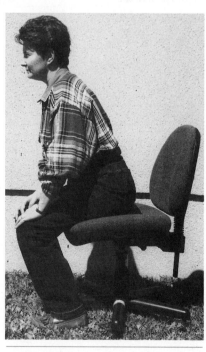

Figure 11-14

Exercise 11-5 continued on page 220

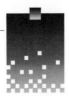

■ *Exercise 11-5. Movement and component analysis—cont*

Joints	Movement	Specific muscles	Nerves
Hip	1. _____	1. _____	1. _____
		2. _____	2. _____
		3. _____	3. _____
		4. _____	
		5. _____	
		6. _____	
Knee	1. _____	1. _____	1. _____
		2. _____	2. _____
		3. _____	3. _____
		4. _____	4. _____
		5. _____	5. _____
		6. _____	
		7. _____	
		8. _____	
		9. _____	
		10. _____	
Knee	1. _____	1. _____	1. _____
		2. _____	2. _____
		3. _____	3. _____
		4. _____	
		5. _____	
		6. _____	
Ankle	1. _____	1. _____	1. _____
		2. _____	
		3. _____	
		4. _____	
Ankle	1. _____	1. _____	1. _____
		2. _____	2. _____
		3. _____	
		4. _____	
		5. _____	
		6. _____	
		7. _____	
		8. _____	

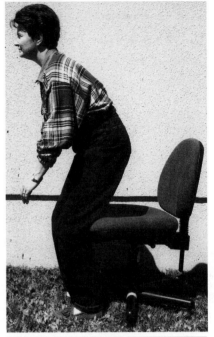

Figure 11-15

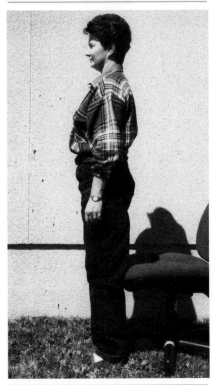

Figure 11-16

■ ■ **Exercise 11-6. *Movement and component analysis***

Stand with weight on both feet, and place left foot on a stair step (Fig. 11-17).

Joints	Movement	Specific muscles	Nerves
Trunk, Vertebral column	1._____	1._____	1._____
		2._____	2._____
		3._____	
		4._____	
		5._____	
		6._____	
		7._____	
		8._____	
		9._____	
Hip	Left— _____	1._____	1._____
		2._____	2._____
		3._____	3._____
		4._____	4._____
		5._____	
		6._____	
		7._____	
		8._____	
		9._____	
		10._____	
		11._____	
Hip	Right— _____	1._____	1._____
		2._____	2._____
		3._____	3._____
		4._____	
		5._____	
		6._____	
Hip	Right (on fixed femur)— _____	1._____	1._____
		2._____	2._____
		3._____	
		4._____	
		5._____	
Knee	Left— _____	1._____	1._____
		2._____	2._____
		3._____	3._____
		4._____	4._____
		5._____	5._____
		6._____	
		7._____	
		8._____	
		9._____	
		10._____	

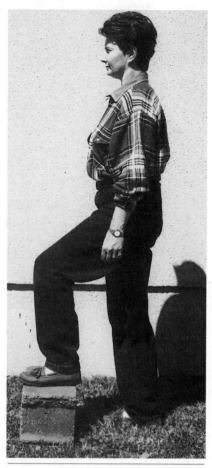

Figure 11-17

221

Exercise 11-6 continued on page 222

■ *Exercise 11-6. Movement and component analysis—cont*

Joints	Movement	Specific muscles	Nerves
Knee	Right—	1. _____	1. _____
	_____	2. _____	2. _____
		3. _____	3. _____
		4. _____	
		5. _____	
		6. _____	
Ankle	Left—	1. _____	1. _____
	_____	2. _____	
		3. _____	
		4. _____	
Ankle	Right—	1. _____	1. _____
	_____	2. _____	2. _____
		3. _____	
		4. _____	
		5. _____	
		6. _____	
		7. _____	
		8. _____	

■ *Exercise 11-7. Movement and component analysis*

While seated in a wheelchair, reach back, grasp the wheel rims, and propel the chair forward; use only the trunk and upper extremities. (Figs. 11-18 and 11-19)

Joints	Movement	Specific muscles	Nerves
Trunk, Vertebral column	1. _____	1. _____	1. _____
		2. _____	2. _____
		3. _____	
Trunk, Vertebral column	1. _____	1. _____	1. _____
		2. _____	2. _____
		3. _____	
		4. _____	
		5. _____	
		6. _____	
		7. _____	
		8. _____	
		9. _____	
Scapulo-thoracic	Adduction Elevation Downward rotation	1. _____	1. _____
		2. _____	2. _____
		3. _____	
		4. _____	
		5. _____	

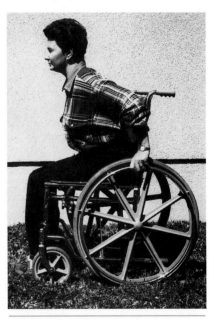

Figure 11-18

■■ ■ **Exercise 11-7. Movement and component analysis—cont**

Joints	Movement	Specific muscles	Nerves
Scapulo-thoracic	Abduction Depression Upward rotation	1._____ 2._____ 3._____	1._____ 2._____
Shoulder	Abduction Extension (hyper-) Lateral rotation	1._____ 2._____ 3._____ 4._____ 5._____ 6._____ 7._____	1._____ 2._____ 3._____ 4._____ 5._____
Shoulder	Adduction Flexion Medial rotation	1._____ 2._____ 3._____ 4._____ 5._____ 6._____ 7._____ 8._____	1._____ 2._____ 3._____ 4._____ 5._____ 6._____ 7._____
Elbow	1._____	1._____ 2._____ 3._____ 4._____ 5._____ 6._____ 7._____ 8._____	1._____ 2._____ 3._____ 4._____
Elbow	1._____	1._____ 2._____	1._____
Wrist	Extension Radial deviation	1._____ 2._____ 3._____ 4._____ 5._____ 6._____ 7._____ 8._____	1._____

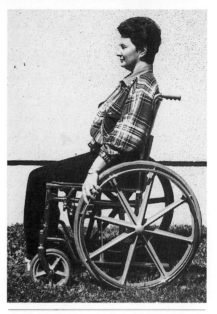

Figure 11-19

Exercise 11-7 continued on page 224

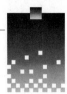

Exercise 11-7. Movement and component analysis—cont

Joints	Movement	Specific muscles	Nerves
Wrist	Flexion Ulnar deviation	1. _____ 2. _____ 3. _____ 4. _____ 5. _____ 6. _____ 7. _____	1. _____ 2. _____
Hand	Thumb— 1. _____ 2. _____	1. _____ 2. _____ 3. _____ 4. _____ 5. _____	1. _____ 2. _____
Hand	Digits II-IV— 1. _____	1. _____ 2. _____ 3. _____ 4. _____ 5. _____ 6. _____ 7. _____ 8. _____	1. _____ 2. _____

Exercise 11-8. Movement and component analysis

While seated, reach down and grasp an object lying beside the left foot with the right hand (Figs. 11-20 and 11-21). Be sure to follow hand with the eyes.

Joints	Movement	Specific muscles	Nerves
Trunk, Vertebral column	1. _____	1. _____ 2. _____ 3. _____ 4. _____ 5. _____ 6. _____ 7. _____ 8. _____ 9. _____	1. _____ 2. _____

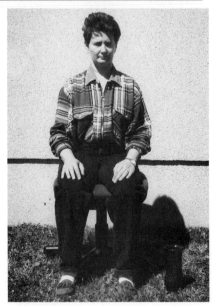

Figure 11-20

■ ■ *Exercise 11-8. Movement and component analysis—cont*

Joints	Movement	Specific muscles	Nerves
Trunk, Vertebral column	1. _____	1. _____ 2. _____ 3. _____ 4. _____ 5. _____ 6. _____ 7. _____ 8. _____ 9. _____ 10. _____	1. _____ 2. _____ 3. _____
Trunk, Vertebral column	1. _____	1. _____ 2. _____ 3. _____	1. _____
Shoulder	1. _____	1. _____ 2. _____ 3. _____ 4. _____	1. _____ 2. _____ 3. _____ 4. _____
Shoulder	1. _____ _____	1. _____ 2. _____ 3. _____ 4. _____ 5. _____	1. _____ 2. _____ 3. _____ 4. _____ 5. _____ 6. _____
Shoulder	1. _____	1. _____ 2. _____ 3. _____ 4. _____	1. _____ 2. _____ 3. _____ 4. _____ 5. _____ 6. _____
Elbow	1. _____	1. _____ 2. _____ 3. _____ 4. _____ 5. _____ 6. _____ 7. _____ 8. _____	1. _____ 2. _____ 3. _____
Elbow	1. _____	1. _____ 2. _____	1. _____
Radio-ulnar	1. _____	1. _____ 2. _____ 3. _____	1. _____ 2. _____

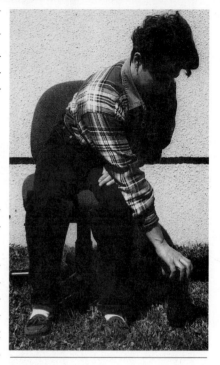

Figure 11-21

225

Exercise 11-8 continued on page 226

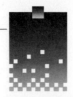

Exercise 11-8. Movement and component analysis—cont

Joints	Movement	Specific muscles	Nerves
Wrist, hand	1._____	1._____	1._____
		2._____	2._____
		3._____	3._____
		4._____	
		5._____	
		6._____	
		7._____	
		8._____	
		9._____	
		10._____	
		11._____	

Identify the muscles indicated in Figures 11-22 and 11-23.

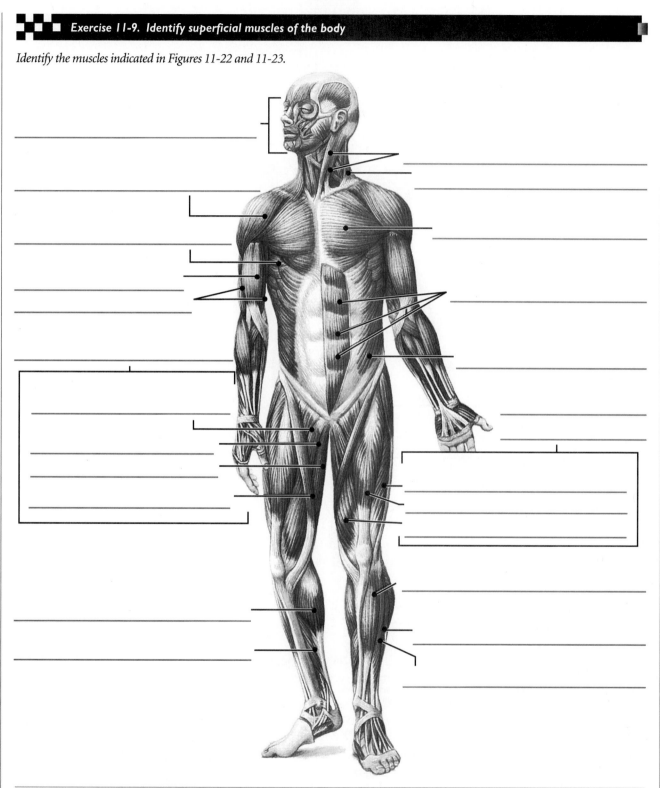

Figure 11-22. Major superficial muscles of the body (anterior view).
From Thibodeau, Patton: Structure & function of the body, *ed 10, 1997, Mosby.*

227

Exercise 11-9 continued on page 228

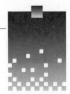

Exercise II-9. Identify superficial muscles of the body—cont

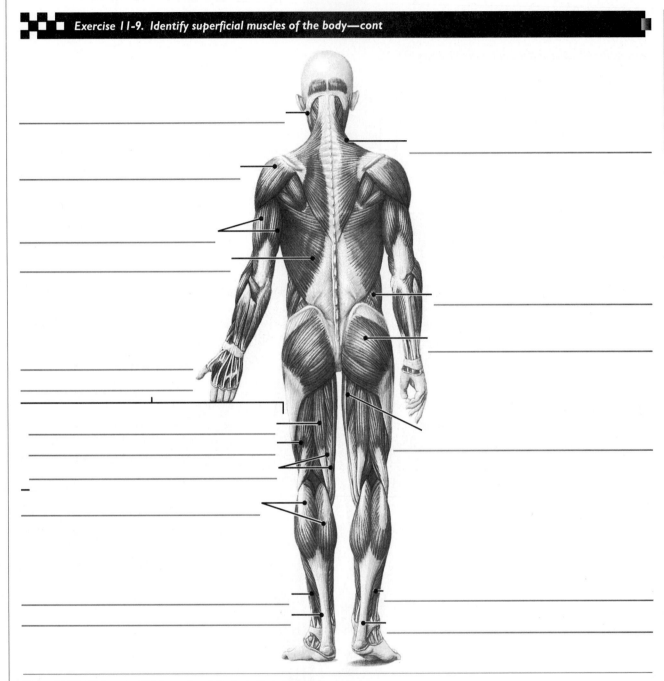

Figure II-23. Major superficial muscles of the body (anterior view).
From Thibodeau, Patton: Structure & function of the body, *ed 10, 1997, Mosby.*

Key Words

activities of daily living
biomechanics
concentric muscle contractions
eccentric muscle contractions
fixators

functional ability
functional movement
functional muscle groups
isometric contractions
isotonic contractions

kinesiology
kinetic
normal movement

Bibliography

Broer MR: *Efficiency of human movement,* Philadelphia, 1966, WB Saunders.

Chusid JG: *Correlative neuroanatomy & functional neurology,* ed 18, Los Altos, Calif, 1982, Lange Medical Publications.

Cooper JM, Glassow RB: *Kinesiology,* ed 2, St Louis, 1968, Mosby–Year Book.

Cramer GD, Darby SA: *Basic and clinical anatomy of the spine, spinal cord, and ANS,* St Louis, 1995, Mosby–Year Book.

Dorland's illustrated medical dictionary, ed 26, Philadelphia, 1981, WB Saunders.

Gamble JG: *The musculoskeletal system,* New York, 1988, Raven Press.

Gould JA, Davies GJ: *Orthopaedic and sports physical therapy,* vol 2, St Louis, 1985, Mosby–Year Book.

Gray H: *Anatomy, descriptive and surgical (Gray's anatomy),* Philadelphia, 1974, Running Press.

Guyton AC: *Human physiology and mechanisms of disease,* ed 5, Philadelphia, 1992, WB Saunders.

Hole JW: *Human anatomy & physiology,* ed 6, Dubuque, 1993, WC Brown.

Kendall FP, McCreary EK, Provance PG: *Muscles: testing and function,* ed 4, Baltimore, 1993, Williams & Wilkins.

Kisner C, Colby LA: *Therapeutic exercise: foundations and techniques,* ed 2, Philadelphia, 1990, FA Davis.

Magee KR, Saper JR: *Clinical and basic neurology for health professionals,* Chicago, 1981, Mosby–Year Book.

Marieb EN: *Human anatomy and physiology,* Redwood City, Calif, 1989, Benjamin/Cummings.

Norkin CC, Levangie PK: *Joint structure and function: a comprehensive analysis,* Philadelphia, 1983, FA Davis.

Palastanga N, Field D, Soames R: *Anatomy and human movement: structure and function,* ed 2, Oxford, 1994, Butterworth-Heinemann.

Pratt NE: *Clinical musculoskeletal anatomy,* Philadelphia, 1991, JB Lippincott.

Rothstein JM: *Measurement in physical therapy,* New York, 1985, Churchill Livingstone.

Seeley RR, Stephens DT, Tate P: *Essentials of anatomy and physiology,* St Louis, 1991, Mosby–Year Book.

Smith LK, Weiss EL, Lehmkuhl LD: *Brunnstrom's clinical kinesiology,* ed 5, Philadelphia, 1996, FA Davis.

Spence AP: *Basic human anatomy,* Menlo Park, Calif, 1982, Benjamin/Cummings.

Trombly CA: *Occupational therapy for physical dysfunction,* ed 4, Baltimore, 1995, Williams & Wilkins.

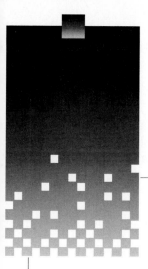

Glossary

abdominal region Lower anterior trunk

abduction To move away from midline of the body or body part; opposite of adduction

acetabular labrum Reinforcing piece of fibrocartilage that surrounds the acetabulum, making it a deeper, more stable articular surface for the head of femur

acetabulum Large fossa of the coxal bone where the head of femur articulates

acetylcholine Neurotransmitter necessary to stimulate skeletal muscle

acromial region Area of the acromion process of scapula

actin filament One of two types of myofilaments that make up the contractile unit of muscle tissue; attaches to myosin filament during muscle contraction

action Movement or work accomplished by skeletal muscle; described by using movement terminology

action potential Sequential depolarization of a neuron whereby it conducts a nerve impulse

active transport system Sodium-potassium pump; mechanism by which ions are returned to their original locations in sufficient quantity to conduct an impulse along a neuron

activities of daily living Any tasks commonly performed by an individual

adduction To move toward the midline of the body or body part; opposite of abduction

adipose tissue Fat

afferent neuron Sensory neuron that carries impulses from sensory receptors throughout the body to the central nervous system via the peripheral nervous system

agonist Muscle serving as the primary initiator for a specific action; prime mover

"all-or-none response" Quality of muscle and nerve tissues whereby a contraction or impulse occurs completely or not at all

ambulate To walk

amphiarthrosis Joint that allows only a slight degree of movement

anatomic position Arrangement of the human body in an upright standing posture, arms outstretched and downward, palms forward

anatomic regions Specific areas of the body that are named for a significant structure or landmark within the area

antagonist Muscle that opposes the prime mover

antebrachial region Area between the elbow and forearm

antecubital region Area anterior to the elbow

anterior To the front of; opposite of posterior

anterior horn Portion of gray matter central to the spinal cord; location of the cell bodies of motor neurons

anterior tilt Scapular movement whereby superior portion of the bone is pulled anteriorly toward the thorax; pelvic movement whereby the reference landmark is pulled anteriorly

anterolateral Diagonally to the front and away from midline

anteromedial Diagonally to the front and toward midline

apex Inferior tip of the heart or patella

appendicular skeleton Bones of the upper and lower extremities, including the shoulders and hips

articular cartilage Hyaline cartilage that covers the ends of bones that form a joint

articulate To join; to form a joint; point where two or more bones are attached or are movable

association neurons Neurons that communicate impulses between other neurons

atlas First cervical vertebra; C_1

autonomic nervous system Portion of the nervous system that is responsible for innervation of involuntary activities, such as heart and respiration rates, blood pressure, and digestion

axial skeleton Bones of the cranium, face, vertebral column, sternum, and ribs, including the hyoid bone

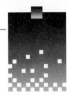

axillary region Area directly below the shoulder; the armpit

axis Second cervical vertebra; C_2

axon Trunk of a neuron that carries a nerve impulse

ball-and-socket joint Round sphere that fits into a cup; spheroid joint; multiplanar joint; diarthrotic or freely movable joint

basal ganglia Area of the brain that controls voluntary motor function

base Superior portion of the heart or patella

biconcave Having two sides that dip inward toward the center

bifid Divided into two parts

bilateral Occurring on two sides of the body; action that occurs as the result of right and left components of a muscle acting at the same time

biomechanics Analysis of human movement involving elements such as gravity, mass, weight, force, levers, and direction of movement

biplanar joint Joint that allows movement only in two planes; example: condyloid and saddle joints

bone marrow Substance contained within the medullary cavity of long bones and within the cavities of cancellous bones; red marrow performs hematopoiesis or blood cell production, whereas yellow marrow is primarily fat storage

brachial region Area between the shoulder and elbow

bradycardia Slow heart rate; less than 60 bpm

buccal region Facial area of the cheek

bursa Fluid-filled sac that provides padding for tendons near a joint; associated with synovial joints

calcaneal region Heel of the foot

calcium salts Common form of the most abundant mineral in the body; primary component of bone

cancellous bone Spongy bone; resists compressive forces; found in the epiphyses of long bones

cardiac output Measurement of overall efficiency of the heart; taken by multiplying heart rate by stroke volume

cardinal planes Three geometric divisions of the body; sagittal, frontal, and transverse planes

carpal Area and bones of the wrist

cartilaginous joint Joint where bones are attached via strong connective tissues such as hyaline, elastic, or fibrocartilage; immovable or slight movement only

caudal Toward or inferior to the tail; opposite of cephal

cell body Central portion of a neuron through which impulses must travel

central nervous system Brain and spinal cord

cephal Toward or superior to the head; opposite of caudal

cephalic region Area of the head

cerebellum Separate portion of the brain in the occipital region that processes sensory and motor information; controls posture, repetitive motion, and accuracy of skeletal movement

cerebral cortex Outer gray matter area of the brain

cerebrum Two large hemispheres of the brain

cervical region Area of vertebral column near the neck or throat; cervical vertebrae C_{1-7}

chamber Open area, similar to a room; one of four such areas within the heart

choroid plexus Specialized cells within the brain that produce cerebrospinal fluid

cilia Hairlike projections that carpet the membranes of the upper respiratory tract

circumduction Moving the body or body part in a large circle; combination of many individual movements

collagen fibers Semiflexible organic matrix made of protein molecules; framework for the skeleton

compact bone Dense, tightly packed bone tissue; found in the diaphysis of long bones and in a thin layer of other bones; resists bending; cortical bone

compliance Ease with which the lungs can be inflated and its tissues remain open in response to the surface tension created by a thin layer of serous or watery fluid between the two moist pleural membranes

compressive forces Pressure exerted on body tissues, such as from weight bearing

concave Hollow interior of a curved surface

concentric contraction Muscle contraction whereby the muscle belly is shortening

conductivity Quality of nerve tissue whereby it is capable of transmitting or carrying an impulse or signal to other tissues

condyle Type of bony landmark; rounded projection on the epiphysis of a long bone

condyloid joint Oval condyle that fits into an elliptical groove (biconcave into biconvex); biplanar joint; diarthrotic or freely movable joint

convex Rounded exterior of a curved surface

coronal suture Attachment between the frontal and parietal bones of the cranium

cortical bone Dense, tightly packed bone tissue; found in the diaphysis of long bones and in a thin layer of other bones; resists bending; compact bone

costal cartilage Dense, avascular tissue; hyaline cartilage; attaches the ribs to the sternum

costal facet Oval area on thoracic vertebrae where the head and tubercles of the ribs attach

coxal bone Three fused bones that make up one half of the pelvis; ilium, ischium, and pubis

coxal region Lateral area of the hips

cranial nerves Twelve pairs of nerves that branch directly off the brain; nerves that carry motor and sensory neurons to control certain body functions and receive feedback

cranial region Area of the head or skull

cranium Skull; made up of eight bones

crest Type of bony landmark; angular ridge on the diaphysis or on the edge of an irregular bone

cross section Horizontal division through the body or body part; transverse plane

crural region Area of the anterior lower leg between the knee and ankle

deep Below the surface; opposite of superficial

degree of movement Direction of movement; more than one degree of movement; more than one direction of possible movement

dendrites Branches of a neuron that receive incoming impulses

depolarization Stimulation of a polarized muscle fiber or a muscle fiber at rest

depression To move body part inferiorly; opposite of elevation

dermatome Area of innervation by a specific sensory nerve

diaphysis Long shaft of a long bone; primarily made up of compact bone

diarthrosis Joint that is freely movable; synovial joint

diastolic pressure Lowest normal pressure within the aorta, approximately 70-80 mm Hg; occurs when the aortic semilunar valve temporarily closes, preventing blood from flowing into the aorta

digital region Area of the fingers or toes

digits Fingers or toes; made up of either two or three phalanges

directional terms Words that describe a location or direction from a known reference point

distal Farther from a known reference point, usually the head; opposite of proximal

dorsal Toward the back; opposite of ventral

dorsiflexion To flex the ankle; from anatomic position to pointing the toe in a superior fashion or skyward; opposite of plantar flexion

eccentric contraction Muscle contraction whereby the muscle belly is lengthening

edema Interstitial fluid that accumulates in tissues, unable to be adequately removed by the vascular and lymphatic systems

efferent neuron Motor neuron that carries impulses from the muscles to the central nervous system via the peripheral nervous system

elastic recoil Quality of lung and connective tissues; promotes the expulsion of air from the lungs after having been stretched

elevation To move a body part superiorly as in shrugging the shoulders or hiking the hip; opposite of depression

endochondral bone Early stage of bone formation when its composition is primarily hyaline cartilage, later replaced by osteoblasts

endomysium Connective tissue that covers a single muscle fiber

endosteum Layer of bone tissue that lines the medullary cavity

epicondyle Type of bony landmark; a raised and usually rough area; proximal to a wide epiphysis of a long bone

epimysium Connective tissue that covers a group of fascicles to form a single muscle

epiphyseal plate Layer of cartilage that separates the diaphysis and epiphysis of long bones; location of bone growth; also called the growth plate

epiphysis Ends of a long bone; made up primarily of spongy bone

esophagus Passage for food that extends from the pharynx to the stomach

eversion To turn the sole of the foot until it faces outward, away from midline of the body; opposite of inversion

excitability Quality of muscle and nerve tissues in which the tissue responds to stimulation

expiration Exhalation; expelling air from the lungs by increasing the pressure in the thoracic cavity

expiratory reserve volume Quantity of air that can be forcibly exhaled beyond the tidal volume

extension When the angle between two body parts increases; bringing the humerus back toward the trunk within the sagittal plane after flexing at the shoulder; opposite of flexion

external auditory meatus Bony landmark on temporal bone; the canal leading from the exterior of the cranium to the inner ear

external rotation To pivot around an internal axis away from midline; synonymous with lateral rotation; opposite of internal rotation;

extracapsular Existing outside a synovial joint

facet Type of bony landmark; small, flat face; smooth and usually circular; area of articulation

facial region Area of the eyes, nose, mouth, and ears

false ribs Distal five pairs of ribs that attach onto the sternum via heavy costal cartilages

fascicle Collection of muscle fibers; wrapped by the connective tissue layer called the perimysium

femoral region Area between the hip and knee

fibrous connective tissue Dense, nonvascular connective tissue; collagen fibers; very few elastic fibers

fibrous joint Bony articulation attached by fibrous connective tissue; allows no movement

first class lever Simple mechanical machine whereby the fulcrum is central to force and resistance; seesaw; muscles of the neck that pull the cranium backward

fixator Muscle whose activity is to hold a bone in place; immobilizes a body part; stabilizes the skeleton; does not directly cause movement

flat bone Platelike bone that has a broad, smooth surface; located in the cranial, thoracic, and coxal regions

flexion Decreased angle between two body parts; from anatomic position, the humerus moves anteriorly in the sagittal plane; opposite of extension

floating ribs Last two pairs of false ribs that have no sternal attachment

foramen Type of bony landmark; round hole completely through a bone

foramen magnum Landmark of the occipital bone; large opening through which the spinal cord attaches to the brain

forefoot Portion of the foot that consists of metatarsals and phalanges

fossa Type of bony landmark; round, cuplike depression

frontal plane Vertical division of the body, separating anterior from posterior

functional ability Individual skill level with respect to activities of daily living

functional movement Any activity that results in the performance of a purposeful task; any voluntary movement that requires planning and coordination with specific intent by the individual

functional muscle group Categorization of muscles according to their similarities in action

functional reserve capacity Quantity of air that can be calculated by adding the expiratory reserve volume to the residual volume

glenoid labrum Reinforcing piece of fibrocartilage that surrounds the glenoid fossa, making it a deeper, more stable articular surface for the head of humerus

gliding joint Two semiflat surfaces that face one another; multiplanar joint; diarthrotic or freely movable joint

gluteal region Posterior area of the hips; the buttocks

golgi tendon organs Specialized receptors in the tendons of skeletal muscle, which return sensory information concerning the degree of strain on the tendon to the central nervous system

gomphosis Area where the root of a tooth attaches to either the maxilla or mandible by ligaments; immovable joint

gray matter Areas of concentrated neuron cell bodies within the central nervous system; thin layer covering outer surface of cerebrum; inner butterfly-shaped region of spinal cord

groove Type of bony landmark; long, shallow depression or trough

hand Distal end of the upper extremity; consists of carpals, metacarpals, and phalanges

hard palate Bony portion of roof of the mouth formed by the pair of maxillary bones

haversian canal Microscopic vertical opening within compact bone tissue; the center of the lamellae

haversian system Group of structures that make up compact bone that includes the lamellae, osteocytes, lacuna, haversian and Volkmann's canals, and canaliculi; also known as the osteon structure

head Type of bony landmark; blunt, hammerlike protrusion, often round and smooth

hematopoiesis Process of blood cell production by bone marrow

hinge joint Concave surface on a convex surface; uniplanar joint; diarthrotic or freely movable joint

hip hike Elevation of the pelvis; action of quadratus lumborum

horizontal plane Cross section or division of the body that separates superior from inferior; transverse plane

hyaline cartilage Firm, flexible tissue made up primarily of collagen fibers

hyperextension Excessive increase in angle between two body parts; movement common to hip, shoulder, and wrist

hypertension Abnormally high blood pressure

hyperventilation Pattern of deeper and increased rate of breathing, greater than normal

hypotension Abnormally low blood pressure

hypothalamus Area of the brain that regulates body temperature, appetite, gastrointestinal activity, sleep, release of hormones from the pituitary gland, and some emotions

hypothenar eminence Raised portion at the base of the palm on the side of the fifth metacarpal; muscles of the fifth digit

inferior Below; opposite of superior

inferolateral Diagonally below and away from midline

inferomedial Diagonally below and toward midline

inguinal region Area of the anterior hip

innervation Method by which tissue receives impulses from the central and peripheral nervous systems; neuron carrying impulses

innominate bones Two bony halves of the pelvic girdle by which the lower extremities attach to the axial skeleton; made up of the fused sets of ilium, ischium, and pubis

insertion Movable attachment of skeletal muscle

inspiration Inhalation; drawing air into the lungs after a temporary decrease in pressure or vacuum within the thoracic cavity

inspiratory capacity Quantity of air that can be forcibly inhaled beyond the tidal volume

inspiratory reserve volume Quantity of air that can be actively and forcibly inhaled beyond the tidal volume

internal rotation To pivot around an internal axis toward midline; synonymous with medial rotation; opposite of external rotation

intervertebral disk Cushion made of fibrous connective tissue and filled with clear fluid found between the vertebral bodies; absorbs pressure during weight bearing

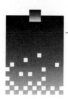

intervertebral foramen Opening created between two adjacent vertebrae through which a spinal nerve root passes; formed by the vertebral notches of adjacent vertebrae

intracapsular Existing inside a synovial joint

inversion To turn sole of foot until it faces inward or toward midline of the body; opposite of eversion

irregular bone Bone without a simple or common pattern; located in the facial, vertebral, and sacral regions

irritability Quality of nerve tissues; capability of tissues to be sensitive and responsive to stimuli

isokinetic contraction Muscle motion whereby resistance is applied in opposition to a movement, maintaining a constant rate of movement

isometric contraction Muscle motion whereby the muscular tone changes as muscle length remains constant

isotonic contraction Muscle motion whereby the muscle length changes as muscular tone remains constant

joint capsule Enclosed sac that surrounds the structures of a synovial joint

joint receptor Specialized sensory component within the tissues of a synovial joint that relays information regarding body position

kinesiology Study of human movement

kinetic Motion; movement; change in position

lacuna Microscopic open spaces in compact bone

lambdoidal suture Attachment between the parietal and occipital bones of the cranium

lamellae Microscopic layers of compact bone

lamina Bony attachment between the transverse and spinous processes on a thoracic or lumbar vertebra

landmark Reference point that has a specific name

lateral Away from midline; opposite of medial

lateral flexion To bend the vertebral column away from midline to the right or left

lateral rotation To pivot around an axis away from midline; synonymous with external rotation; opposite of medial rotation

lever Simple mechanical machine designed to accomplish work; consists of a rigid bar, a fulcrum where movement takes place, an applied force to cause movement, and some form of resistance

ligament Very strong connective tissue that attaches bone to bone

long bone Bone that has a diaphysis with an epiphysis at each end; found only in the extremities

lower extremity Leg, including the hip, knee, ankle, and foot

lumbar region Area of the lower posterior trunk; low back; vertebrae L_{1-5}

malleolus Bony landmarks on either side of ankle; distal aspect of both tibia and fibula

mandible Facial bone of the lower jaw

mastication Act of chewing food

medial Toward midline; opposite of lateral

medial rotation To pivot around an internal axis toward midline; synonymous with internal rotation; opposite of lateral rotation

medullary cavity Hollow central canal of a long bone; contains bone marrow

meninges Multiple layered protective covering that surrounds the brain and spinal cord

meniscus Cushion made of fibrocartilage that is generally circular; pair found in the knee; improves the mobility of the articulating bones while keeping them properly aligned

mental region Area of the lower jaw

midsagittal plane Vertical division of the body, separating right and left halves equally

motor end plate Specialized area on a skeletal muscle fiber where neurotransmitters are received thus initiating an impulse that causes the fiber to contract

motor neuron Nerve tissue that carries impulses from the central and peripheral nervous systems to an effector or muscle

motor unit Neuromuscular components required to cause skeletal muscle fiber contraction; includes motor neuron, synaptic vesicles, neurotransmitter, synapse, synaptic cleft, motor end plate, and motor fiber

movement Change in position of a body part or substance from one location to another

multiplanar joint Joint that allows movement in all three planes; example: ball-and-socket joint

muscle Contractile connective tissue that is responsible for causing movement of and within the body; types: skeletal, cardiac, smooth

muscle fiber Collection of many myofibrils; wrapped by a thin layer of connective tissue called the endomysium

muscle spindle Component within skeletal muscle that relates sensory information to the central nervous system; information includes muscle length, speed of contraction, and degree of stretch

muscle tone Constant, sustained contraction that exists in all normal skeletal muscle

myelin sheath Insulation-like lipid material that surrounds the axon of some neurons; serves to speed up impulse transmission by saltatory conduction

myofibril Component of muscle tissue; collection of sarcomere arranged end to end

myofilament Microscopic, interlocking, rodlike portion of muscle tissue; actin and myosin

myosin filament One of two types of myofilaments that make up the contractile unit of muscle tissue; attaches to actin filament during muscle contraction

myotome Area of innervation by a specific motor nerve

nasal region Area of the nose

neurilemma Outer membrane of Schwann's cells, making up the myelin sheath, which covers the axon of a neuron

neuromuscular junction Area where motor neuron communicates with muscle fiber; portion of the motor unit where the terminal branch releases neurotransmitters into the synaptic cleft near a motor end plate

neuron Simplest component of the nervous system; motor, sensory, or association

neurotransmitter Chemical substance released from the terminal branches of a neuron and received by a receptor or postsynaptic neuron, causing a response

nodes of Ranvier Intermittent gaps or thin areas of the myelin sheath that surround the axon of a neuron at which ionic changes occur during conduction of a nerve impulse

nomenclature Method of describing a body of information by similar categories

normal movement Motion accomplished by the otherwise healthy individual in a manner common to other healthy individuals

nucleus pulposus Structure central to the intervertebral disk; contained within the annulus fibrosus

oblique plane Any diagonal division of the body

obturator foramen Round hole through the right and left sides of the pelvic girdle; created by the fused portions of ischium and pubis

occipital condyle Pair of bony landmarks on the inferior aspect of occipital bone; articulates with first cervical vertebra

occipital protuberance Raised, roughened area on posterior aspect of occipital bone

occipital region Area of the posterior cranium; back of the head

odontoid facet Flattened area on the anterior aspect of the vertebral canal of the first cervical vertebra (atlas); articulates with odontoid process of second cervical vertebra (axis)

odontoid process Raised projection on the superior aspect of the second cervical vertebra (axis); articulates with the odontoid facet of first cervical vertebra (atlas)

opposition Medial rotation of the first metacarpal combined with flexion and abduction; movement of the thumb toward the midline of the hand; opposite of reposition

oral region Area of the mouth

orbit Large depression that contains the eye; formed by the frontal, zygomatic, maxillary, lacrimal, ethmoid, and sphenoid bones

orbital region Area of the eye

organic matrix Complex network of semiflexible collagen fibers made up of chains of protein molecules; primary substance of bone and other connective tissues

origin Fixed attachment of skeletal muscle

os coxae Hip bones; pelvic girdle made up of the paired and fused ilium, ischium, and pubis

ossification Process whereby calcium is deposited onto the organic matrix to form bone

osteoblast Bone-forming cell

osteocyte Microscopic bone cell

osteon structure Group of structures making up compact bone that includes the lamellae, osteocytes, lacuna, haversian and Volkmann's canals, and canaliculi; also known as the haversian system

otic region Area of the ear

P wave Change in electrical activity within the heart; monitored on an electrocardiogram (ECG); represents the depolarization of the atria

palmar region Anterior area of the hand

parasympathetic nervous system Portion of the autonomic nervous system that is responsible for calming the body after stimulation by the sympathetic nervous system; responsible for decreasing the heart rate, respiration, blood pressure, and other events

parietal region Lateral area of the cranium

patellar region Area of the patella or knee-cap; anterior to the knee

pectoral region Area of the anterior chest; the breast

pedicle Thoracic or lumbar vertebral landmark; bony bridge, connecting the vertebral body to transverse process

perimysium Connective tissue that covers a fascicle

perineal region Genital area

periosteum Outermost layer of bone; attachment for muscle, tendon, ligament, and other connective tissue

peripheral nerves Thirty-one pairs of nerves that branch off the spinal cord and carry motor and sensory neurons to control the body and receive feedback

peripheral nervous system Nerves outside of the central nervous system that innervate body systems; consists of the cranial and spinal nerves; divided into the autonomic, somatic, and sensory nervous systems

peroneal region Lateral area of the lower leg between the knee and ankle

phalanges Individual bones that make up the digits

pivot joint One bone that rotates on a fixed landmark; uniplanar joint; diarthrotic or freely movable joint

plantar flexion To extend the ankle from anatomic position, pointing the toe inferiorly or toward the ground; opposite of dorsiflexion

plantar region Bottom of the foot

polarity Biochemical state; has a positive or negative charge, depending on the location and quantity of ions

polarization Resting state of muscle tissue; precedes stimulation and contraction

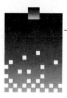

polarized neuron Unstimulated neuron that has a balance between its positive- and negative-charged ions

popliteal region Posterior area of the knee

posterior In back; opposite of anterior

posterior horn Portion of the gray matter that is central to the spinal cord; location of the cell bodies of sensory neurons

posterolateral Diagonally to the back of and away from midline

posteromedial Diagonally to the back of and toward midline

prime mover Muscle that serves as a primary initiator for a specific action; agonist

pronation To turn that hand palm down; radius rotates medially around ulna; foot turns until lateral edge is raised; opposite of supination

proprioception Quality of joint posture sense; awareness of the location of body parts in space; quality of the neuromuscular regulation of human movement

protraction To move body part anteriorly; thrust jaw, head, or shoulders forward

proximal Closer to the head; opposite of distal

pubic region Anterior midline area between the legs

pubic symphysis Point of articulation for left and right pubic bones; composed of hyaline cartilage

QRS complex Change in electrical activity within the heart; monitored on an electrocardiogram (ECG); represents the depolarization of the ventricles

radial deviation To laterally flex the wrist until thumb moves toward radius

ramus Flat bridge between two bones; thick branch of an irregular bone

ray Component of the hand that includes the metacarpal and its corresponding phalanges

receptor Recipient of neurotransmitters from a communicating neuron

recruitment Increase in the quantity of motor units being stimulated within a muscle

reference point Specific location

reflex arc Direct transmission of a nerve impulse from a sensory neuron to an association neuron in the spinal cord to a motor neuron

refractory period Brief moment when a neuron is unable to conduct an impulse after being depolarized; just before repolarization

remodeling Development of bone tissue in response to the body activity, such as weight bearing

repolarized neuron Reset phase of a neuron by which the ion charge realigns to its polarized state before becoming depolarized

reposition Lateral rotation of first metacarpal combined with extension and adduction; movement of the thumb away from the midline of the hand; opposite of reposition

residual volume Quantity of air that remains unchanged in the lungs and maintains the inflation of the lungs

resorption Physiologic removal of calcium from bone

respiration Collection of oxygen, its efficient transport to the cellular level where it is exchanged for carbon dioxide, and the removal of the carbon dioxide from the body

respiratory capacity Elements used to evaluate the quality of respiratory effort of an individual

resting potential Natural polarity of a neuron before becoming depolarized when conducting a nerve impulse

retraction To move body part posteriorly; to pull jaw, head, or shoulders backward

ribs Twelve pairs of flat bones that give shape to the thoracic region

sacral region Posterior midline area between the hips

sacroiliac joint Articulation between the sacrum and ilium

saddle joint Each bone concave in one direction and convex in another; biplanar joint; diarthrotic or freely movable joint

sagittal plane Division of the body, separating right from left

sagittal suture Attachment between the two parietal bones of the cranium

saltatory conduction Conduction of a nerve impulse along an axon covered by a myelin sheath; ionic changes occur only at the nodes of Ranvier

sarcolemma Cell membrane of a sarcomere

sarcomere Interlocking myofilaments; smallest unit of muscle contraction; portion of a myofibril

Schwann's cells Repeating segments of the myelin sheath that surrounds some axons; increases impulse transmission when ionic changes in axon skip myelinated segments

second class lever Simple mechanical machine whereby the resistance is central to the force and fulcrum; wheelbarrow; lifting the body weight on tiptoes

sensory neuron Afferent neuron that carries impulses from sensory receptors throughout the body to the central nervous system via the peripheral nervous system

sesamoid bone Usually small, round bones located within tendons; often serves as the fulcrum to improve mechanical advantage of a muscle or joint; most common sesamoid bone is the patella

short bone Round, smooth bone that has no diaphysis or epiphysis; carpals and tarsals

sinus Enclosed cavern in a bone; commonly found in the facial bones; serves to reduce weight and improve voice resonance

sinus rhythm Normal pattern of electrical activity in the heart; monitored on an electrocardiogram (ECG)

sodium-potassium pump Active transport system; mechanism by which ions are returned to their original locations in sufficient quantity to conduct an impulse along a neuron

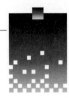

somatic nervous system Portion of the nervous system that is responsible for innervation of voluntary skeletal muscles through large myelinated axons

spheroid joint Round sphere that fits into a cup; ball-and-socket joint; multiplanar joint; diarthrotic or freely movable joint

sphygmomanometer Device used to monitor blood pressure; has an inflatable cuff that is wrapped around the upper extremity; monitors the blood flow in an artery; along with a stethoscope, the change in sound can be heard after the pressure from inflating the cuff is sharply increased and then slowly decreased

spinous process Thin projection; usually found on the posterior aspect of vertebrae

spirometry Measurement of respiratory capacity by a sophisticated instrument; measured in cubic centimeters

spongy bone Cancellous bone; resists compressive forces; found in the epiphyses of long bones

squamosal suture Attachment between the parietal and temporal bones of the cranium

sternal region Anterior midline area between the breasts

stethoscope Device used to listen to a variety of sounds that correspond to events that occur within the body

stroke volume Volume of blood pumped out of the heart through the aorta with each contraction; recorded in milliliters per beat

styloid process Bony landmark; small tip or tubercle; bulb-like protrusion

superficial Near the surface; opposite of deep

superior Above; opposite of inferior

superolateral Diagonally above and away from midline

superomedial Diagonally above and toward midline

supination To turn hand palm up; forearm in anatomic position; to turn foot until medial edge is raised

sural region Area of the posterior lower leg between the knee and ankle

surface tension Quality given to membranes within the body by a thin layer of fluid, causing surfaces to become attracted to one another

surfactant Substance produced by the body and excreted into the fluid that covers membranes within the respiratory system; causes decreased surface tension; prevents collapse of fragile airways that is due to surface tension

suture Area where two flat bones meet side to side, often interlocking; jointed by dense fibrous connective tissue; immovable joint or synarthrotic; attachment between bones of the cranium; irregular area where bones interlock

sympathetic nervous system Portion of the autonomic nervous system responsible for preparing the body to protect itself; responsible for increasing heart rate, respiration, blood pressure, and other events

symphysis Cartilaginous joint; slightly movable or amphiarthrotic

synapse Location at which neurons communicate impulses with a receptor

synaptic cleft Space between the terminal branch of a neuron and its receptor site

synarthrosis Type of joint that allows no movement

synchondrosis Cartilaginous joint; absorbs calcium in adulthood; loses its flexibility

syndesmosis Joint where bones are joined by long fibrous connective tissue, allowing slight movement

synergist Muscle that assists another in accomplishing similar work or movement

synovial capsule Enclosed sac that surrounds the structures of a synovial joint; joint capsule

systolic pressure Highest normal pressure within the aorta; approximately 120 mm Hg; occurs during contraction of the left ventricle, forcing blood into the aorta with great force

T wave Change in electrical activity within the heart; monitored on an electrocardiogram (ECG); represents the repolarization of the ventricles

tachycardia Rapid heart rate; greater than 100 bpm

tarsal Area and bones of the ankle

temporal region Anterolateral area of the cranium

tendon Rigid connective tissue that attaches muscle to bone

tendon sheath Long, thin cylindrical tissue that surrounds tendons; helps reduce friction

tensile strength Quality of bone that allows slight bending before breaking; made possible by the collagen fibers of the organic matrix

terminal branch Branch of neuron through which impulses travel to the next receptor

thalamus Area of the brain that directs sensory information in the brain

thenar eminence Raised portion at the base of the palm on the side of the first metacarpal; muscles of the thumb

third class lever Simple mechanical machine whereby the force is central to the resistance and fulcrum; use of a broom; most common lever of the musculoskeletal system

thoracic region Area of the vertebral column between the scapulae; thoracic vertebra T_{1-12}

threshold stimulus Minimum level of stimulus required to change the resting potential of a neuron

tidal volume Air exchanged during normal breathing, such as occurs when sitting quietly

total lung capacity Greatest volume of air that can be possibly contained by the lungs and respiratory system

trabeculae Irregular web of cancellous branches that make up spongy bone

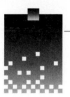

transverse foramen Pathway for the vertebral artery through the cervical vertebrae between the transverse process and superior articulating facet

transverse plane Cross section or division of the body, separating superior from inferior; horizontal plane

transverse processes Horizontal bony projection that extends laterally from vertebrae

true ribs Most proximal seven pairs of ribs that attach directly onto the sternum

tubercle Type of bony landmark; small, round, bulblike protrusion

tuberosity Type of bony landmark; large, rough, bulblike protrusion

ulnar deviation To laterally flex the wrist until fifth digit moves toward ulna

umbilical region Area central to the abdomen; commonly known as the navel

unilateral Occurring on one side of the body; action occurring as the result of the right or left component of a muscle acting alone

uniplanar joint Joint that allows movement in one plane only; examples: hinge and pivot joints

upper extremity Arm, including the shoulder, elbow, wrist, and hand

vasoconstriction Contraction of the smooth muscle or tunica media, causing the narrowing of vessel diameter

vasodilation Relaxation of the smooth muscle or tunica media in a blood vessel, causing enlargement of vessel diameter

ventilation Event of air that enters and exits the body

ventral Toward the belly; opposite of dorsal

ventricle Open area in the brain; contains cerebrospinal fluid

vertebral canal Open area central to the vertebrae through which the spinal cord passes

vertebral region Area of the vertebrae or spinal column

visceral Pertains to an organ; lying in close proximity to a body organ

vital capacity Quantity of air calculated by adding the value of the tidal volume and both the inspiratory and expiratory reserve volumes

Volkmann's canal Pathway between the haversian canal within compact bone tissue

white matter Area of concentrated myelinated axons within the central nervous system; central portion of the brain; outer portion of the spinal cord that surrounds the gray matter

Z line Separating boundary between individual sarcomere

Answer Key

Chapter 1

Exercise 1-1. Directional terms

1. Medial
2. Lateral
3. Proximal
4. Distal
5. Superior (cephal)
6. Inferior (caudal)
7. Posterior (dorsal)
8. Anterior (ventral)
9. Cephal (superior)
10. Caudal (inferior)
11. Distal
12. Proximal
13. Lateral
14. Medial
15. Anterior (ventral)
16. Posterior (dorsal)

Exercise 1-2. Anatomic regions

1. Digital (foot)
2. Tarsal
3. Crural
4. Patellar
5. Femoral
6. Peroneal
7. Pubic
8. Inguinal
9. Umbilical
10. Abdominal
11. Coxal
12. Axillary
13. Cubital
14. Brachial
15. Carpal
16. Digital (hand)
17. Cephalic
18. Frontal
19. Orbital
20. Otic
21. Oral
22. Buccal
23. Sternal
24. Acromial
25. Pectoral
26. Antecubital
27. Antebrachial
28. Palmar
29. Temporal
30. Nasal
31. Mental
32. Parietal
33. Occipital
34. Cervical
35. Vertebral
36. Thoracic
37. Lumbar
38. Sacral
39. Gluteal
40. Perineal
41. Popliteal
42. Sural
43. Calcaneal
44. Plantar

Exercise 1-3. Cardinal planes

1. Frontal
2. Transverse
3. Sagittal
4. Oblique

Exercise 1-4. Directional terminology

1. Lateral
2. Superficial
3. Posterior
4. Distal
5. Inferior
6. Medial
7. Anterosuperior
8. Deep
9. Superior
10. Proximal
11. Posterior
12. Distal
13. Anterior
14. Inferior
15. Inferior
16. Anterior
17. Proximal
18. Lateral
19. Proximal
20. Inferior

Exercise 1-5. Cardinal planes defined

1. Sagittal
2. Transverse
3. Midsagittal
4. Frontal or coronal
5. Transverse
6. Sagittal; frontal
7. Frontal

Exercise 1-6. Anatomic locations

Results are dependent on student performance.

Exercise 1-7. Anatomic locations by region

Results are dependent on student performance.

Exercise 1-8. Anatomic directions

Results are dependent on student performance.

Chapter 2

Exercise 2-1. Bone tissue

1. k or t	9. m	17. u
2. v	10. x	18. q
3. e	11. w	19. b
4. p	12. j	20. r
5. l	13. t	21. h
6. f	14. n	22. g
7. s	15. i	23. d
8. c	16. a	24. o

Exercise 2-2. Functions of bone tissue

Function 1: Shape and framework
Description: Solid, interlocking parts; foundation for soft tissues to attach and cover bone
Function 2: Mineral storage
Description: Calcium attached to organic matrix
Function 3: Muscle attachment
Description: Muscle attached to bone via tendon; contracts and moves the bone
Function 4: Protection
Description: Body armor that covers the brain and internal organs
Function 5: Blood cell production
Description: Through hematopoiesis, blood cells are produced in the marrow of bones, inside the medullary canal
Function 6: Filtration
Description: Blood, circulating through bone, deposits materials in the skeleton
Function 7: Fat storage
Description: Specialized cells in the bone marrow, responsible for storing fat

Exercise 2-3. Bone tissue

See Figures 2-1, 2-2, and 2-3.

Exercise 2-4. Terminology of bone shapes

1. d	4. c
2. e	5. b
3. a	

Exercise 2-5. Bone identity by shape

See Figure 2-7.

Exercise 2-6. Bones of the cranium

Frontal	1	Superior portions of right and left orbits	Flat
		Supraorbital foramen	
Ethmoid	1	Cribriform plates	Irregular
		Perpendicular plate	
		Superior and middle nasal conchae	
		Crista galli	
Sphenoid	1	Deepest portion of orbit	Irregular
		Sella turcica	
Parietal	2	None	Flat
Temporal	2	External auditory meatus	Irregular
		Mastoid process	
		Styloid process	
		Mandibular fossa	
		Zygomatic process	
Occipital	1	Foramen magnum	Irregular
		Occipital condyles	
		Occipital crest	
		Occipital protuberance	
		Superior curved line	
		Inferior curved line	

Exercise 2-7. Sutures of the cranium

Coronal	Frontal and parietal
Sagittal	Right parietal and left parietal
Squamosal	Temporal and parietal
Lambdoidal	Parietal and occipital

Exercise 2-8. Cranium

See Figures 2-10, 2-11, 2-12, and 2-13.

Exercise 2-9. Bones and landmarks of the face

See Figures 2-10, 2-12, and 2-13.

Exercise 2-10. Bones of the face

Maxilla	2	Hard palate
Nasal	2	Forms bridge of nose
Vomer	1	Forms nasal septum
Lacrimal	2	Between orbit and nasal cavity
Zygomatic	2	Cheek bone
		Temporal process
Palatine	2	Forms hard palate and floor of nasal cavity
Inferior nasal conchae	2	Covered by nasal membrane
Mandible	1	Only movable bone of the face
		Ramus
		Body
		Angle
		Mandibular condyle
		Coronoid process

Exercise 2-11. Vertebrae and vertebral landmarks

C_1 (Atlas)	1	Superior articulating facets (2)
		Inferior articulating facets (2)
		Anterior arch
		Vertebral canal
		Odontoid facet
		Transverse processes (2)
		Transverse foramen (2)
C_2 (Axis)	1	Odontoid facet
		Body
		Superior articulating facets (2)
		Inferior articulating facets (2)
		Transverse processes (2)
		Transverse foramen (2)
		Bifid spinous process
Thoracic	12	Body
		Vertebral foramen
		Costal facets for head of rib
		Costal facets for tubercle of rib
		Pedicle
		Transverse processes (2)
		Superior articulating facet (2)
		Inferior articulating facets (2)
		Lamina
		Downward-angled spinous process
Cervical	7	Body
		Vertebral foramen
		Transverse processes (2)
		Superior articulating facets (2)
		Inferior articulating facets (2)
		Lamina
		Downward-angled spinous process
Lumbar	5	Largest body
		Vertebral canal
		Pedicle
		Transverse processes (2)
		Superior articulating facet (2)
		Inferior articulating facets (2)
		Lamina
		Downward-angled spinous process
Sacrum	5 (fused)	Sacral promontory
		Superior articulating facets (2)
		Sacral canal
		Ala of sacrum
		Sacroiliac facets
		Sacral foramen (4 pairs)
		Sacral hiatus
Coccyx	4 (fused)	None

Exercise 2-12. Vertebrae and vertebral landmarks

See Figures 2-25, 2-26, 2-27, and 2-28

Exercise 2-13. Vertebral comparison

1. Lumbar
2. Cervical
3. Transverse foramen
4. Costal facets
5. Vertebral foramen
6. Bifid, pointed inferiorly
7. Short wide, pointed posteriorly
8. Cervical-aligned horizontally; thoracic- and lumbar-aligned vertically
9. Cervical—thin and rounded; thoracic—thin and long; lumbar—thick, short
10. C_1 (Axis); C_2 (Atlas)

Exercise 2-14. Components of the ribs and sternum

True ribs	14 (7 pairs)	Head, tubercle, attaches anteriorly directly onto the sternum
False ribs	10 (5 pairs)	Head, tubercle, attaches anteriorly indirectly via costal cartilages
Floating ribs	4 (2 pairs)	Head; tubercle, no anterior attachment
Sternum	1	Manubrium, body, xiphoid process

Exercise 2-15. Identify components of the ribs and sternum

See Figures 2-33 and 2-34.

Exercise 2-16. Components of the axial skeleton

Cranium	Frontal	Parietal
	Ethmoid	Temporal
	Sphenoid	Occipital
Face	Maxillary	Lacrimal
	Zygomatic	Palatine
	Nasal	Inferior nasal conchae
	Vomer	Mandible
Anterior cervical region	Hyoid	
Vertebrae	Atlas	Cervical
	Axis	Thoracic
	Lumbar	Sacrum
	Coccyx	
Thoracic cage	Ribs	Sternum

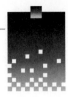

Exercise 2-17. Palpating landmarks of the axial skeleton

Results are dependent on student performance.

Exercise 2-18. Pectoral girdle and upper extremity

1. Clavicle; scapula
2. Manubrium of sternum
3. Humerus
4. Ulna; radius
5. Humerus
6. Ulna
7. Radius
8. First metatarsal
9. Pisiform; triquetrum; lunate; scaphoid; hamate; capitate; trapezoid; trapezium
10. Metatarsals

Exercise 2-19. Landmarks of pectoral girdle and upper extremity

Clavicle:	Sternal end (proximal)
	Acromial end (distal)
Scapula:	Superior angle
	Inferior angle
	Vertebral (medial) border
	Axillary (lateral) border
	Spine of scapula
	Root of scapula
	Acromion process
	Coracoid process
	Glenoid fossa
	Supraspinous fossa
	Infraspinous fossa
	Subscapular fossa
	Supraglenoid tubercle
	Infraglenoid tubercle
	Subscapular notch
Proximal humerus:	Head of humerus
	Anatomical neck
	Surgical neck
	Greater tubercle
	Lesser tubercle
	Bicipital groove
	Deltoid tuberosity
Distal humerus:	Radial fossa
	Coronoid fossa
	Capitulum
	Trochlea
	Olecranon fossa
	Medial epicondyles
	Lateral epicondyles
	Medial supracondylar ridges
	Lateral supracondylar ridges

Proximal ulna:	Olecranon process
	Trochlear notch
	Coronoid process
	Radial notch
	Ulnar tuberosity
	Supinator crest
	Interosseous border
Distal ulna:	Head
	Styloid process
Proximal radius:	Head
	Radial tuberosity
	Interosseous border
Distal radius:	Styloid process
	Dorsal tubercle
Carpals:	Pisiform
	Triquetrum
	Lunate
	Scaphoid
	Hook of hamate
	Capitate
	Trapezoid
	Trapezium

Exercise 2-20. Landmarks and directional terms

1. Posterior
2. Anterior
3. Medial
4. Proximal
5. Proximal
6. Distal
7. Inferior
8. Superior
9. Anterior
10. Medial
11. Lateral
12. Posterodistal
13. Proximal
14. Anterior
15. Medial
16. Distal
17. Distal
18. Distal
19. Anterior
20. Proximal
21. Anterior
22. Distal
23. Distal
24. Proximal
25. Proximal

Exercise 2-21. Bones and landmarks of the pectoral girdle and upper extremity

See Figures 2-38 through 2-43.

Exercise 2-22. Palpate landmarks of the pectoral girdle and upper extremity

Results are dependent on student performance.

Exercise 2-23. Pelvic girdle and lower extremity

1. Ilium; ischium; pubis
2. Sacrum
3. Femur
4. Femur
5. Tibia
6. Fibula
7. Talus; calcaneus, first, second, and third cuneiforms; navicular; cuboid
8. Talus
9. Metatarsals; phalanges
10. 14

Exercise 2-24. Landmarks of the pelvic girdle and lower extremity

Ilium:
Ala of ilium
Iliac crest
Anterior superior iliac spine
Posterior superior iliac spine
Anterior inferior iliac spine
Posterior inferior iliac spine
Greater sciatic notch
Auricular surface
Iliac fossa

Ischium:
Obturator foramen
Ischial spine
Lesser sciatic notch
Ischial tuberosity
Ischial ramus

Pubis:
Body of pubis
Pubic symphysis
Superior rami of pubis
Inferior rami of pubis
Pelvic tuberosity

Proximal femur:
Head of femur
Fovea capitis
Neck of femur
Intertrochanteric fossa
Greater trochanter
Intertrochanteric line
Intertrochanteric crest
Lesser trochanter
Gluteal tuberosity

Distal femur:
Linea aspera
Medial and lateral epicondyles of femur
Medial and lateral condyles of femur
Intercondylar fossa
Patellar groove

Patella:
Superior border
Apex of patella
Articulating surface for femur

Proximal tibia:
Tibial plateau
Intercondylar eminence
Medial and lateral condyles of tibia
Soleal line
Tibial tuberosity

Distal tibia:
Interosseous border
Medial malleolus

Fibula:
Head of fibula
Interosseous border of fibula
Styloid process of fibula
Lateral malleolus of fibula
Neck of fibula
Diaphysis of fibula

Foot:
Talus
Calcaneus
First, second, third cuneiforms
Navicular bone
Cuboid
Metatarsals (5)—base, head
Phalanges (15)—proximal, middle, distal

Exercise 2-25. Landmarks and directional terms

1. Superior
2. Anterior
3. Medioproximal
4. Distal
5. Superior
6. Proximal
7. Inferior
8. Inferomedial
9. Distal
10. Anterior
11. Superior
12. Distal
13. Inferior
14. Proximomedial
15. Posterior
16. Proximal
17. Inferior (distal)
18. Anterior
19. Lateral
20. Proximal
21. Distal
22. Medial
23. Distal
24. Distal
25. Lateral

Exercise 2-26. Pelvic girdle and lower extremity

See Figures 2-51 through 2-54 and Figures 2-56 through 2-58.

Exercise 2-27. Palpate landmarks of pelvic girdle and lower extremity

Results are dependent on student performance.

Exercise 2-28. Landmark terminology

Condyle *Location:* Femur, humerus
   Definition: Rounded projection on epiphysis
Crest *Location:* Ilium
   Definition: Angular ridge
Epicondyle *Location:* Femur, humerus
   Definition: Raised, rough area proximal to epiphysis of long bone
Facet *Location:* Vertebrae
   Definition: Small, flat, circular face
Foramen *Location:* Coxal bone
   Definition: Round hole through bone
Fossa *Location:* Scapula, coxal bone
   Definition: Round, cuplike depression
Groove *Location:* Humerus
   Definition: Long, shallow depression or trough
Head *Location:* Radius, humerus, femur
   Definition: Blunt, hammerlike protrusion
Ramus *Location:* Coxal bones
   Definition: Flat bridge between two bones
Sinus *Location:* Facial bones
   Definition: Enclosed cavern
Tubercle *Location:* Vertebrae, ribs
   Definition: Small, rough bulblike protrusion
Tuberosity *Location:* Radius, ulna
   Definition: Large, rough bulblike protrusion

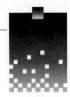

Chapter 3

Exercise 3-1. Joints—structure and movement

1. Amphiarthrotic
2. Symphysis (cartilaginous) joint, pubic symphysis
3. Fibrous connective
4. Fibrous, syndesmosis
5. Pivot
6. Synovial
7. Articular cartilage, hyaline cartilage
8. Slightly movable
9. Syndesmosis (fibrous) joint
10. Synchondrosis
11. Synovial or diarthrotic
12. Saddle
13. Ball and socket
14. Two
15. Elbow, knee
16. Fibrous
17. Amphiarthrotic, slight
18. Bursa
19. Ball and socket
20. Gliding

Exercise 3-2. Joint structures

Fibrous

Fibrous connective	1. Sutures	1. Immovable
ligaments	2. Syndesmoses	2. Slightly movable
	3. Gomphoses	3. Immovable

Cartilaginous

| Cartilage— | 1. Synchondrosis | 1. Immovable |
| strong, flexible | 2. Symphysis | 2. Slightly movable |

Synovial

Articular cartilage	1. Shoulder	1. Freely movable
Joint cavity	2. Hip	
Joint capsule	3. Knee	
Synovial membrane	4. Interphalange	
Synovial fluid		
Ligaments		

Exercise 3-3. Joint movements

Synarthrotic	Fibrous	Immovable
Amphiarthrotic	Cartilaginous	Slightly movable
Diarthrotic	Synovial	Freely movable

Exercise 3-4. Components of joint structures

See Figures 3-1, 3-2, and 3-3.

Exercise 3-5. Synovial (diarthrotic) joints

Ball and socket

Description Round sphere that fits into a cup

Examples Shoulder—humerus on glenoid fossa of scapula; hip—head of femur on acetabulum

Degrees and planes of motion Multiplanar—sagittal, frontal, transverse

Hinge

Description Concave surface on a convex surface

Examples Elbow—humerus on ulna; knee—femur on tibia

Degrees and planes of motion Uniplanar—sagittal

Pivot

Description One bone turns on a fixed landmark

Examples Atlas on Axis; proximal radius on ulna

Degrees and planes of motion Uniplanar—transverse

Saddle

Description Each bone concave in one direction and convex in the other direction

Examples First metacarpal on trapezium

Degrees and planes of motion Biplanar—sagittal, frontal

Gliding

Description Two semiflat surfaces facing one another

Examples Articular facets of vertebrae; intercarpal (very slight movement

Degrees and planes of motion Multiplanar—sagittal, frontal, transverse, oblique

Condyloid

Description Oval condyle fits into an elliptical groove

Examples Mandibular condyle on temporal bone; metacarpal on proximal phalanx

Degrees and planes of motion Biplanar—sagittal, frontal

Exercise 3-6. Types of synovial (diarthrotic) joints

See Figure 3-4.

Exercise 3-7. Movement definitions

1. n	7. t	13. u	19. g
2. e	8. c	14. f	20. b
3. q	9. l	15. r	21. h
4. k	10. i	16. m	22. o
5. a	11. d	17. v	23. p
6. w	12. j	18. s	

Exercise 3-8. Movements

See Figures 3-9 through 3-20.

Exercise 3-9. Joint structures of the shoulder and upper extremity

Sternoclavicular

Bones and landmarks Manubrium of sternum; proximal clavicle
Type of joint Gliding
Ligaments and soft tissues Sternoclavicular ligaments; costo-clavicular ligaments
Movements Slight movement

Acromioclavicular

Bones and landmarks Distal clavicle; acromion processes of scapula
Type of joint Gliding
Ligaments and soft tissues Acromioclavicular ligaments; cora-coclavicular ligaments; coracoacro-mial ligaments
Movements Slight movement

Glenohumeral

Bones and landmarks Glenoid fossa of scapula, head of humerus
Type of joint Ball and socket
Ligaments and soft tissues Glenohumeral ligaments' coraco-humeral ligaments; transverse humeral ligament; glenoid labrum; rotator cuff group
Movements Flexion; extension; hyperextension; rotation; abduction; adduction; horizontal abduction and adduction; circumduction

Scapulothoracic

Bones and landmarks Scapula; humerus
Type of joint Ball and socket
Ligaments and soft tissues Muscle attaching scapula to trunk
Movements Abduction; adduction; elevation; depression; medial/lateral; rotation; anterior tilt

Elbow

Bones and landmarks Trochlea of humerus; trochlear notch of ulna; capitulum of humerus; head of radius
Type of joint Hinge
Ligaments and soft tissues Ulna collateral ligament; annular ligament; radial collateral ligament; interosseous ligament
Movements Flexion; extension

Radioulnar

Bones and landmarks Radial notch of ulna; head of radius; diaphysis of radioulnar; ulnar notch of radius; head of ulna
Type of joint Pivot
Ligaments and soft tissues Interosseous ligament
Movements Supination; pronation

Wrist

Bones and landmarks Distal ends of radius and ulna; proxi-mal row of carpals; distal row of carpals; metacarpals
Type of joint Gliding (and condyloid)
Ligaments and soft tissues Ulnar and radial collateral liga-ments; dorsal and palmar radio-carpal ligaments; palmar ulnocarpal ligaments; intercarpal ligaments; flexor and extensor retinacula
Movements Flexion; extension; hyperextension; radial/ulnar deviation

Hand

Bones and landmarks Carpometacarpal joint; intermetacarpal joint; metacarpophalangeal joint; inter-phalangeal joint
Type of joint Ball and socket
Ligaments and soft tissues Dorsal and palmar carpo-metacarpal ligaments; inter-metacarpal ligaments; palmar and collateral ligaments
Movements Various

Exercise 3-10. Structures of the pectoral girdle and upper extremity

See Figures 3-34, 3-35, 3-36, and 3-38.

Exercise 3-11. Ligaments of the pectoral girdle and upper extremity

1. e	5. d, f	9. f	13. a
2. c	6. d, f	10. g	14. b
3. c	7. d	11. a	15. b
4. c	8. f	12. f	16. b

Exercise 3-12. Joint structures of the hip and lower extremity

Hip

Bones and landmarks Acetabulum of coxal bone; head of femur
Type of joint Ball and socket
Ligaments and soft tissues Iliofemoral; ischiofemoral; pubofemoral; ligamentum teres; acetabular labrum
Movements Flexion; extension; hyperextension; rotation; abduction; adduction; circumduction

Knee

Bones and landmarks Distal femur at medial and lateral condyles; tibia; patellar groove of femur; tibial plateau; tibial tuberosity

Type of joint Hinge

Ligaments and soft tissues Anterior and posterior cruciate ligaments; tibial and fibular collateral ligaments; oblique popliteal ligament; transverse ligament; medial and lateral menisci; quadriceps tendon; patellar tendon ligament

Movements Flexion; extension; slight rotation when flexed

Ankle

Bones and landmarks Tibia; fibula; medial—malleolus of tibia; lateral—malleolus of fibula; talus; cuboid; navicular bone; three cuneiforms

Type of joint Hinge

Ligaments and soft tissues Deltoid ligament; fibulocalcaneal ligament

Movements Dorsiflexion; plantar flexion

Exercise 3-13. Ligaments of the hip and lower extremity

1. b	5. c	9. b	13. b
2. a	6. b	10. c	14. a
3. b	7. b	11. a	
4. a	8. a	12. b	

Exercise 3-14. Identify structures of the hip and lower extremity

See Figures 3-43, 3-44, 3-45, 3-46, 3-47, and 3-48.

Chapter 4

Exercise 4-1. Types of muscle tissue

Skeletal

Voluntary or involuntary Voluntary

Resulting activity Moves the skeleton
Holds the skeleton in place
Posture

Cardiac

Voluntary or involuntary Involuntary

Resulting activity Cardiac muscle
Pumps blood

Smooth

Voluntary or involuntary Involuntary

Resulting activity Moves substances through the arteries, veins, stomach, and intestines

Exercise 4-2. Principles of skeletal muscle contraction

1. e	5. k	9. d
2. i	6. j	10. f
3. l	7. b	11. a
4. h	8. c	12. g

Exercise 4-3. Components of muscle contraction

See Figure 4-4.

Exercise 4-4. Types of levers

First

Mechanical description Seesaw; crowbar; scissors

Anatomic example Cranium on Atlas; humerus on ulna in elbow extension

Second

Mechanical description Wheelbarrow

Anatomic example Rising on tips of toes (plantar flexion)

Third

Mechanical description Broom

Anatomic example Most skeletal movement; humerus on ulna in elbow flexion; tibia on femur in knee extension

Exercise 4-5. Identification of levers

See Figures 4-9, 4-10, and 4-12.

Exercise 4-6. Types of muscle contractions

1. d	6. e	11. b
2. f	7. k	12. a
3. g	8. m	13. c
4. i	9. l	
5. j	10. h	

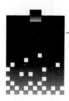

Chapter 5

Exercise 5-1. Movement analysis: scapular stabilizers

Movement	Trapezius upper	Trapezius middle	Trapezius lower	Rhomboids	Levator scapulae	Serratus anterior	Pectoralis minor
Scapular elevation	X				X		
Scapular depression			X				
Scapular rotation—upward	X		X				
Scapular rotation—downward				X	X		
Scapular adduction		X		X			
Scapular abduction						X	
Scapular tilt—anterior							X
Cervical extension	X				X		
Cervical rotation					X		
Cervical lateral flexion	X				X		
Assists inspiration						X	X

Exercise 5-2. Innervation analysis: scapular stabilizers

Movement	Trapezius upper	Trapezius middle	Trapezius lower	Rhomboids	Levator scapulae	Serratus anterior	Pectoralis minor
Spinal accessory	X	X	X				
Dorsal scapular				X	X		
Long thoracic						X	
Medial pectoral							X

Exercise 5-3. Movement analysis: shoulder and rotator cuff

Movement	Flexion	Extension	Abduction	Adduction	Medial rotation	Lateral rotation
Pectoralis major	X			X	X	
Coracobrachialis	X			X		
Biceps brachii	X		X			
Deltoid	X	X	X		X	X
Latissimus dorsi		X		X	X	
Triceps brachii		X		X		
Teres major		X		X	X	
Supraspinatus			X			
Infraspinatus						X
Teres minor						X
Subscapularis					X	

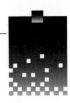

Exercise 5-4. Innervation analysis: shoulder and rotator cuff

Muscles	Pectoral	Musculocutaneous	Axillary	Thoracodorsal	Radial	Suprascapular	Subscapular
Pectoralis major	X						
Coracobrachialis		X					
Biceps brachii		X					
Deltoid			X				
Latissimus dorsi				X			
Triceps brachii					X		
Teres major							X
Supraspinatus						X	
Infraspinatus						X	
Teres minor			X				
Subscapularis							X

Exercise 5-5. Scapular stabilizer muscles

See Figure 5-1.

Exercise 5-6. Shoulder muscles

See Figure 5-6.

Exercise 5-7. Movement analysis: elbow and forearm

Muscles that cross the shoulder and elbow	Elbow flexion	Elbow extension	Pronation	Supination
Biceps brachii	X			X
Triceps brachii		X		

Muscles that cross the elbow only	Elbow flexion	Elbow extension	Pronation	Supination
Brachialis	X			
Brachioradialis	X		X	X
Anconeus		X		
Supinator				X
Pronator teres			X	

Exercise 5-8. Innervation analysis: elbow and forearm

Muscles that cross the shoulder and elbow	Radial	Musculocutaneous	Median
Biceps brachii		X	
Triceps brachii	X		

Muscles that cross elbow only	Radial	Musculocutaneous	Median
Brachialis	X	X	
Brachioradialis	X		
Anconeus	X		
Supinator	X		
Pronator teres			X

Exercise 5-9. **Movement analysis: radioulnar joint**

Muscles	Supination	Pronation
Supinator	X	
Pronator teres		X
Pronator quadratus		X

Exercise 5-10. **Innervation analysis: radioulnar joint**

Muscles	Radial	Median
Supinator	X	
Pronator teres		X
Pronator quadratus		X

Exercise 5-11. **Muscles of the shoulder and elbow**

See Figures 5-4 and 5-8.

Exercise 5-12. **Movement analysis: muscles of the wrist and muscles extrinsic to the hand**

Muscles that cross the elbow and wrist	Flexion	Extension	Radial deviation	Ulnar deviation
Flexor carpi radialis	X		X	
Flexor carpi ulnaris	X			X
Palmaris longus	X			
Flexor digitorum superficialis	X			
Extensor carpi radialis longus		X	X	
Extensor carpi radialis brevis		X	X	
Extensor carpi ulnaris		X		X
Extensor digitorum		X		

Muscles that cross the wrist	Flexion	Extension	Radial deviation	Ulnar deviation
Flexor digitorum profundus	X			
Flexor pollicis longus	X			
Abductor pollicis longus			X	
Extensor indicis				
Extensor pollicis brevis			X	
Extensor pollicis longus		X	X	

Exercise 5-13. *Innervation analysis: muscles of the wrist and muscles extrinsic to the hand*

Muscles that cross the elbow and wrist	Median	Radial	Ulnar
Flexor carpi radialis	X		
Flexor carpi ulnaris			X
Palmaris longus	X		
Flexor digitorum superficialis	X		
Extensor carpi radialis longus		X	
Extensor carpi radialis brevis		X	
Extensor carpi ulnaris		X	
Extensor digitorum		X	
Extensor digiti minimi		X	

Muscles that cross only the wrist	Median	Radial	Ulnar
Flexor digitorum profundus	X		X
Flexor pollicis longus	X		
Abductor pollicis longus		X	
Extensor indicis		X	
Extensor pollicis brevis		X	
Extensor pollicis longus		X	

Exercise 5-14. *Movement analysis: intrinsic muscles of the hand*

Muscles	Extension MCPs	Flexion MCPs	Extension IPs	Flexion IPs	Abduction	Adduction
Lumbricals		X	X			
Dorsal interossei		X	X		X	
Palmar interossei		X	X			X
Abductor digiti minimi		X	X		X	
Flexor digiti minimi		X				
Opponens digiti minimi		X				
Flexor pollicis brevis		X				
Abductor pollicis brevis					X	
Opponens pollicis					X	
Adductor pollicis		X				X

Exercise 5-15. Innervation analysis: intrinsic muscles of the hand

Muscles	Ulnar	Median
Lumbricals	X	X
Dorsal interossei	X	
Palmar interossei	X	
Abductor digiti minimi	X	
Flexor digiti minimi	X	
Opponens digiti minimi	X	
Flexor pollicis brevis	X	X
Abductor pollicis brevis		X
Opponens pollicis		X
Adductor pollicis	X	

Exercise 5-16. Extensor muscles of the forearm, wrist, and hand

See Figures 5-12, 5-11, and 5-20.

Exercise 5-17. Illustrate muscles of the shoulder and upper extremity

Results are dependent on student performance.

Exercise 5-18. Palpate muscles of the shoulder and upper extremity

Results are dependent on student performance.

Exercise 5-19. Review muscles of the shoulder and upper extremity

1. Posterior cervical region and posterior to clavicle.
2. Lower trapezius.
3. No, serratus anterior inserts on the costal surface of the scapula.
4. Levator scapula can perform cervical extension when contracting bilaterally; the insertion is fixed.
5. Deep.
6. Musculocutaneous innervates both coracobrachialis and biceps brachii.
7. Latissimus dorsi and teres major perform shoulder adduction and extension.
8. The tendon of the long head of biceps brachii lies along the bicipital groove.
9. Supraspinatus.
10. Supraspinatus, infraspinatus, teres minor, subscapularis.
11 Musculocutaneous innervates biceps brachii and brachialis.
12 The radial nerve innervates triceps brachii and anconeus.
13. Supinator originates on the posterior aspect of the ulna and inserts on the anterior radius. The pronators originate anteriorly on the ulna and insert on the posterior and lateral aspect of the radius.
14. Flexors of the wrist and hand.
15. Extrinsic; its origin lies on the posterior aspect of the radius.
16. Lateral epicondyle of humerus.
17. Radial nerve.
18. Ulnar nerve.
19. Palmaris longus performs wrist flexion and assists with elbow flexion.
20. Extensor pollicis longus and extensor pollicis brevis.
21. Extensor indicis.
22. Lumbricals.
23. Ulnar nerve.
24. Adductor pollicis.
25. Dorsal interossei.

Chapter 6

Exercise 6-1. Movement analysis: muscles of the hip

Muscles that cross the hip	Flexion	Extension	Abduction	Adduction	Lateral rotation	Medial rotation
Psoas major and minor	X					
Iliacus	X					
Gluteus medius	X	X	X		X	X
Gluteus minimus	X		X			X
Piriformis			X		X	
Gemellus superior			X		X	
Obturator internus			X		X	
Gemellus inferior			X		X	
Obturator externus				X	X	
Quadratus femoris				X	X	
Pectineus	X			X		
Adductor longus	X			X		
Adductor brevis	X			X		
Adductor magnus				X		
Muscles that cross the hip						
Sartorius	X		X		X	
Tensor fasciae latae	X		X			X
Rectus femoris	X					
Gluteus maximus		X			X	
Gracilis				X		X
Biceps femoris—long head		X			X	
Semitendinosus		X				X
Semimembranosus		X				X

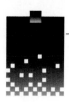

Exercise 6-2. Innervation analysis: muscles of the hip

Muscles that cross the low back and hip	Lumbar Plexus	Femoral	Gluteal	Sacral Plexus	Obturator	Sciatic
Psoas major and minor	X					
Iliacus		X				
Gluteus medius			X			
Gluteus minimus			X			
Piriformis				X		
Gemellus superior				X		
Obturator internus				X		
Gemellus inferior				X		
Obturator externus					X	
Quadratus femoris				X		
Pectineus		X				
Adductor longus					X	
Adductor brevis					X	
Adductor magnus					X	X
Muscles that cross the hip and knee						
Sartorius		X				
Tensor fasciae latae			X			
Rectus femoris		X				
Gluteus maximus			X			
Gracilis						X
Biceps femoris—long head						X
Semitendinosus						X
Semimembranosus						X

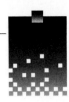

Exercise 6-3. Movement analysis: muscles of the knee

Muscles that cross the knee and hip	Knee flexion	Knee extension	Knee rotation
Sartorius	X		
Tensor fasciae latae		X	
Rectus femoris		X	
Gluteus maximus		X	
Gracilis	X		
Biceps femoris—long head	X		
Semitendinosus	X		X
Semimembranosus	X		X
Muscles that cross the knee only			
Biceps femoris—short head	X		X
Vastus intermedius		X	
Vastus medialis		X	
Vastus lateralis		X	
Popliteus	X		X
Muscles that cross the knee and ankle			
Gastrocnemius	X		
Plantaris	X		

Exercise 6-4. Innervation analysis: muscles of the knee

Muscles that cross the knee and hip	Femoral	Gluteal	Obturator	Sciatic	Tibial
Sartorius	X				
Tensor fasciae latae		X			
Rectus femoris	X				
Gluteus maximus		X			
Gracilis			X		
Biceps femoris—long head				X	
Semitendinosus				X	
Semimembranosus				X	
Muscles that cross the knee only					
Biceps femoris—short head				X	
Vastus intermedius	X				
Vastus medialis	X				
Vastus lateralis	X				
Popliteus					X
Muscles that cross the knee and ankle					
Gastrocnemius					X
Plantaris					X

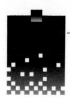

Exercise 6-5. Muscles of the hip and knee

See Figures 6-2, 6-5, 6-6, and 6-10.

Exercise 6-6. Movement analysis: muscles of the ankle and those extrinsic to the foot

Muscles	Plantar flexion	Dorsiflexion	Inversion	Eversion
Gastrocnemius	X			
Plantaris	X			
Soleus	X			
Tibialis posterior	X		X	
Flexor digitorum longus	X		X	
Flexor hallucis longus	X		X	
Tibialis anterior		X	X	
Extensor digitorum longus		X		X
Extensor hallucis longus		X	X	
Peroneus tertius		X		X
Peroneus longus	X			X
Peroneus brevis	X			X

Exercise 6-7. Innervation analysis: muscles of the ankle and those extrinsic to the foot

Muscles	Tibial	Deep peroneal	Superficial peroneal
Gastrocnemius	X		
Plantaris	X		
Soleus	X		
Tibialis posterior	X		
Flexor digitorum longus	X		
Flexor hallucis longus	X		
Tibialis anterior		X	
Extensor digitorum longus		X	
Extensor hallucis longus		X	
Peroneus tertius		X	
Peroneus longus			X
Peroneus brevis			X

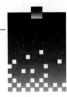

Exercise 6-8. Movement analysis: intrinsic muscles of the foot

Muscles	Flexion of MTP joints	Extension of MTP joints	Flexion of IP joints	Extension of IP joints	Abduction	Adduction
Flexor digitorum brevis	X		X			
Flexor hallucis brevis	X					
Extensor digitorum brevis		X		X		
Extensor hallucis brevis		X				
Lumbricals	X			X		
Abductor hallucis	X				X	
Adductor hallucis						X
Flexor digiti minimi brevis	X					
Quadratus plantae	X		X			

Exercise 6-9. Innervation analysis: intrinsic muscles of the foot

Muscles	Deep peroneal	Medial plantar	Lateral plantar	Tibial
Flexor digitorum brevis		X		
Flexor hallucis brevis		X		
Extensor digitorum brevis	X			
Extensor hallucis brevis	X			
Lumbricals		X	X	
Abductor hallucis		X		
Adductor hallucis			X	
Flexor digiti minimi brevis			X	
Quadratus plantae				X

Exercise 6-10. Muscles of the knee, lower leg, and foot

See Figures 6-14, 6-15, 6-22, 6-26.

Exercise 6-11. Muscles of the hip and lower extremity

Results are dependent on student performance.

Exercise 6-12. Palpate the muscles of the hip and lower extremity

Results are dependent on student performance.

Exercise 6-13. Muscles of the hip and lower extremity

1. Psoas major, psoas minor, and iliacus.
2. Sartorius, tensor fasciae latae, gluteus medius, and gluteus minimus.
3. Biceps femoris—long and short heads.
4. Tensor fasciae latae and gluteus maximus.
5. Lateral rotation of femur.
6. Gracilis.
7. Rectus femoris, vastus intermedius, vastus medius, and vastus lateralis.
8. Hamstrings: biceps femoris—long and short heads, semitendinosus, and semimembranosus.
9. Sartorius.
10. Lateral rotation of femur.
11. Sagittal.
12. Femoral nerve.
13. Tibial tuberosity.

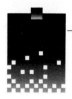

14. Vastus medialis.

15. Gastrocnemius, plantaris, and soleus.

16. Popliteus.

17. Tibial nerve.

18. Tibialis anterior.

19. Flexor digitorum longus.

20. Peroneus tertius.

21. Peroneus longus.

22. Flexor digiti minimi.

23. Flexion of the MTP joints while extending the IP joints of digits II-V.

24. Extensor digitorum brevis.

25. Quadratus plantae.

Chapter 7

Exercise 7-1. Movement and innervation analysis: abdominal muscles

Muscles	Trunk flexion	Lateral trunk extension	Rotation same side	Rotation opposite side	Trunk stabilization	Nerves
Rectus abdominis	X					spinal nerve
External oblique	X	X		X		spinal nerve
Internal oblique	X	X	X			spinal nerve
Transverse abdominis					X	spinal nerve

Exercise 7-2. Movement and innervation analysis: vertebral column

Muscles	Extension	Flexion	Rotation same side	Rotation opposite side	Lateral flexion	Assists with inspiration	Nerves
Sternocleidomastoid		X		X	X	X	spinal accessory
Scalenus (anterior, medial, posterior)		X			X	X	branches of C_{6-8}
Trapezius (upper)	X			X	X	X	spinal accessory
Levator scapulae	X				X		dorsal scapular
Splenius (capitis, cervicis)	X		X		X		C_{4-8}
Semispinalis (capitis, cervicis, thoracis)	X		X		X		C_{1-2}
Quadratus lumborum	X				X		lumbar plexus
Multifidus							spinal nerves
Rotatores							spinal nerves
Interspinales	X				X		spinal nerves
Intertransversarii					X		spinal nerves
Iliocostalis (cervicis, thoracic, lumborum)	X		X		X	X	spinal nerves
Longissimus (capitis, cervicis, thoracis)	X		X		X	X	spinal nerves
Spinalis (capitis, cervicis, thoracis)	X				X	X	spinal nerves

Exercise 7-3. Identify muscles of the abdomen and trunk

See Figure 7-2.

Exercise 7-4. Movement and innervation analysis: respiratory muscles

Muscles	Inspiration	Expiration	Nerves
Diaphragm	X		phrenic
External intercostals	X		intercostal
Internal intercostals	X		intercostal

Accessory muscles

Sternocleidomastoid	X		spinal accessory
Scalenes (anterior, medial, posterior)	X		branches of C_{4-8}
Serratus anterior	X		long thoracic
Pectoralis major	X		pectoral
Pectoralis minor	X		pectoral
Trapezius (upper, middle)	X		accessory
Erector spinae	X		spinal
Rectus abdominis		X	spinal
External oblique		X	spinal
Internal oblique		X	spinal
Transversus abdominis		X	spinal

Exercise 7-5. Movement and innervation analysis: facial muscles

Muscles	Movement	Nerves
Buccinator	Compresses cheeks	facial
Depressor anguli oris	Pulls angle of mouth downward	facial
Levator anguli oris	Pulls angle of mouth upward	facial
Mentalis	Protrudes lower lip, pouting muscle	facial
Orbicularis oris	Closes lips, whistling muscle	facial
Platysma	Pulls bottom lip down and flattens it	facial
Risorius	Pulls angle of mouth straight backward	facial
Zygomaticus major	Raises angle of mouth, smiling muscle	facial
Corrugator	Pulls eyebrows together	facial
Frontalis	Raises eyebrows, wrinkles forehead	facial
Nasalis	Flares nostrils	facial
Orbicularis oculi	Closes eye, winking muscle	facial
Procerus	Wrinkles up nose	facial

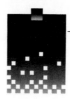

Exercise 7-6. Muscles of the face and temporomandibular joint

See Figures 7-14, 7-15, and 7-16.

Exercise 7-7. Movement and innervation analysis: muscles of the temporomandibular joint

Muscles	Elevation	Depression	Retraction	Protraction	Lateral movement	Nerves
Temporalis	X		X			Trigeminal
Masseter	X			X		Trigeminal
Medial pterygoid	X			X		Trigeminal
Lateral pterygoid		X			X	Trigeminal

Exercise 7-8. Illustrate the muscles of the abdomen and trunk

Results are dependent on student performance. See Figures 7-2 through 7-16.

Exercise 7-9. Palpate the muscles of the abdomen, trunk, and face

Results are dependent on student performance. Compare student's work against that of the study partner. See Figures 7-2 through 7-16.

Exercise 7-10. Review the muscles of the abdomen, trunk, and face

1. Rectus abdominis
2. Linea alba
3. External oblique
4. Levator scapulae
5. Performs lateral flexion of the trunk in the lumbar region; assists with trunk extension; elevates the pelvis
6. Multifidus
7. Extends the vertebral column; performs lateral flexion
8. Phrenic nerve
9. Contracted
10. Protracts the lower lip as in pouting
11. Superior to and between the orbits
12. Flattens the bottom lip; tightens the skin over the throat
13. From the angle of the mouth to the zygomatic arch
14. Wrinkles the nose
15 Close the eye (winking muscle)
16 Trigeminal nerve
17. Temporalis
18. Lateral pterygoid
19. Palatine bone and maxilla
20. Angle of mandible

Chapter 8

Exercise 8-1. Elements of nerve tissue and impulse transmission

1. Irritability, conductivity
2. Dendrites
3. Efferent neurons
4. Afferent neurons
5. Myelin sheath
6. Terminal branches; receptor
7. Synapse
8. Neurotransmitters
9. Acetylcholine
10. Motor end plate
11. Motor unit
12. Multipolar
13. Unipolar
14. Polarized
15. Threshold stimuli
16. Depolarized
17. Action potential
18. Repolarization
19. Sodium-potassium pump; active transport system
20. Schwann's cells
21. Nodes of Ranvier
22. Refractory period
23. Neurilemma
24. Saltatory conduction
25. Nervous system

Exercise 8-2. Structure of a neuron
See Figures 8-2, A, 8-2, B, and 8-4.

Exercise 8-3. Nerve impulse transmission
See Figures 8-5, A and 8-5, B.

Exercise 8-4. Central nervous system
1. Central nervous system; peripheral nervous system
2. Brain; spinal cord
3. Cerebrum; cerebellum
4. Cerebrum
5. Cerebellum
6. Longitudinal fissure
7. Corpus callosum
8. White matter
9. Frontal
10. Temporal
11. Basal ganglia
12. Hypothalamus
13. Choroid plexus; ventricles
14. Cerebellum
15. L$_2$
16. Conus medullaris
17. Cauda equina
18. 31; 26
19. Gray matter
20. Anterior horns
21. Posterior horns
22. Ascending tracts
23. Descending tracts
24. Dura mater
25. Pia mater

Exercise 8-5. Structures of the brain and spinal cord
See Figures 8-9, A, 8-10, A, and 8-11.

Exercise 8-6. Peripheral nervous system
1. Cranial nerves
2. Spinal nerves
3. Vestibulocochlear (auditory)
4. X vagus nerve
5. Brachial plexus
6. Sympathetic
7. Parasympathetic
8. Somatic
9. Reflex arc
10. Golgi tendon organs
11. Muscle spindle
12. Proprioception
13. Muscle spindles; golgi tendon organs; joint receptors

Exercise 8-7. Identify components of the reflex arc
See Figures 8-17 and 8-21.

Chapter 9

Exercise 9-1. Structures of the heart
1. Inferior and superior vena cava
2. Mediastinum
3. Four
4. Ventricles
5. Interventricular septum
6. Myocardium
7. Endocardium
8. Skeleton of the heart
9. Bicuspid (mitral valve)
10. Pulmonary trunk; pulmonary arteries
11. Pulmonary semilunar valve
12. Left atrium
13. Left ventricle
14. Chordae tendinea
15. Aorta
16. Papillary muscles
17. Stethoscope
18. Heart rate
19. Quantity of blood present; strength of contractions; peripheral resistance in vascular system
20. Tachycardia
21. Sphygmomanometer
22. Systolic pressure
23. Cardiac output
24. Diastolic pressure
25. Hypertension

Exercise 9-2. Internal anatomy of the heart
See Figures 9-1 and 9-2, A.

Exercise 9-3. Path of a blood through the heart
1. Inferior and superior venae cavae
2. Right atrium
3. Right atrioventricular valve (tricuspid)
4. Right ventricle
5. Pulmonary trunk
6. Pulmonary semilunar valve
7. Pulmonary arteries
8. Lungs
9. Pulmonary veins
10. Left atrium
11. Left atrioventricular valve (bicuspid or mitral)
12. Left ventricle
13. Aortic semilunar valve
14. Aorta

Exercise 9-4. Cardiac impulse transmission

1. Intercalated disks
2. QRS complex
3. Atrioventricular node
4. Electrocardiogram
5. Sinoatrial node
6. Direction of the apex of the heart
7. T wave
8. P wave
9. Sinus rhythm
10. Repolarization of the atria

Exercise 9-5. Identification of cardiac impulse activity

See Figure 9-6.

Exercise 9-6. Electrocardiographic wave pattern

See Figure 9-7.

Exercise 9-7. Cardiac electrical activity

1. Sinoatrial node
2. Atria
3. Atrioventricular node (bundle of His)
4. Purkinje's fibers
5. Ventricular myocardium
6. Ventricles

Exercise 9-8. Blood vessels

1. Arterioles
2. Tunica media
3. Capillaries

4. Valves
5. Intermittent surge in the pressure against the walls of the arteries with the contraction of the ventricles
6. Capillary bed
7. Lumen
8. Vasoconstriction
9. Coronary arteries
10. Coronary veins; coronary sinus

Exercise 9-9. Blood vessels

See Figure 9-12.

Exercise 9-10. Blood

1. Round, biconcave
2. Erythrocyte
3. Carry oxygen and carbon dioxide
4. Hematopoiesis
5. Leukocytes
6. Phagocytosis
7. Neutrophils; eosinophils; basophils; monocytes; lymphocytes
8. Initiate the clotting process
9. Serotonin
10. Water

Exercise 9-11. Lymphatic system

1. Water; waste products
2. Capillaries; lymph nodes; lymphatic trunks; ducts
3. Subclavian vein
4. Edema
5. Thymus gland; spleen

Chapter 10

Exercise 10-1. Anatomy of the respiratory system

1. Respiration
2. Ventilation
3. Cilia; mucus
4. Warm the inhaled air
5. Nasopharynx; oropharynx; laryngopharynx
6. Epiglottis
7. Larynx
8. Nasopharynx
9. Oropharynx; laryngopharynx
10. Trachea
11. Bronchial tree
12. 3; 2
13. Visceral pleura

14. Space between the visceral and parietal pleura
15. Alveolar ducts, alveoli
16. Alveoli
17. Compliance
18. Surfactant
19. Diaphragm; phrenic nerve
20. Capillary network
21. Nose; nasal cavity; pharynx; larynx; trachea
22. Bronchial tree; bronchioles; alveolar ducts; alveoli

Exercise 10-2. Identification of the anatomy of the respiratory system

See Figures 10-1 and 10-2.

Exercise 10-3. Respiration

1. Inspiration
2. Expiration
3. Downward; upward
4. Passive
5. Elastic recoil
6. Diaphragm; external intercostals
7. Pectoralis major
   Pectoralis minor
   Sternocleidomastoid
   Scalenes
   Serratus anterior
8. Trapezius
   Rhomboids
   Levator scapula
   Erector spinae
   Quadratus lumborum
9. Rectus abdominus
   Internal and external obliques
   Transverse abdominus
   Latissimus dorsi
10. Respiratory volumes
11. Tidal volume
    Inspiratory reserve volume
    Expiratory reserve volume
    Residual volume
12. Inspiratory capacity
    Vital capacity
    Functional reserve capacity
    Total lung capacity
13. Tidal volume
14. Inspiratory reserve volume
15. Residual volume
16. Expiratory reserve volume
    Residual volume
17. Tidal volume
    Inspiratory reserve volume
    Expiratory reserve volume
18. Pons; medulla
19. Hypothalamus
20. Hyperventilation

Exercise 10-4. Respiratory system

See Figure 10-8.

Chapter 11

Exercise 11-1. Joint movement identification

1. a. Flexion
   b. Extension
   c. Dorsiflexion
2. a. Flexion
   b. Flexion
   c. Internal rotation
   d. Adduction
3. a. Extension
   b. Flexion
   c. Lateral rotation
   d. Adduction
4. a. Elbow—flexion
   b. Radioulnar—supination to neutral
   c. Shoulder—flexion
   d. Shoulder—medial rotation
   e. Wrist—extension
   f. Metacarpal and interphalangeal—extension
5. a. Hip—pelvis flexes forward on fixed femurs
   b. Shoulder—abduction
   c. Shoulder—medial rotation
   d. Elbow—flexion
   e. Metacarpal and interphalangeal—extension
   f. Radioulnar—supination

Exercise 11-2. Muscle and nerve analysis

Joints	Movement	Specific muscles	Nerves
Knee	Extension	1. Rectus femoris 2. Vastus intermedius 3. Vastus medialis 4. Vastus lateralis 5. Tensor fasciae latae 6. Gluteus maximus	1. Femoral 2. Superior gluteal 3. Inferior gluteal
Hip	Flexion	1. Psoas major 2. Psoas minor 3. Iliacus 4. Rectus femoris 5. Sartorius 6. Tensor fasciae latae 7. Gluteus medius 8. Gluteus minimus 9. Pectineus 10. Adductor longus 11. Adductor brevis	1. Lumbar plexus 2. Femoral 3. Superior gluteal 4. Obturator
Hip	Lateral rotation	1. Piriformis 2. Gemellus superior 3. Obturator internus 4. Gemellus inferior 5. Obturator externus 6. Quadratus femoris 7. Sartorius 8. Gluteus maximus 9. Gluteus medius 10. Biceps femoris—long head	1. Sacral plexus 2. Obturator 3. Femoral 4. Superior gluteal 5. Inferior gluteal 6. Sciatic
Hip	Adduction	1. Pectineus 2. Adductor longus 3. Adductor brevis 4. Adductor magnus 5. Gracilis 6. Gluteus maximus 7. Obturator externus 8. Quadratus femoris	1. Femoral 2. Obturator 3. Sciatic 4. Inferior gluteal

Exercise 11-3. Muscle and nerve analysis

Joints	Movement	Specific muscles	Nerves
Elbow	Flexion	1. Brachialis 2. Biceps brachii 3. Brachioradialis 4. Pronator teres 5. Flexor carpi radialis 6. Flexor carpi ulnaris 7. Palmaris longus 8. Extensor carpi radialis longus	1. Musculocutaneous 2. Radial 3. Median 4. Ulnar

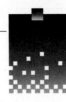

Exercise 11-3. Muscle and nerve analysis—cont

Joints	Movement	Specific muscles	Nerves
Radio-ulnar	Supination to neutral	1. Supinator 2. Biceps brachii 3. Brachioradialis	1. Musculocutaneous 2. Radial
Shoulder	Flexion	1. Pectoralis major 2. Coracobrachialis 3. Anterior deltoid 4. Biceps brachii	1. Medial pectoral 2. Lateral pectoral 3. Axillary 4. Musculocutaneous
Shoulder	Medial rotation	1. Pectoralis major 2. Anterior deltoid 3. Latissimus dorsi 4. Teres major 5. Subscapularis	1. Medial pectoral 2. Lateral pectoral 3. Axillary 4. Thoracodorsal 5. Superior subscapular 6. Inferior subscapular
Wrist	Extension	1. Extensor carpi radialis longus 2. Extensor carpi radialis brevis 3. Extensor carpi ulnaris 4. Extensor pollicis longus 5. Extensor pollicis brevis	1. Radial
MCP joints (I-V)	Extension	1. Extensor pollicis longus 2. Extensor pollicis brevis 3. Extensor digitorum 4. Extensor indicis 5. Extensor digiti minimi	1. Radial
IP joints (I-V)	Extension	1. Extensor pollicis longus 2. Extensor digitorum 3. Extensor indicis 4. Extensor digiti minimi 5. Lumbricals 6. Dorsal interossei 7. Palmar interossei 8. Abductor digiti minimi	1. Radial 2. Ulnar 3. Median

MCP, Metacarpophalangeal; *IP,* interphalangeal.

Exercise 11-4. Muscle and nerve analysis

Joints	Movement	Specific muscles	Nerves
Trunk, Vertebral column	Maintain extension	1. Upper trapezius 2. Levator scapulae 3. Splenius group 4. Semispinales group 5. Erector spinae 6. Quadratus lumborum 7. Multifidus 8. Rotatores 9. Interspinales	1. Spinal accessory 2. Dorsal scapular
Hip	Pelvis moves on fixed femurs	1. Psoas major 2. Psoas minor 3. Iliacus 4. Rectus femoris 5. Sartorius 6. Tensor fasciae latae 7. Gluteus medius 8. Gluteus minimus 9. Pectineus 10. Adductor longus 11. Adductor brevis	1. Lumbar plexus 2. Femoral 3. Superior gluteal 4. Obturator
Shoulder	Abduction	1. Supraspinatus 2. Deltoid	1. Suprascapular 2. Axillary
Shoulder	Medial rotation	1. Pectoralis major 2. Anterior deltoid 3. Latissimus dorsi 4. Teres major 5. Subscapularis	1. Medial pectoral 2. Lateral pectoral 3. Axillary 4. Thoracodorsal 5. Superior subscapular 6. Inferior subscapular
Elbow	Flexion	1. Brachialis 2. Biceps brachii 3. Brachioradialis 4. Pronator teres 5. Flexor carpi radialis 6. Flexor carpi ulnaris 7. Palmaris longus 8. Extensor carpi radialis longus	1. Musculocutaneous 2. Radial 3. Median 4. Ulnar
Wrist	Extension	1. Extensor carpi radialis longus 2. Extensor carpi radialis brevis 3. Extensor carpi ulnaris 4. Extensor pollicis longus 5. Extensor pollicis brevis	1. Radial
MCP joints (I-V)	Extension	1. Extensor pollicis longus 2. Extensor pollicis brevis 3. Extensor digitorum 4. Extensor indicus 5. Extensor digiti minimi	1. Radial

Exercise 11-4. Muscle and nerve analysis—cont

Joints	Movement	Specific muscles	Nerves
IP joints (I-V)	Extension	1. Extensor pollicis longus 2. Extensor digitorum 3. Extensor indicus 4. Extensor digiti minimi 5. Lumbricals 6. Dorsal interossei 7. Palmar interossei 8. Abductor digiti minimi	1. Radial 2. Ulnar 3. Median
Radio-ulnar	Supination	1. Supinator 2. Biceps brachii 3. Brachioradialis	1. Radial 2. Musculocutaneous

MCP, Metacarpophalangeal; *IP,* interphalangeal.

Exercise 11-5. Movement and component analysis

Joints	Movement	Specific muscles	Nerves
Trunk, Vertebral column	Extension	1. Upper trapezius 2. Levator scapulae 3. Splenius group 4. Semispinales group 5. Erector spinae 6. Quadratus lumborum 7. Multifidus 8. Rotatores 9. Interspinales	1. Spinal accessory 2. Dorsal scapular
Hip	Pelvis—moves on fixed femurs	1. Psoas major 2. Psoas minor 3. Iliacus 4. Rectus femoris 5. Sartorius 6. Tensor fasciae latae 7. Gluteus medius 8. Gluteus minimus 9. Pectineus 10. Adductor longus 11. Adductor brevis	1. Lumbar plexus 2. Femoral 3. Superior gluteal 4. Obturator
Hip	Extension	1. Gluteus maximus 2. Gluteus medius 3. Biceps femoris—long head 4. Semimembranosus 5. Semitendinosus 6. Tensor fasciae latae	1. Superior gluteal 2. Inferior gluteal 3. Sciatic

Exercise 11-5. Movement and component analysis—cont

Joints	Movement	Specific muscles	Nerves
Knee	Flexion	1. Biceps femoris—long head 2. Biceps femoris—short head 3. Semimembranosus 4. Semitendinosus 5. Popliteus 6. Gastrocnemius 7. Plantaris 8. Sartorius 9. Tensor fasciae latae 10. Gracilis	1. Sciatic 2. Tibial 3. Temoral 4. Superior gluteal 5. Obturator
Knee	Extension	1. Rectus femoris 2. Vastus intermedius 3. Vastus medialis 4. Vastus lateralis 5. Tensor fasciae latae 6. Gluteus maximus	1. Femoral 2. Superior gluteal 3. Inferior gluteal
Ankle	Dorsiflexion	1. Tibialis anterior 2. Peroneus tertius 3. Extensor digitorum longus 4. Extensor hallucis longus	1. Deep peroneal
Ankle	Flexion	1. Gastrocnemius 2. Plantaris 3. Soleus 4. Tibialis posterior 5. Flexor digitorum longus 6. Flexor hallucis longus 7. Peroneus longus 8. Peroneus brevis	1. Tibial 2. Superficial peroneal

Exercise 11-6. Movement and component analysis

Joints	Movement	Specific muscles	Nerves
Trunk, Vertebral column	Extension	1. Upper trapezius 2. Levator scapulae 3. Splenius group 4. Semispinales group 5. Erector spinae 6. Quadratus lumborum 7. Multifidus 8. Rotatores 9. Interspinales	1. Spinal accessory 2. Dorsal scapular

Exercise 11-6. Movement and component analysis—cont

Joints	Movement	Specific muscles	Nerves
Hip	Left—flexion	1. Psoas major 2. Psoas minor 3. Iliacus 4. Rectus femoris 5. Sartorius 6. Tensor fasciae latae 7. Gluteus medius 8. Gluteus minimus 9. Pectineus 10. Adductor longus 11. Adductor brevis	1. Lumbar plexus 2. Femoral 3. Superior gluteal 4. Obturator
Hip	Right—extension	1. Gluteus maximus 2. Gluteus medius 3. Biceps femoris—long head 4. Semimembranosus 5. Semitendinosus 6. Tensor fasciae latae	1. Superior gluteal 2. Inferior gluteal 3. Sciatic
Hip	Right (on fixed femur)—abduction	1. Gluteus medius 2. Gluteus minimus 3. Sartorius 4. Tensor fasciae latae 5. Gluteus maximus	1. Superior gluteal 2. Femoral
Knee	Left—flexion	1. Biceps femoris—long head 2. Biceps femoris—short head 3. Semimembranosus 4. Semitendinosus 5. Popliteus 6. Gastrocnemius 7. Plantaris 8. Sartorius 9. Tensor fasciae latae 10. Gracilis	1. Sciatic 2. Tibial 3. Femoral 4. Superior gluteal 5. Obturator
Knee	Right—extension	1. Rectus femoris 2. Vastus intermedius 3. Vastus medialis 4. Vastus lateralis 5. Tensor fasciae latae 6. Gluteus maximus	1. Femoral 2. Superior gluteal 3. Inferior gluteal
Ankle	Left—dorsiflexion	1. Tibialis anterior 2. Peroneus tertius 3. Extensor digitorum longus 4. Extensor hallucis longus	1. Deep peroneal

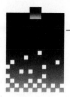

Exercise 11-6. Movement and component analysis—cont

Joints	Movement	Specific muscles	Nerves
Ankle	Right— plantar flexion	1. Gastrocnemius 2. Plantaris 3. Soleus 4. Tibialis posterior 5. Flexor digitorum longus 6. Flexor hallucis longus 7. Peroneus longus 8. Peroneus brevis	1. Tibial 2. Superficial peroneal

Exercise 11-7. Movement and component analysis

Joints	Movement	Specific muscles	Nerves
Trunk, Vertebral column	Flexion	1. Rectus abdominus 2. External oblique 3. Internal obliques	1. Thoracic 2. Spinal accessory
Trunk, Vertebral column	Extension	1. Upper trapezius 2. Levator scapulae 3. Splenius group 4. Semispinales group 5. Erector spinae 6. Quadratus lumborum 7. Multifidus 8. Rotatores 9. Interspinales	1. Spinal accessory 2. Dorsal scapular
Scapulo-thoracic	Adduction Elevation Downward rotation	1. Rhomboids 2. Levator scapulae 3. Upper trapezius 4. Middle trapezius 5. Lower trapezius	1. Spinal accessory 2. Dorsal scapular
Scapulo-thoracic	Abduction Depression Upward rotation	1. Serratus anterior 2. Upper trapezius 3. Lower trapezius	1. Long thoracic 2. Spinal accessory
Shoulder	Abduction Extension (hyper-) Lateral rotation	1. Supraspinatus 2. Deltoid 3. Latissimus dorsi 4. Teres major 5. Triceps brachii 6. Infraspinatus 7. Teres minor	1. Suprascapular 2. Axillary 3. Thoracodorsal 4. Inferior subscapular 5. Radial

Exercise 11-7. Movement and component analysis—cont

Joints	Movement	Specific muscles	Nerves
Shoulder	Adduction Flexion Medial rotation	1. Pectoralis major 2. Coracobrachialis 3. Latissimus dorsi 4. Teres major 5. Triceps brachii 6. Anterior deltoid 7. Biceps brachii 8. Subscapularis	1. Medial pectoral 2. Lateral pectoral 3. Axillary 4. Musculocutaneous 5. Thoracodorsal 6. Inferior subscapular 7. Radial
Elbow	Flexion	1. Brachialis 2. Biceps brachii 3. Brachioradialis 4. Pronator teres 5. Flexor carpi radialis 6. Flexor carpi ulnaris 7. Palmaris longus 8. Extensor carpi radialis longus	1. Musculocutaneous 2. Radial 3. Median 4. Ulnar
Elbow	Extension	1. Triceps brachii 2. Anconeus	1. Radial
Wrist	Extension Radial deviation	1. Extensor carpi radialis longus 2. Extensor carpi radialis brevis 3. Extensor carpi ulnaris 4. Flexor carpi radialis 5. Abductor pollicis longus 6. Extensor pollicis longus 7. Extensor pollicis brevis 8. Extensor digitorum	1. Radial
Wrist	Flexion Ulnar deviation	1. Flexor carpi ulnaris 2. Flexor carpi radialis 3. Extensor carpi ulnaris 4. Palmaris longus 5. Flexor digitorum superficialis 6. Flexor digitorum profundus 7. Flexor pollicis longus	1. Median 2. Ulnar

Hand	Thumb—
	    flexion
	    opposition
		1. Flexor pollicis longus
		2. Flexor pollicis brevis
		3. Opponens pollicis
		4. Adductor pollicis
		5. Abductor pollicis brevis
			1. Median
			2. Ulnar

Hand	Digits II-IV— flexion	1. Flexor digitorum superficialis 2. Flexor digitorum profundus 3. Flexor digiti minimi 4. Opponens digiti minimi 5. Lumbricals 6. Dorsal interossei 7. Palmar interossei 8. Abductor digiti minimi	1. Median 2. Ulnar

Exercise 11-8. Movement and component analysis

Joints	Movement	Specific muscles	Nerves
Trunk, Vertebral column	Extension	1. Upper trapezius 2. Levator scapulae 3. Splenius group 4. Semispinales group 5. Erector spinae 6. Quadratus lumborum 7. Multifidus 8. Rotatores 9. Interspinales	1. Spinal accessory 2. Dorsal scapular
Trunk, Vertebral column	Rotation	1. External oblique 2. Internal oblique 3. Sternocleidomastoid 4. Upper trapezius 5. Levator scapulae 6. Splenius group 7. Semispinales group 8. Erector spinae 9. Rotatores 10. Multifidus	1. Spinal accessory 2. Dorsal scapular 3. 11th cranial nerve
Trunk, Vertebral column	Flexion	1. Rectus abdominus 2. External oblique 3. Internal oblique	1. Spinal accessory
Shoulder	Flexion	1. Pectoralis major 2. Coracobrachialis 3. Anterior deltoid 4. Biceps brachii	1. Medial pectoral 2. Lateral pectoral 3. Axillary 4. Musculocutaneous
Shoulder	Medial rotation	1. Pectoralis major 2. Anterior deltoid 3. Latissimus dorsi 4. Teres major 5. Subscapularis	1. Medial pectoral 2. Lateral pectoral 3. Axillary 4. Thoracodorsal 5. Superior subscapular 6. Inferior subscapular
Shoulder	Adduction	1. Pectoralis major 2. Coracobrachialis 3. Latissimus dorsi 4. Teres major	1. Medial pectoral 2. Lateral pectoral 3. Musculocutaneous 4. Thoracodorsal 5. Superior subscapular 6. Inferior subscapular

Exercise 11-8. Movement and component analysis—cont

Joints	Movement	Specific muscles	Nerves
Elbow	Flexion	1. Brachialis 2. Biceps brachii 3. Brachioradialis 4. Pronator teres 5. Flexor carpi radialis 6. Flexor carpi ulnaris 7. Palmaris longus 8. Extensor carpi radialis longus	1. Radial 2. Median 3. Ulnar
Elbow	Extension	1. Triceps brachii 2. Anconeus	1. Radial
Radio-ulnar	Pronation	1. Pronator teres 2. Pronator quadratus 3. Brachioradialis	1. Median 2. Radial
Wrist, hand	Extension	1. Extensor carpi radialis longus 2. Extensor carpi radialis brevis 3. Extensor pollicis longus 4. Extensor pollicis brevis 5. Extensor digitorum 6. Extensor indicus 7. Extensor digiti minimi 8. Lumbricals 9. Dorsal interossei 10. Palmar interossei 11. Abductor digiti minimi	1. Radial 2. Ulnar 3. Median

Exercise 11-9. Identify superficial muscles of the body

See Figures 11-9 and 11-10.

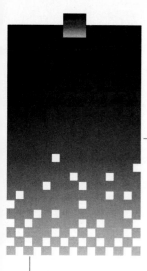

Index

A

Abdominal muscles, 143-144, 145t
    functional significance, 144
    importance in correct posture, 144
    layers of, 143
Abdominal region, 4
Abducens nerves, 170t, *171*
Abduction, definition of movement, 62, *63*
Abductor digiti minimi muscles, *103*, 107, 109t
Abductor hallucis muscles, 133, *134*, 135t
Abductor pollicis brevis muscles, *103*, 107, 109t
Abductor pollicis longus muscles, *98, 101, 103*-105
Acetabular labrum, 71
Acetabulum, 41
Acetylcholine, 160
Achilles tendon; *see* Tendocalcaneus
Acromial, anatomic location, 4
Acromial end, of clavicle, 35, *36*
Acromioclavicular joints, 65
Acromioclavicular ligaments, 65, *66*
Acromion process
    and muscle attachment, 90, *92*
    of scapula, 35, 36, *36, 37*
Actin filaments, 80-81
Action, as nomenclature in muscles, 89, 90t
Action potential, of neurons, 161, *163*
Active transport system, 161
Adduction, definition of movement, 62, *63*
Adductor brevis muscles, 118, 120
Adductor hallucis muscles, 133, *134*, 135t
Adductor longus muscles, 118, 120
Adductor magnus muscles, 118, 120
Adductor muscles, of the hip, 118, 120
Adductor pollicis muscles, *103*, 107, 109t
Afferent (sensory) neurons, 159-160, 170
    function, 159
    and movement, 175, *176*
Agonist muscles, 86
Air, cycle of, 203; *see also* Breathing
Ala of ilium, 45

Ala of sacrum, 28
"All-or-none" response
    in the heart, 184
    within muscle fiber, 81-82
    in neurons, 161
Alveolar ducts, 198, *199*
Alveolar sac, 198, *199*
Alveoli, 198, *199*
Ambulation, 119, 121, 134
Amphiarthrotic joint movement, 56
Anatomic neck, of humerus, 37, *38*
Anatomic reference points
    anatomic model, *2*
    anatomic position, 2-4
    regions, 3-4, *4*
Anconeus muscles, 94, *94*, 98
Angle of mandible, *18, 19*, 23
Ankle
    joints, 73, *75*
    muscles, 131-135
Annular ligaments, 67
Annulus fibrosus, 77
Antagonist muscles, 86
Antebrachial, anatomic location, 4
Antecubital, anatomic location, 4
Anterior (anatomical reference), definition, 2-3
Anterior arch, on atlas vertebrae, 24, *28*
Anterior cruciate ligaments, 72, *73, 74*
Anterior horns, 167-168
Anterior inferior iliac spine (AIIS), 45
Anterior longitudinal ligaments, 78
Anterior superior iliac spine (ASIS), 45
Anterolateral, definition, 3
Anteromedial, definition, 3
Aorta, 180-182
    muscles surrounding, *150*
    pressure within, 182
Aortic semilunar valves, 180-181
Apex
    of the heart, 179, *180*
    of patella, 47

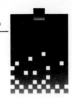

Arachnoid mater, 168
Arm region
    anatomic reference point, 4
    muscles in, 98-101
Arteries, *181,* 188-189
    blood flow within, 188-190
    smooth muscle tissue's role in, 80
Arterioles, *181,* 188-189
Articular cartilage, 58
Articulation, 15
Ascending tracks, of spinal cord, *167,* 168
Association neurons, 159-160
Atlas, 24, *28*
    posterior tubercle on, 24, *28*
    tubercle on, 24, *28*
Atria, 179-182
    electrical stimulation of, 184, *185*
    location, 179-180
Atrioventricular (AV) bundle, 184, *185*
Atrioventricular (AV) node, 184, *185*
Atrioventricular (AV) valves, 180
Auricular surface, 45
Autonomic nervous system (ANS), 174-175
    controlling cardiac muscle contractions, 184
    definition and subsystems, 174
    and involuntary body functions, 174-175
Axial skeleton; *see also* Bones
    definition, 17
Axillary, anatomic location, 4
Axillary nerves, 171
Axis vertebra, 26, *28*
Axons
    in neurons, 160-163
    in white matter, 165

B

Back muscles, 145-148; *see also* Vertebral column
Ball-and-socket joints, 57t
    in hip, 71
    in shoulder, 65
Basal ganglia, 165, 167
Base, of the heart, 179, *180*
Basophils, 193
Biceps brachii muscles, *91, 92, 93,* 95t, *96,* 98, 99t, *100*
Biceps femoris—long head muscles, 118-119, *121,* 122, *123,* 124t, 125t
Biceps femoris-short head muscles, 122, *123,* 124t, 125t
Bicipital groove, 37, *38*
Biconcave, definition, 192
Bicuspid valves, 180
Bifid, definition, 26, *28*
Bilateral muscle contraction, definition, 144-145
Biomechanics, definition, 209
Bipolar neurons, 160-161; *see also* Neurons
Blood
    carried by arteries, 188-189
    clotting, 193
    components of, 192
    description of, 192-193
    flow through heart valves, 180
    flow within the circulatory system, 181
    function of, 192

Blood—*cont'd*
    pathway through the heart, 179-181
    platelets, 192-193
    pressure gradients in flow, *190*
    viscosity, 182
Blood plasma, 192, 193
Blood pressure
    definition, 182
    degrees of, in different vessels, 188-190
    gradients in flow, *190*
Blood vessels, 188-190
    coronary, 190, *191*
    pressure on, 182
Body of mandible, *19,* 23
Body of pubis, *45,* 46
Body of sternum, *33, 34*
Bone cells; *see* Osteocytes
Bone marrow, 11, 12
Bones
    compounds found in, 9
    flexibility, 9
    forces on, 11-12
    formation, 10
    functions, 11-12
    as living tissue, 9
    maintenance of strength, 12
    minerals in, 12
    prenatal development of, 9-10
    terminology of shapes, 14-15
    terminology of skeletal landmarks, 15-17
    types, 10-11
Brachial, anatomic location, 4
Brachial plexus nerves, 171, *173*
Brachialis muscles, 98, 99t
Brachioradialis muscles, 98, 99t
Bradycardia, 182
Brain, 165, *166,* 167
Breathing, 204, *206; see also* Respiration
    diaphragm's role in, 150-152
    mechanics of, 202
Bronchi, 198
Bronchial tree, 198
Bronchioles, 198
Buccal, anatomic location, 4
Buccinator muscles, *153,* 154t
Bursae, definition, 59

C

Calcaneal, anatomic location, 4
Calcaneus bones, 48
Calcium, in bones, 12
Calcium ions, in muscle fiber, 82
Calcium salts, 9
Canaliculus, definition, 10
Cancellous; *see* Spongy bone
Capillaries, *181,* 188-189
Capillary beds, 189
Capillary network, 197-198
Capitate bones, 39, *40*
Capitulum of humerus, 37, *38*
Cardiac muscle fibers, composition of, 184
Cardiac muscles

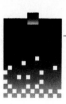

Cardiac muscles—*cont'd*
  contraction of, 180
  definition, 79
  electrical stimulation of, 184, *185*
  structure, 179
Cardiac output (CO), formula, 182
Cardinal planes
  description of, 4-5
  movements along, 63
Cardiovascular system, 179-191
  blood pathway through the heart, 181
  blood vessels, 188-190
  internal anatomy of the heart, 179-180
  monitoring blood pressure, 182, 188-190
  relationship to lymphatic system, 194
Carpal bones, 15, 39, *40,* 67
Carpal joints, 68
Carpal region, anatomic location, 4
Carpometacarpal joints, 68
Cartilaginous joints, definition, 56
Cauda equina, definition, 167
Caudad (anatomical reference), definition, 2-3
Cell bodies
  blood, 192-193
  in gray matter, 165
  of neurons, 160
Central canal, of spinal cord, 167
Central nervous system (CNS), 165-168
  brain, 165, *166,* 167
  major regions, 165
  and muscle contraction, 82
  nutrients to, 167
  spinal cord, 167-168
Cephalic, anatomic location, 4
Cerebellum, 165, *166,* 167
Cerebral cortex, 165, 204
Cerebrospinal fluid, 167
Cerebrum, 165, *166,* 167
Cervical, anatomic location, 4
Cervical plexus nerves, 171
Cervical spine, muscles surrounding, 91
Cervical vertebrae, 24, 26, *28*
Chambers; *see also* Heart, internal anatomy
  of the heart, 179-180
Cheek muscles, 152, *153,* 154t; *see also* Facial region
Chemical balances, in neurons, 161
Chewing, 152, 154t
Chin, muscles surrounding, 154t
Chordae tendineae, 180, *180*
Choroid plexus, 167
Cilia, 197
Circulatory system; see also Blood
  blood flow within, 181
  blood vessels in, 188-190
Circumduction, definition of movement, 63
Clavicle, sternal end of, 35, *36*
Clavicles, 35, *36*
  joints surrounding, 65
  muscle attachment, 90
Coccyx, *27, 28*
Collagen fibers, in bone, 9
Common carotid artery, 182, *188*
Common peroneal nerves, 171, *172, 173*

Compact bone, 10
Compliance, 200
Compression forces, 9, 12
Concave curve, 24
Concentric muscle contraction, 85-86, 213
Conductivity, in nerve tissue, 159
Condyles, definition, 17t
Condyloid joints, 57t, *58*
Conus medullaris, 167
Convex curve, 24
Coracobrachialis muscles, *91,* 92, 95t, *96*
Coracoclavicular ligaments, 65, *66*
Coracohumeral ligaments, 65
Coracoid process of scapula, 36, *37*
Coronal sutures, *18, 19,* 20
Coronary arteries, 190, *191*
Coronary sinus, 190, *191*
Coronary veins, 190, *191*
Coronoid fossa of humerus, 37, *38*
Coronoid process of mandible, *19,* 23
Coronoid process of ulna, 38
Corpus callosum, 165
Corrugator muscles, *153,* 154t
Cortical bone; *see* Compact bone
Corticospinal tract, 168
Costal cartilage, 34
Costoclavicular ligaments, 65
Coxal
  anatomic location, 4
  bones, 41, *45,* 46
Cranial nerves
  definition, 170
  and the senses, 170
  types, 170t, *171*
Cranial region, 4; *see also* Cranium
Cranium, 17-23, *18, 19*
  ethmoid bone, 20
  frontal bone, 17, *19*
  occipital bone, 20
  parietal bone, 17, *18, 19*
  sphenoid bone, 17, *18, 19*
  sutures, 20
  temporal bone, 20
Crest, definition, 17t
Cricoid cartilage, 24
Cross sections, 5
Crural, anatomic location, 4
Cubital, anatomic location, 4
Cuboid bones, 49
Cuneiform bones, 49

D

Deep (anatomical reference), definition, 2-3
Deep muscles, of vertebral column, 146, *147*
Deltoid ligaments, 73, *75*
Deltoid muscles, *90, 91, 92,* 93, 95t, *96*
Deltoid tuberosity, 37, *38*
Dendrites, 160
Deoxygenated blood, 181, 189
Depolarization
  of muscle fibers, 82
  of neurons, 161, *163*

Depression, definition of movement, 63
Depressor anguli oris muscles, *153*, 154t
Dermatome, 171, *172*
Descending tracks, of spinal cord, *167*, 168
Diaphragm
    muscles, 150-151, 152t
    role in respiratory system, *199, 200, 202, 203*
Diaphysis, definition, *11*, 15
Diaphysis of fibula, 47
Diarthrotic joints; *see* Synovial joints
Diastolic pressure, 182, *190; see also* Blood pressure
Digestive system, smooth muscle tissue's role in, 80
Digital, anatomic location in arm and leg region, 4
Digits (fingers), 39, 107
Digits (toes), 49, 132-134
Directional terminology
    combination of, 3
    definition, 2
    practice of, 3
    uses of, 2-3
Distal (anatomic reference), definition, 2-3
Distal row, of carpal bones, 39
Dorsal (anatomic reference), definition, 2-3
Dorsal interossei muscles, *103*, 107-108
Dorsal radiocarpal ligaments, 67
Dorsal tubercle, on radius, 39
Dorsiflexion, definition of movement, 62, *63*
Dura mater, 168

E

Ears, nerves controlling hearing, 170
Eccentric muscle contraction, 85-86, 213
Edema, 194
Efferent (motor) neurons
    function, 159-160, 170
        in the autonomic nervous system, 174
    and movement, 175, *176*
    in muscle fiber, 84
    role in respiration, 204
Elastic recoil, 202
Elbow, 67, *68*
    functional significance of muscles, 99
    muscles, 93-94, 98-100
    muscles as synergists, 99
Electrocardiogram (ECG), 184, *186*
Elevation, definition of movement, 62
Endocardium, 179
Endochondral bone, definition, 10
Endosteum, 11
Eosinophils, 193
Epicardium, 179
Epicondyle, definition, 17t
Epiglottis, 197
Epimysium, 80
Epiphyseal plate, *11*, 15
Epiphysis, *11*, 15
Erector spinae muscles
    assisting respiration, 203
    definition, 146, 149, 149t
Erythrocytes, 192; *see also* Red blood cells
Esophagus
    location, *24*

Esophagus—*cont'd*
    muscles surrounding, *150*
    role in respiratory system, 197-198
Ethmoid bones, *18*, 20
Eversion, definition of movement, 62, *63*
Excitability, in muscle fiber, 82
Exhalation; *see* Expiration
Expiration
    definition, 202, *203*
    muscles used in, 150, *151*
Expiratory reserve volume, 203, *204*
Extension
    definition of movement, 62, *63*
    of lower leg, 85
Extensor carpi radialis longus muscles, *98, 101,* 103-105
Extensor carpi ulnaris muscles, *94, 98, 101,* 103-105
Extensor digiti minimi muscles, *98, 101,* 104-105
Extensor digitorum brevis muscles, 133, *134,* 135t
Extensor digitorum longus muscles, 131-132, *134*
Extensor digitorum muscles, *98, 101,* 104-105
Extensor expansion, 104
Extensor hallucis brevis muscles, 133, *134,* 135t
Extensor hallucis longus muscles, 131-132, *134*
Extensor hood mechanism, 104
Extensor indicis muscles, *98, 101,* 104-105
Extensor pollicis brevis muscles, *98, 101,* 103-105
Extensor pollicis longus muscles, *98, 101,* 103-105
Extensor retinaculum
    of ankle, 132, *134*
    of hand, 68, 104
External auditory meatus bones, *19,* 20
External intercostal muscles, 150-151
External oblique muscles, 143-144, 145t, 203
External rotation, definition of movement, 62, *63*
Extracapsular, 73
Extrafusal muscle fibers, innervation of, 175
Extrinsic muscles
    definition, 103-105
    of the foot, 131-135
Eyes
    bone orbits, 17
    muscles and movement of, 152, *153,* 154t
    nerves controlling, 170

F

Facets
definition, 17t
on vertebrae, 24, 26-28
Facial muscles and verbal communication, 152, 154t
Facial region
    anatomic location, 4
    bones, 23
    muscles, 152, *153,* 154t
    nerves, 170t, *171*
    nerves controlling movement, 170
False ribs, *33,* 34
Fascicles, 80, 84; *see also* Muscle tissue
Fast twitch muscle fibers, 82
Femoral, anatomic location, 4
Femoral nerves, 171, *173*
Femur, 46-47
    intertrochanteric crest of, 46

Femur—*cont'd*
    intertrochanteric fossa of, 46
    intertrochanteric line of, 46
    lateral condyles of, 46
    lateral epicondyles of, 46
    lesser trochanter of, 46
    linea aspera of, 46
    medial condyles of, 46
    muscles controlling, 116, 118-119
    neck of, 46
Fibrous connective tissue, 55
Fibrous joints, types of, 55-56
Fibrous sheaths, 103-104
Fibula
    interosseous border of, 47
    lateral malleolus of, 47
    neck of, 47
    styloid process of, 47
Fibula bone, 47-48
    joints attached to, 73, *74*
Fibular (lateral) collateral ligaments, 73
Fibulocalcaneal ligaments, 73, *75*
Filtration of contaminants by bones, 12
Fingers; *see* Digits
First class levers
    anatomic examples of, 83
    definition, 83
Fixator, 90
Fixator muscles, 86
Fixed objects *versus* movable, 96, 115
Flat bones, 14-15
Flexion
    definition of movement, 62, *63*
    of lower leg, 85
Flexor carpi radialis muscles, *101,* 103-105
Flexor carpi ulnaris muscles, *98, 101,* 103-105
Flexor digiti minimi brevis muscles, 133, *134,* 135t
Flexor digiti minimi muscles, 107-108
Flexor digitorum brevis muscles, 133, *134,* 135t
Flexor digitorum longus muscles, 131, 134t
Flexor digitorum profundus muscles, *101,* 103-105
Flexor digitorum superficialis muscles, *101,* 103-105
Flexor hallucis brevis muscles, 133, *134,* 135t
Flexor hallucis longus muscles, 131, 134t
Flexor pollicis brevis muscles, 107-108
Flexor pollicis longus muscles, *101,* 103-105
Flexor retinaculum
    of ankle, 131
    of hand, 68, 103-104
Floating ribs, *33,* 34
Foot
    bones, 48-49
    muscles, 133-134
Foramen, definition, 17t
Foramen magnum, *19,* 20
    connection to neural tissue, 167
Forces, in levers, 83
Forearm
    muscles, 98-101
    muscles as synergists, 99
Forefoot, 49
Forehead, muscles surrounding, 154t
Fossa, definition, 17t

Fovea capitis, 46
Frontal, anatomic location, 4
Frontal bones, 17, *18, 19*
    definition, 17
    muscles surrounding, *153,* 154t
Frontal lobes, 165, *166*
Frontal planes, 4-5
Frontalis muscles, *153,* 154t
Fulcrum, in lever system, 83
Functional ability, in activities of daily living, 209
Functional movement, definition, 209
Functional muscle groups, activity in, 213
Functional reserve capacity, 203, *204*

G

Gastrocnemius muscles, 123, 124t, 131, *132,* 134t
Gemellus inferior muscles, 116, 118-119
Gemellus superior muscles, 116, 118-119
Glenohumeral joints, 65
    function of, 66
    and muscle movement, 95t
Glenohumeral ligaments, 65, *66*
Glenoid fossa, 36, *37*
Glenoid labrum, 65
Gliding joints, 57t, *58,* 65
Glossopharyngeal nerves, 170t, *171*
Glottis, 197-198
Gluteal, anatomic location, 4
Gluteal muscle group, 116-119
Gluteal tuberosity, 46
Gluteus maximus muscles, 116-119
    connection to knee muscle, 122, 124t
    description of, 116
Gluteus medius muscles, 116-119
Gluteus minimus muscles, 116-119
Golgi tendon organs, 175
Gomphoses, 56
Gracilis muscles, 118, 120, *121,* 122, 124t
Gray matter, 165, 167-168
Great toe, 49; *see also* Hallucis
Greater sciatic notch, 45
Greater trochanter, of femur, 46
Greater tubercle of humerus, 37, *38*
Groove, definition, 17t

H

Hallucis, 131
Hamate bones, 39, *40*
Hamstring muscles, 118-119, *121,* 125t
Hands
    bones, 39
    joints in, 68
l   igaments, 68
    movement of, 68
    muscles, 103-105, 107
Hard palate, 23
Haversian canals, 10
Haversian system, 10
Head
    definition (landmark term), 17t
    of femur, 46

Head of femur—*cont'd*
 joints surrounding, *72*
 of fibula, 47
 of humerus, 37, *38*
 muscles, 144-148
 of radius, 38
 of ulna, 38
Hearing, nerves controlling, 170
Heart, 179-191
 base of, 179, *180*
 blood vessels, 181
 chambers, 179-180
 electrical activity in, 184, *185, 186*
 internal anatomy of, 179-181
 location in body, 179
 monitoring activity in, 181-183
 muscles in, 79
 primary structures, 179-180
 skeleton, 180
 sounds, 182
Heart chambers, 179-180
Heart rate (HR)
 adult normal resting rate, 182
 definition, 181-182
 rapid, 182
Heart valves, 179-181
Heel bones, 48
Hematopoiesis, 12, 192
Hemispheres, cerebral, 165, *166*
Hemoglobin, 192, 200
High blood pressure; *see* Hypertension
Hinge joints, 57t, *58*
Hip hiking, 146-148
Hips, 41, 45, 46, 71-72
 adductor muscles, 118, 120
 anterior muscles, 115-117
 bones, 145-148
 lateral rotator muscles, 116, 118-119
 ligaments, 72
 muscles, 115-121
  functional significance, 119, 121
 region in body, 4
Homeostasis, 175
Hook of hamate, 39
Horizontal planes, 5; *see also* Transverse planes
Horse's tail nerves, 167
Human anatomy, complexity of, 89
Humerus, 37, *38*
 fractures of, 37
 lateral epicondyles of, 37, *38*
 lesser tubercle of, 37, *38*
 medial epicondyles of, 37, *38*
 movements of, 66-67
 olecranon fossa of, 37, *38*
 radial fossa of, 37, *38*
 surgical neck of, 37, *38*
 trochlea of, 37, *38*
Hyaline cartilage, 58
 definition, 9-10
Hyoid bones, 23, *24*
Hyperextension, definition of movement, 62, *63*
Hypertension, 182
Hyperventilation, definition, 204

Hypoglossal nerves, 170t, *171*
Hypotension, 182
Hypothalamus, 165, 167, 204, *206*
Hypothenar eminence, 107

I

Iliac crest, 45
Iliac fossa, 45
Iliacus muscles, 115-117
Iliocostalis muscles (cervicis, thoracis, and lumborum), 146, 149
Iliofemoral ligaments, 72
Iliopsoas muscles, 115-117
Iliotibial band, 115-117, *118*
Ilium, 45
Immune system and white blood cells, 192-193
Inferior (anatomical reference), definition, 2-3
Inferior gluteal nerves, 171, *173*
Inferior nasal conchae, *18, 23*
Inferior pubic ramus, *45*, 46
Inferior venae cavae, 181, 189, *190*
Inferolateral, definition, 3
Inferomedial, definition, 3
Infraglenoid tubercle, of scapula, 37
Infraorbital foramen, *19*
Infraspinatus muscles, *90, 93*, 94, 95t, *96*
Infraspinous fossa of scapula, 36, *37*
Inguinal, anatomic location, 4
Inhalation; *see* Inspiration
Inner ear, 20
Innervation
 of muscles, 82-83
 as nomenclature in muscles, 89, 90t
Innominate bones, 41
Insertion, as nomenclature in muscles, 89, 90t
Inspiration, 150, *151*
 definition, 202, *203*
Inspiratory capacity, 203, *204*
Inspiratory reserve volume, 203, *204*
Interatrial septum, 179, *180*
Intercalated disks, 184
Intercarpal ligaments, 67
Intercellular fluid, 193
Intercondylar eminence, 47
Intercondylar fossa, of femur, 46
Intercostal muscles, 202
Intermetacarpal joints, 68
Internal intercostal muscles, 150-151
Internal oblique muscles, 143-144, 145t
 assisting respiration, 203
 function of, 143
Internal rotation, definition of movement, 62, *63*
Interosseous border of fibula, 47
Interosseous border of radius, *38*, 39
Interosseous border of tibia, 47
Interosseous border of ulna, 38
Interosseous ligaments, 56
Interphalangeal joints (IP), 68, 131
Interspinales muscles, 146-149
Interspinous ligaments, 78
Interstitial fluid, 193
Intertransversarii muscles, 146-149
Intertransverse ligaments, 78

Intertrochanteric crest of femur, 46
Intertrochanteric fossa of femur, 46
Intertrochanteric line of femur, 46
Interventricular septum, 179, *180*
Intervertebral disks, 24, 77
Intervertebral foramen, 27
  nerves in, 171
Intervertebral joints, 77-78
Intracapsular, definition, 72
Intrafusal muscle fibers, innervation of, 175
Intrinsic muscles
  definition, 107
  of the foot, 131-135
Inversion, definition of movement, 62, *63*
Involuntary body functions, 159
controlled by the autonomic nervous system, 174-175
Involuntary muscle contraction, 80
Ions in neurons, 161
Irregular bones, 14-15
Irritability, in nerve tissue, 159
Ischial ramus, *45,* 46
Ischial spine, *45,* 46
Ischial tuberosity, *45,* 46
Ischiofemoral ligaments, 72
Ischium, 46
Isokinetic contraction in muscles, 85-86
Isometric contraction in muscles, 85-86
Isotonic contraction in muscles, 85-86

J

Jaw; *see also* Facial region
  muscles surrounding, 152, *153,* 154t
Joint capsules, 58
Joint cavity, 58
Joint posture sense; *see* Proprioception
Joint receptors, 175
Joints, 55-78
  cartilaginous, 56
  definition, 55
  degree of movement, 55
  interphalangeal, 131
  intervertebral, 77
  lower extremity, 71-75
  metatarsophalangeal, 131
  nerves and receptors in, 175
  of the pectoral girdle, 65-67
  of the pelvic girdle, 71-72
  and shoulder muscle movement, 95t
  structural categories
    cartilaginous, 56
    fibrous, 55-56
    synovial, 56-59
  tissue types, 55
  of the upper extremity, 65-68

K

Kinesiology, definition, 209
Kinetic, definition, 209
Knee
  bones in, 47
  functional significance of muscles, 125

Knee—*cont'd*
  joints, 72-73, *74*
  ligaments, 72-73
  movement capabilities, 72
  muscles, 122-125
Kneecap, 47; *see also* Patella

L

Labra (*sing.* labrum), definition, 59
Lacrimal bones, *18, 19,* 23
Lacuna, definition, 10
Lambdoidal sutures, *18, 19,* 20
Lamellae, of bone, 10
Lamina, 26, *28*
Landmarks
  as anatomic reference points, 2-3
  carpal bones, 39
  coxal bones, 41, 45, 46
  on electrocardiogram, 184
  foot bones, 48-49
  frontal bone, 17
  humerus, 37
  leg bones, 46-48
  occipital bones, 20
  practice referring to, 23
  scapulae, 36t
  skeletal, 15, 17t
  temporal bones, 20
  ulna, 38
  vertebral, 26
Laryngopharynx, 197
Larynx, 197-198, *199*
Lateral (anatomic reference), definition, 2-3
Lateral condyles of femur, 46
Lateral condyles of the tibia, 47
Lateral epicondyles of femur, 46
Lateral epicondyles of humerus, 37, *38*
Lateral flexion, definition of movement, 62
Lateral malleolus of fibula, 47
Lateral menisci, 73, *74*
Lateral pterygoid muscles, 152, *153,* 154t
Lateral rotator muscles of the hip, 116, 118-119
Lateral supracondylar ridges, 37, *38*
Latissimus dorsi muscles
  assisting respiration, 203
  movement in, 93, *94,* 95t, 96, 146-148
Leg
  bones, 46-48
  extension and flexion, 85
  muscles in lower, 131-132
Leg region, 4
Lesser sciatic notch, *45,* 46
Lesser trochanter, of femur, 46
Lesser tubercle of humerus, 37, *38*
Leukocytes, 192-193
Levator anguli oris muscles, *153,* 154t
Levator scapulae muscles
  assisting respiration, 203
  and body movement, 145-148
  definition, 90t, 91
Levers
  anatomic examples of, 83-84

Levers—*cont'd*
   definition and description, 83-84
   joints and, 84
   in muscle contraction, *81*
Ligamenta subflava, 78
Ligaments
   definition, 56
   of the elbow, 67
   of the hand, 68
   in hands, 68
   of the hip, 72
   nerves and receptors in, 175
   of the shoulder, 65-67
   of vertebrae, *77, 78*
   of the wrist, 67-68
Linea alba, 143
Linea aspera of femur, 46
Little latissimus muscles; *see* Teres major muscles
Lobes, 165, *166*, 198, *199*
Lobules, 198, *199*
Long bones, 14-15
Longissimus muscles (capitis, cervicis, and thoracis), 146, 149
Longitudinal fissure, 165
Low blood pressure; *see* Hypotension
Lower back muscles, 145-148; *see also* Vertebral column
Lower extremity, 46-49
   anatomic location, 4
   bones in, 46-49
   joints in, 71-73
   muscles, 122-135
   nerves in, 171, *172, 173*
Lower respiratory tract, 197-198
Lower trapezius muscles, 90t, 91
Lumbar
   anatomic location, 4
   muscles supporting, 145-148
Lumbar vertebrae, 27, *30*
   attachment to diaphragm, 150, 152t
Lumbosacral plexus nerves, 171, *172, 173*
Lumbricals
   foot, 133, *134,* 135t
   hand, *104,* 107
Lumen, definition, 188
Lunate bones, 39, *40*
Lung tissue, 198, *199,* 200
Lungs, 197-198, *199*
   location relative to the heart, 179
   working with diaphragm muscles, 150-152
Lymph glands, 193-194
Lymph nodes, 193-194
Lymphatic system, 192-193, 193-194
   edema and, 194
   function of, 193
   principle organs, *194*
Lymphatic trunks, 193-194
Lymphocytes, 193

M

Macrophages, 193
Mandible, *18, 19,* 23
   muscles and movement, 152, 154t
   ramus of, *18, 19*

Mandibular condyles, *19,* 23
Mandibular fossa, *19,* 20, 23
Mandibular ramus, 23
Manubrium, *33, 34*
Masseter muscles, 152, *153,* 154t
Mastication, 152
Mastoid process
   definition, *19,* 20
   muscles surrounding, *153,* 154t
Maxilla, *18, 19*
Maxillary bones, 23
Medial (anatomic reference), definition, 2-3
Medial condyles of femur, 46
Medial epicondyles
   of femur, 46
   of tibia, 47
Medial epicondyles of humerus, 37, *38*
Medial knee, *122*
Medial malleolus of tibia, 47
Medial menisci, 73, *74*
Medial pterygoid muscles, 152, *153,* 154t
Median nerves, 171
Median sagittal planes; *see* Midsagittal planes
Mediastinum, 179
Medulla, monitoring respiration, 204, *206*
Medullary cavity, 11
Meninges, 168
Menisci, definition, 59
Mental, anatomic location, 4
Mental foramen, *18, 19*
Mentalis muscles, *153,* 154t
Metacarpal bones, 39, *40*
Metacarpal joints, 67, *68*
Metacarpophalangeal joints, 68
Metatarsal bones, 49
Metatarsophalangeal joints (MTP), 131
Midbrain, monitoring respiration, 204, *206*
Middle trapezius muscles, 90t, 91
Midsagittal planes, 4
Minerals, in bones, 9, 12
Mitral valves, 180
Monocytes, 193
Motion, range of, 210
Motor end plate on muscle fiber, 160
Motor neurons; *see* Efferent neurons
Motor units, 160-161
Mouth, 23, *24*
   bones of, 23
   muscles, 152, *153,* 154t
Movable objects *versus* fixed, 83, 96, 115
Movement
   definition, 79
   degree of in joints, 58
   and function, 209
   identification of, 209
   in joints, 55-59
   and the nervous system, 175
   normal *versus* abnormal, 213
   between planes, 58
   terminology, 62-64
   therapeutic practice of, 210
Mucus, 197
Multifidus muscles, 146-149

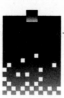

Multipolar neurons, 160-161
Muscle contraction, 79-86
Muscle fiber, 80
    abdominal, 143-144
    cardiac, 184
    components of, *81*
    depolarization of, 82
    in the heart, 179-180
    innervation of, 82-83, 175
    myofibrils in, 80
    and the nervous system, 160-161
    polarization of, 82
    stimulation of, 84-85
    structure of, *80*
Muscle spindles, 175
Muscle tissue
    components of, 80
t   ypes of, 79-80
Muscle tone, 85
Muscles
    abdomen, 143-144, 145t
    ankle, 131-135
    attachment to bones, 12
    cardiac, 179
    extrinsic to the hand, 103-105
    intrinsic to the hand, 107
    and joint actions, 95t
    knee, 122-125
    of lower back, 145-148
    major, *214, 215*
    neuromuscular regulation of movement, 175
    of respiration, 202-203
    and rib movement, 150-152
    sartorius, 115, 117t
    shoulder, 95t
    skeletal attachment, 115-125, 131-135
    in synovial joints, 59
    use in daily living, 209, 210, 213
    wrist, 103-105
Musculocutaneous nerves, 171
Musculoskeletal lever system, 83-84; *see also* Levers
Myelin sheath, 160-162
Myocardium, 179-181; *see also* Cardiac muscle
Myofibrils, 80, *81*
Myofilaments, 80-81
Myosin buds, 81
Myosin filaments, 80-81
Myotomes, 171

N

Nasal, anatomic location, 4
Nasal bones, *18, 19,* 23
Nasal cavity, 197-198
Nasal conchae, 197
Nasalis muscles, *153,* 154t
Nasopharynx, 197
Navicular bones, 49
Neck of femur, 46
Neck of fibula, 47
Necrosis, 194
Nerve impulse transmission, 160-163, *163*
Nerve impulses, 160-163

Nerve tissue
    in the brain, 165, 167
    definition, 159
    qualities of, 159
Nerves
    lower extremities, 171, *172, 173*
    upper extremities, 171, *172, 173*
Nervous system, 159-176
    autonomic, 174-175
    central, 165-168
    definition, 159
    function and structure, 159-161
    nerve impulse transmission, 161, *163*
    neuromuscular regulation, 175, *176*
    peripheral, 170-171, *172, 173*
    saltatory conduction, 162, *163*
    somatic, 175
Neurilemma, *160,* 162
Neuromuscular junctions, 160, *161*
Neuromuscular regulation of movement, 175, *176*
Neurons
    composition of, 160
    functions of, 159-160
    repolarized, 161, *163*
    structure of, 160-161
    types of, 159-160
Neurotransmitters, definition, 160
Neutrophils, 193
Nodes of Ranvier, 162
Nomenclature, definition, 89
Nonverbal communication and facial muscles, 152, 154t
Nose
    bones of, *18, 19,* 23
    muscles surrounding, *153,* 154t
    nerves controlling sense of smell, 170
    role in respiratory system, 197-198
Nucleus pulposus, 77

O

Oblique planes, 1
Oblique popliteal ligaments, 73
Obturator externus muscles, 116, 118-119
Obturator foramen, 46
Obturator internus muscles, 116, 118-119
Obturator nerves, 171, *173*
Occipital, anatomic location, 4
Occipital bones, *18, 19,* 20
Occipital condyles, *19,* 20
Occipital lobes, 165, *166*
Occipital protuberances, *18, 19,* 20
Oculomotor nerves, 170t, *171*
Odontoid facet, 24, *28*
Odontoid processes, 26, *28*
Olecranon fossa of humerus, 37, *38*
Olecranon process of ulna, 38
Olfactory nerves, 170t, *171*
Opponens digiti minimi muscles, *103,* 107, 109t
Opponens pollicis muscles, *103,* 107, 109t
Opposition, definition of movement, 63
Optic nerves, 170t, *171*
Oral, anatomic location, 4
Orbicularis oculi muscles, *153,* 154t

Orbicularis oris muscles, *153*, 154t
Orbital, anatomic location, 4
Orbits, 17, *18; see also* Eyes
    muscles surrounding, *153*, 154t
Organic matrix, 9
Organs
    control by spinal nerves, 171
    protection by skeleton, 12
Origin, as nomenclature in muscles, 89, 90t
Oropharynx, 197
Os coxae, 41
Ossification
    definition, 10
    in joints, 56
Osteoblasts, definition, 10
Osteocytes, definition, 10
Osteon structure, 10
Otic, anatomic location, 4
Oxygen
    in blood, 181
    in respiratory system, 197, 200

P

P waves, 184, *186*
Pacemaker of the heart, 184, *185*
Pain and reflex, 175
Palatine bones, *19*, 23
Palmar, anatomic location, 4
Palmar interossei muscles, *103*, 107-108
Palmar radiocarpal ligaments, 67
Palmar ulnocarpal ligaments, 67
Palmaris longus muscles, *101*, 103-105
Papillary muscles, 180
Paraspinal muscles, 145-149
Parasympathetic nervous system, 174-175
Parietal, anatomic location, 4
Parietal bones, 17, *18, 19*
    muscles surrounding, *153*, 154t
Parietal lobes, 165, *166*
Parietal pericardium, 179
Parietal pleura, 198, *199*
Patella, superior border of, 47
Patella bones, 47
Patellar, anatomic location, 4
Patellar grooves, 46
Patellar ligament, 122
Pectineus muscles, 118, 120
Pectoral, anatomic location, 4
Pectoral girdle
    bones, 35-37
    joints, 65-67
    muscles surrounding, 91
Pectoralis major muscles, *91*, 92, 93, 95t, 96
    assisting respiration, 203
    description of, 92
Pectoralis minor muscles
    assisting respiration, 203
    location of, 90t, 91
Pedicles of vertebral column, 26
Pelvic girdle
    bones of, 41, 45-46
    joints of, 71-72

Pelvic girdle—*cont'd*
    muscles surrounding, 115-121
Pelvis, muscles surrounding, 144
Pelvis region, 4
Per anserinus, 122, *132*
Pericardium, 179
Perimysium, 80
Perineal, anatomic location, 4
Periosteum, 58
    definition, 10
Peripheral nervous system, 170-171, *172, 173*
    cranial nerves in, 170
    and muscle contraction, 82
    spinal nerves in, 171
Peroneal, anatomic location, 4
Peroneal retinaculum, *131*, 132
Peroneus brevis muscles, 132
Peroneus longus muscles, 132
Peroneus tertius muscles, 132, *134*
Phagocytic cells, 194
Phagocytosis, 192
Phalanges
    of foot, 49
    hand, 39
Pharynx, 197-198
Phrenic nerves, *199*, 200
Pia mater, 168
Piriformis muscles, 116, 118-119
Pisiform bones, 39, *40*
Pivot joints, 57t, *58*
Planes of motion in synovial joints, 57-58
Plantar, anatomic location, 4
Plantar flexion, definition of movement, 62, *63*
Plantaris muscles, 123, 124t, 131, *132*, 134t
Plasma, 192, 193; *see also* Blood
Platelets, 192, 193; *see also* Blood
Platysma muscles, 152, *153*, 154t
Pleura, 198, *199*
Pleural cavity, 198, *199*
Plexus, 171
Polarization
    of muscle fiber, 82
    of neurons, 161, *163*
Pollicis, 131
Pons, monitoring respiration, 204, *206*
Popliteal, anatomic location, 4
Popliteus muscles, 123, 124t, *131*
Posterior (anatomic reference), definition, 2-3
Posterior cruciate ligaments, 72, *73, 74*
Posterior horns, 167-168
Posterior inferior iliac spine (PIIS), 45
Posterior longitudinal ligaments, 78
Posterior superior iliac spine (PSIS), 45
Posterior tubercle,on atlas, 24, *28*
Posterolateral, definition, 3
Posteromedial, definition, 3
Postural muscles
    erector spinae, 149
    lower back, 144
Posture, 11-12
    muscle weakness and, 149
    muscles benefiting, 144
Potassium ions in neurons, 161

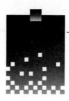

Primary respiration muscles, 150-151, 152t
Prime mover muscles, definition, 86
Procerus muscles, *153*, 154t
Pronation, definition of movement, 62, *63*
Pronator quadratus muscles, 99, *100, 101*
Pronator teres muscles, 99, *100, 101*
Proprioception, 175
Protraction, definition of movement, 63
Proximal (anatomic reference), definition, 2-3
Proximal row, of carpal bones, 39
Psoas major muscles, 115-117
Psoas minor muscles, 115-117
Pubic, anatomical location, 4
Pubic tubercle, *45, 46*
Pubis bones, *45, 46*
Pubis symphysis, *45, 46*
Pubofemoral ligaments, 72
Pudendal, 171, *173*
Pulmonary arteries, 180-181
Pulmonary Function Test, 203
Pulmonary semilunar valves, 180-181
Pulmonary trunk, 180-181
Pulmonary veins, 181
Pulmonary ventilation volumes, *204*
Pulse, 182
Purkinje's fibers, 184, *185*

Q

QRS complex, 184, *186*
Quadratus femoris muscles, 116, 118-119
Quadratus lumborum muscles, 145-148
    assisting respiration, 203
    importance of, 145
Quadratus plantae muscles, 133, *134,* 135t
Quadriceps femoris muscles, 122, 123t
Quadriceps muscles, 84-85
Quadriceps tendons, 73, 122

R

Radial artery, 182, *188*
Radial collateral ligaments, 67, *68*
Radial deviation, definition of movement, 62, *63*
Radial fossa of humerus, 37, *38*
Radial (lateral) collateral ligaments, 67
Radial nerves, 171
Radial notch of ulna, 38
Radial tuberosity, *38,* 39
Radioulnar diaphysis, 67
Radioulnar joints, *68*
Radius, 38-39
Radius
    interosseous border of, *38,* 39
    neck of, 39
    styloid process of, 39
Ramus, 17t, *19,* 46
Ramus, definition, 46
Ramus of mandible, *18, 19*
Range of motion, 210
Rapid heart rate; *see* Tachycardia
Rays, 39
Receptor, definition, 160

Recruitment in muscle motor movements, 85
Rectus abdominis muscles
    assisting respiration, 203
    location of, 143-145
Rectus femoris muscles, 116-117, 122, 124t, 125t
Red blood cells, 192
in respiratory system, *199,* 200
Reference points, 2-5
Reflex arc, 175, *176*
Reflexes, role of neurons, 175
Refractory period in nerve impulse transmission, 161
Remodeling, definition, 12
Repolarized neurons, 161, *163*
Reposition, definition of movement, 63
Residual volume, 203, *204*
Resistance, in lever system, 83-85
Resorption, 12
Respiration
    accessory muscles of, 151, 203
    control of, 204, *206*
    definition, 197
    nerves controlling, 170
Respiratory capacity, 203, *204*
Resting potential, of neurons, 161, *163*
Retraction definition of movement, 63
Rhomboid muscles, 90t, 91
    assisting respiration, 203
Ribs
    bones of, 33-34
    muscles surrounding, 143-144, 145t, 150-152
Right lymphatic duct, 194
Risorius muscles, *153,* 154t
Root of the spine of scapula, 36, *37*
Rotator cuff group of muscles
    description and function of, 94, 95t, 96
    support of joints, 66
Rotatores muscles, 146-149

S

Sacral, anatomic location, 4
Sacral canal, 27, *30*
Sacral foramen, 28, *30*
Sacral hiatus, 28, *30*
Sacral promontory, 27, *30*
Sacroiliac facets, 29, *30*
Sacroiliac joints, 41, *45*
Sacrum, *27, 27-28, 30*
Saddle joints, 57t, *58*
Sagittal planes, 4-5
Sagittal sutures, *18,* 20
Saltatory conduction, 162, *163*
Sarcolemma, definition, 81
Sarcomere, *80,* 81
Sarcoplasmic reticulum, 82
Sartorius muscles, 115, 117t, 122, 124t
Scalenus muscles
    assisting respiration, 203
    definition (anterior, medius, and posterior), 145-148
Scaphoid bones, 39, *40*
Scapula
    definition, 35-36
    inferior angles of, 36

Scapula—*cont'd*
  infraglenoid tubercle of, 37
  infraspinous fossa of, 36, *37*
  joints surrounding, 65-67
  movements of, 66, *67*
  muscles supporting, 90-92
  root of the spine of, 36, *37*
  subscapular fossa of, 36, *37*
  superior angles of, 36
  supraglenoid tubercles of, 36, *37*
  supraspinous fossa of, 36, *37*
Scapula spine, 36, *37*
Scapular muscle group, 90-92
Scapular notch, 37
Scapular stabilizers, 90-92
Scapulohumeral rhythm, 66-67
Scapulothoracic joints, 66-67
Schwann's cells, *159, 160, 161,* 162
Sciatic nerves, 171, *172, 173*
Second class levers, 84
Semilunar valves, 180
Semimembranosus muscles, 118-119, *121,* 122, *123,* 124t, 125t
Semispinalis capitis muscles, 145-149
Semispinalis cervicis muscles, 145-149
Semispinalis thoracis muscles, 145-149
Semitendinosus muscles, 118-119, *121,* 122, *123,* 124t, 125t
Senses and nerves, 170
Sensory neurons, 161, 168; *see also* Afferent neurons
    and movement, 175, *176*
Serotonin, 193
Serratus anterior muscles, 90t, 91
  assisting respiration, 203
Sesamoid bones, 14-15
Short bones, 14-15
Shoulder
    anatomic region, 4
    ball-and-socket joints in, 65
    functional significance, 96
    joints, 65-67
    muscles, 89-109
Shoulder blades; *see* Scapula
Sight, nerves controlling, 170
Sinoatrial (SA) node, 184, *185*
Sinus (landmark term), definition, 17t
Sinus rhythm, 184
Skeletal muscle fiber; *see* Muscle fiber
Skeletal muscles
    contraction, 79-86
    definition, 79
    muscle spindles in, 175
    nerves in, 171
    of respiration, 202-203
Skeleton
    functions of, 11-12
    muscle attachment, 12
    protection of organs, 12
Skeleton of the heart, definition, 180
Skull; *see* Cranium
Slow heart rate; *see* Bradycardia
Slow twitch muscle fibers, 82
Smell, nerves controlling sense of, 170
Smooth muscle
    definition, 80

Smooth muscle—*cont'd*
  in digestive system, 80
Sodium ions in neurons, 161
Sodium-potassium pump, 161
Soleal line of tibia, 47
Soleus muscles, 131, *132,* 134t
Somatic nervous system (SNS), 175
Speech, 197-198
  and muscles, 152, 154t
Sphenoid bones, 17, *18, 19*
Spheroid joints, 57t, *58*
Sphygmomanometer, 182
Spinal accessory nerves, 170t, *171*
Spinal cord, 167-168; *see also* Vertebral column
    central canal, 167
    muscles surrounding, 144-149
    nerve branches, 171, *172, 173*
Spinal nerve roots, 171, *172*
Spinal nerves, 171, *172, 173*
Spinalis muscles (capitis, cervicis, and thoracis), 146, 149
Spine region, 4
Spinocervicothalamic tract, 168
Spinous processes, 26, *28*
Spirometry, 203
Spleen, 194
Splenius capitis muscles, 145-149
Splenius cervicis muscles, 145-149
Spongy bone, 10-11
Squamosal sutures, *18, 19,* 20
Sternal, anatomic location, 4
Sternal end of the clavicle, 35, *36*
Sternoclavicular joints, 65
Sternoclavicular ligaments, 65
Sternocleidomastoid muscles, 145-148
  assisting respiration, 203
Sternum, *33,* 34
Stethoscope, 182
Stroke volume (SV), 182
Styloid process, *18, 19,* 20
    of fibula, 47
    muscles surrounding, *153,* 154t
    of radius, 39
    of ulna, 38
Subclavian veins, 194
Subscapular fossa, of scapula, 36, *37*
Subscapularis muscles, 94, 95t, 96
Superficial (anatomic reference), definition, 2-3
Superior (anatomic reference), definition, 2-3
Superior angles of scapulae, 36
Superior border of patella, 47
Superior gluteal nerves, 171, *173*
Superior pubic ramus, *45,* 46
Superior vena cava
    function of, 181, 189, *190*
    muscles surrounding, *150*
Superolateral, definition, 3
Superomedial, definition, 3
Supination, definition of movement, 62, *63*
Supinator crest, 38
Supinator muscles, 98-99, *100*
Supraglenoid tubercles of scapula, 36, *37*
Supraorbital foramen, 17, *18*
Supraorbital notch, *19*

Supraspinatus muscles, *93*, 94, 95t
Supraspinous fossa of scapula, 36, *37*
Supraspinous ligaments, 78
Sural, anatomic location, 4
Surface tension in lung tissue, 198
Surfactant, *199*, 200
Surgical neck of humerus, 37, *38*
Suture joints, definition, 56
Sutures, cranium, 20
Sympathetic nervous system, 174-175
Symphyses, 56
Synapse, 160
Synaptic cleft, 160
Synaptic vesicles, 160
Synarthrosis, 55
Synchondroses, 56
Syndesmoses, definition, 56
Synergist muscles, 86
Synergists, 99
Synovial fluid, 58
Synovial joints, 56-59
    essential elements of, 58
    and levers, 84
    structures found in, 59t
    types of, *58*
Synovial membrane, 58
Systolic pressure, 182, *190*; *see also* Blood pressure

T

T wave, 184, *186*
Tachycardia, 182
Tailor's strap muscles; *see* Sartorius muscles
Talotibial joints, 73
Talus bones, 48
Tarsal, anatomic location, 4
Tarsal bones, 15, 48
Taste, nerves controlling, 170
Temporal, anatomic location, 4
Temporal bones, *18*, *19*, 20
    muscles surrounding, 152, *153*, 154t
Temporal fossa, *18*
Temporal lobes, 165, *166*
Temporal process, 23
Temporalis muscles, 152, *153*, 154t
Temporomandibular joints, 152, *153*, 154t
Tendocalcaneus, 123
Tendon sheaths, definition, 59
Tendons, definition, 12
    in ankle and foot area, 131-135
    in muscle tissue, 80, *81*
    nerves in, 175
Tensile strength, 9, 12
Tensor fasciae latae muscles, 115-117, 122, 124t
Teres major muscles, *90*, 94, 95t, 96
Teres minor muscles, *93*, 94, 95t, 96
Terminology; *see also* Vocabulary
    memory aids, 96
    of movement, 62-64
Thalamus, 165, 167
Thenar eminence, 107
Third class levers, 84
Thoracic, anatomic location, 4

Thoracic cage, 33-34
Thoracic cavity, pressure in, 202
Thoracic duct, 194
Thoracic vertebrae, 26-27, *29*, *30*, 33
Thorax, muscles surrounding, 90, 91
Threshold stimulus, 161
Throat, 23
    muscles surrounding, 154t
    nerves controlling sensations in, 170
Thumb; *see* Pollicis
Thymus gland, 194
Thyroid cartilage, *24*
Tibia
    bones, 47
    interosseous border of, 47
    joints attached to, 73, *74*
    lateral condyles of, 47
    medial condyles of, 47
    medial malleolus of, 47
    muscles surrounding, 122-123
    soleal line of, 47
Tibial (medial) collateral ligaments, 73
Tibial nerves, 171, *172*, *173*
Tibial plateau, 47
Tibial tuberosity, 47
Tibialis anterior muscles, 131-132, *134*
Tibialis posterior muscles, 131, 134t
Tidal volume, 203, *204*
T-lymphocytes, 194
Tongue, 23, *24*
    nerves controlling movement of, 170
Trabeculae, 11
Trachea, 197-198, *199*
Transverse abdominis muscles
    assisting respiration, 203
    contraction of, 143-144, 145t
Transverse foramen, on vertebrae, 26, *28*
Transverse humeral ligaments, 65, *66*
Transverse ligaments, 73, *74*
Transverse planes, 5
Transverse processes, on vertebrae, 24, *28*
Trapezium bones, 39, *40*
Trapezius muscles
    assisting respiration, 203
    definition and description, 90t, 91
    upper, 145-148
Trapezoid bones, 39, *40*
Trendelenburg sign, 121
Triceps brachii muscles, *93*, 94, 95t, 98, 99t
Triceps surae muscle group, 131, *132*
Tricuspid valves, 180-181
Trigeminal nerves, 170t, *171*
Triquetrum bones, 39, *40*
Trochlea of humerus, 37, *38*
Trochlear nerves, 170t, *171*
Trochlear notch, 38
True ribs, *33*, 34
Trunk muscles, 144-149
Trunk region, 4
Tubercle
    on atlas, 24, *28*
    definition, 17t
    of ribs, 33

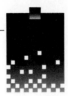

Tuberosity, definition, 17t
Tunica adventitia, 188-189, *190*
Tunica intima, 188-189, *190*
Tunica media, 188-189, *190*

U

Ulna
    definition and description, 37-38, 67-68
    interosseous border of, 38
    olecranon process of, 38
    styloid process of, 38
Ulnar collateral ligaments, 67, *68*
Ulnar deviation, definition of movement, 62, *63*
Ulnar nerves, 171
Ulnar notch of radius, *38, 39*
Ulnar tuberosity, 38
Umbilical, anatomic location, 4
Unilateral muscle contraction, definition, 145
Unipolar neurons, 160-161
Upper extremity
    anatomic location, 4
    bones, 37-40
    joints, 67-68
    muscles, 89-109
    nerves in, 171, *172, 173*
Upper respiratory tract, 197-198
Upper trapezius muscles, 90t, 91

V

Vagus nerves, 170t, *171*
Valves, 179, *180*
Vascular system, 188-190; *see also* Blood vessels
Vasoconstriction, 188
Vasodilation, 188
Vastus intermedius muscles, *122,* 125t
Vastus lateralis muscles, *122,* 125t
Vastus medialis muscles, *122,* 125t
Veins, *181,* 188-189; *see also* Blood vessels
Ventilation, definition, 197
Ventral (anatomic reference), definition, 2-3
Ventricles, 179-182
    within the cerebrum, 167
    muscle tissue innervation in, 184, *185*
Venules, *181,* 188-189
Verbal communication and facial muscles, 152, 154t
Vertebrae
    and corresponding nerve roots, 171, *172*
    joints attached to, 77-78
    transverse foramen on, 26, *28*
    transverse processes on, 24, *28*
Vertebral, anatomic location, 4
Vertebral artery, 26
Vertebral border of scapula, 36
Vertebral canal, nerves in, 167-168
Vertebral column
    bones of, 24-34
    muscles, 144-149
Vestibulocochlear (acoustic) nerves, 170t, *171*
Visceral (organ) activities, 174-175
Visceral pericardium, 179
Visceral pleura, 198, *199*

Vision, nerves controlling, 170
Vocabulary
    of anatomic regions, 3-4
    directional terminology, 2-3
    importance of learning, 3
    memory aids, 96
Vocal cords, 197-198
Volkmann's canals, definition, 10
Voluntary body functions, 159
Voluntary muscle movement, 79
Vomer bones, *19,* 23

W

Walking and hip muscles, 119, 121
Water in blood, 193
White blood cells, 192-193
White matter, 165, 167-168
Windpipe; *see* Larynx
Wolff, Julius, 12
Wormian bones; *see* Sutures
Wrist
    bones of, 39, *40*
    functional significance of muscles, 107
    joints of, 67, *68*
    ligaments of, 67
    muscles, 103-105

X

Xiphoid process, *33, 34*

Z

Z-lines, *80, 81*
Zygomatic arch, 23
    muscles surrounding, 154t
Zygomatic bones, *18, 19,* 20, 23
Zygomatic process, 20
Zygomaticus muscles (major and minor), *153,* 154t